Chronic Lymphocytic Leukemia

BASIC AND CLINICAL ONCOLOGY

Editor

Bruce D. Cheson, M.D.

National Cancer Institute
National Institutes of Health
Bethesda, Maryland

1. Chronic Lymphocytic Leukemia: Scientific Advances and Clinical Developments, *edited by Bruce D. Cheson*

ADDITIONAL VOLUMES IN PREPARATION

Therapeutic Applications of Interleukin-2, *edited by Michael Atkins and James Mier*

Cancer of the Prostate, *edited by Sakti Das and E. David Crawford*

Chronic Lymphocytic Leukemia

Scientific Advances and Clinical Developments

edited by
Bruce D. Cheson

National Cancer Institute
National Institutes of Health
Bethesda, Maryland

Marcel Dekker, Inc.   New York • Basel • Hong Kong

Library of Congress Cataloging-in-Publication Data

Chronic lymphocytic leukemia : scientific advances and clinical
  developments / edited by Bruce D. Cheson.
        p.   cm. -- (Basic and clinical oncology ; v. 1)
    Includes bibliographical references and index.
    ISBN 0-8247-8736-6 (alk. paper)
    1. Chronic lymphocytic leukemia.   I. Cheson, Bruce D.
  II. Series.
    [DNLM: 1. Leukemia, Lymphocytic, Chronic.   WH 250 C55675]
  RC643.C486   1993
  616.99'419--dc20
  DNLM/DLC
  for Library of Congress   92-49857
                                                                 CIP

This book is printed on acid-free paper.

MARCEL DEKKER, INC.
270 Madison Avenue, New York, New York 10016

Current printing (last digit):
10 9 8 7 6 5 4 3 2 1

PRINTED IN THE UNITED STATES OF AMERICA

Series Introduction

The current volume, *Chronic Lymphocytic Leukemia: Scientific Advances and Clinical Developments*, is the first in the Basic and Clinical Oncology series.

Many of the recent advances in oncology have resulted from close interaction between the basic scientist and the clinical researcher. The aim of this new series will therefore be to focus on the advances in cancer research that illustrate the success of this relationship as demonstrated by new therapies and promising areas for scientific research.

As editor of the series, my goal is to recruit volume editors who not only have established reputations based on their outstanding contributions to oncology, but also have an appreciation for the interface between the laboratory and the clinic. I envision state-of-the-art monographs on topics that are of a high level of current interest.

Volumes in progress focus on cancer prevention and control, retinoids as they relate to cancer prevention and therapy, breast cancer, prostate cancer, biological approaches to cancer treatment, notably interleukin-2 and targeted therapy, and supportive care of the cancer patient. I anticipate that these volumes will provide a valuable contribution to the oncology literature.

Bruce D. Cheson, M.D.

Preface

As the editor of *Chronic Lymphocytic Leukemia*, I have certain privileges, one of which is to select those topics I feel are the most important, the other is to provide some controversial speculation. Chronic lymphocytic leukemia (CLL) has traditionally been regarded with conspicuous disinterest. The recent resuscitation of enthusiasm in this disorder reflects the work of a limited number of investigators who, through their persistence, have been successful in advancing our understanding of the biology and immunology of CLL as well as identifying exciting new therapeutic agents. The current volume contains state-of-the-art reviews by many of these investigators, including both previously published and unpublished data. I have also given a charge to the laboratory scientists to speculate on future clinical applications of their research, whereas the clinical scientists were asked to propose future areas for study, in both the laboratory and the clinic. The book clearly demonstrates how we have applied the knowledge derived from the laboratory to the treatment of patients.

Nevertheless, many important issues remain to be resolved. For example, the immunodeficiency that characterizes CLL cannot be explained solely on the basis of a proliferation of malignant B cells, since quantitative and qualitative defects of the other lymphoid subsets are present as well. Possible mechanisms for the diverse variety of immunologic abnormalities are presented in this text. There are significant clinical implications of these immune abnormalities, notably an increased susceptibility to life-threatening infections. An interesting observation is that the spectrum of organisms infecting patients with CLL has changed substantially over the past few years, from primarily encapsulated bacteria to more opportunistic organisms, which is an unfortunate consequence of both the disease and the immunosuppressive properties of newer therapeutic agents.

The marked clinical diversity of CLL patients reflects the biologic and immunologic heterogeneity of this disorder. Ongoing research is directed at determining how the immunophenotype of the CLL cell influences the cellular response to various signals, including growth factors, and how these growth factors and various oncogenes are involved in the disordered proliferation of lymphocytes that results in CLL.

A number of staging systems for CLL have been developed to provide some order to the clinical heterogeneity. Unfortunately, the currently available classification systems neither account for the marked variability within clinical stages nor incorporate newly identified prognostic factors. Prognostic factors not only predict outcome but should allow the treating physician to direct specific therapies at various risk groups. A prerequisite for such an approach is the availability of active therapeutic agents. Newly developed sets of standardized guidelines for diagnosis and response have made studies more interpretable and comparable and, therefore, have enabled us to identify new agents with promising activity in CLL.

The time has come to consider CLL a potentially curable disease. The purine analog—fludarabine, 2'-deoxycoformycin, and 2-chlorodeoxyadenosine—induce complete remissions, a prerequisite for cure, in a substantial number of patients with CLL, at the clinical, cellular, and molecular levels. They have completely altered the direction of therapy for CLL and other indolent lymphoproliferative disorders and will likely redefine what is considered standard treatment. However, if we simply accept these drugs as the new standards and limit ourselves to comparing them either with each other or with conventional agents, we risk falling into a state of scientific hibernation once again. Despite the higher response rates and, perhaps, prolonged survival resulting from these new drugs, CLL is still a fatal disease and additional approaches are needed. We should use these agents as the foundation on which to build innovative therapeutic strategies, including combinations of purine analogs with other cytotoxics and biologics. Other approaches being evaluated include monoclonal antibodies, allogeneic and autologous bone marrow transplantation, manipulation of the cellular pharmacology of CLL cells, and the use of agents with the potential to reverse clinical drug resistance.

The reader will come away from this volume with a sense of the exciting progress that has been made in CLL. More important, however, is the recognition that such progress will continue only with close interaction between basic scientists and clinical researchers. I hope this book will be useful not only as a source of current information about CLL, but also as a guidebook to stimulate future research.

I would like to express my appreciation to Barbara Dunleavy of Marcel Dekker, Inc., who encouraged me to consider this project, as well as the publisher's editorial and production staff.

Most of all, I would like to express my eternal love for Christine and Sara who have put up with me through the years.

Bruce D. Cheson

Contents

Contents

Contributors

E. J. Anaissie   Associate Professor of Medicine, Department of Infectious Diseases, The University of Texas M.D. Anderson Cancer Center, Houston, Texas

Mark Blackstadt   Department of Internal Medicine, Veterans Affairs Medical Center, Minneapolis, Minnesota

G. P. Bodey, M.D.   Chairman, Department of Medical Specialties, and Chief, Section of Infectious Diseases, The University of Texas M.D. Anderson Cancer Center, Houston, Texas

M. K. Brenner, M.B., Ph.D., F.R.C.P., M.R.C.Path.   Director, Division of Bone Marrow Transplantation, Department of Hematology/Oncology, St. Jude Children's Research Hospital, Memphis, Tennessee

Daniel Catovsky, D.Sc., F.R.C.P., F.R.C.Path.   Professor, Academic Hematology and Cytogenetics, Royal Marsden Hospital, Institute of Cancer Research, London, England

Bruce D. Cheson, M.D.   Head, Medicine Section of the Clinical Investigations Branch, Cancer Therapy Evaluation Program, Division of Cancer Treatment, National Cancer Institute, Bethesda, Maryland

Guillaume Dighiero, M.D., Ph.D., Head, Blood Bank, Department of Immunohematology and Immunopathology, Institut Pasteur, Paris, France

Robert Foa, M.D. Associate Professor of Medical Oncology, Department of Biomedical Science and Human Oncology, University of Torino, Torino, Italy

Arnold S. Freedman, M.D. Assistant Professor of Medicine, Division of Tumor Immunology, Dana-Farber Cancer Institute, Boston, Massachusetts

Gösta Gahrton, M.D. Professor, Department of Medicine, Karolinska Institute at Huddinge Hospital, Huddinge, Sweden

Varsha Gandhi, Ph.D. Assistant Professor of Medicine, Department of Medical Oncology, The University of Texas M.D. Anderson Cancer Center, Houston, Texas

Michael L. Grossbard, M.D. Instructor in Medicine, Division of Tumor Immunology, Dana-Farber Cancer Institute, Boston, Massachusetts

H. E. Heslop St. Jude Children's Research Hospital, Memphis, Tennessee

A. V. Hoffbrand, D.M., F.R.C.P., F.R.C.Path., D.Sc. Professor, Department of Hematology, Royal Free Hospital School of Medicine, London, England

Gunnar Juliusson, M.D., Ph.D. Associate Professor, Division of Clinical Hematology and Oncology, Department of Medicine, Karolinska Institute at Huddinge Hospital, Huddinge, Sweden

Neil Kay, M.D. Director of Research, Hybritech, Inc., and Professor, Department of Internal Medicine, University of California, San Diego, La Jolla, California

Michael J. Keating, M.B. Associate Vice-President for Clinical Investigations, Department of Hematology, The University of Texas M.D. Anderson Cancer Center, Houston, Texas

Thomas J. Kipps, M.D., Ph.D. Associate Professor, Department of Medicine, University of California, San Diego, La Jolla, California

D. P. Kontoyianis, M.D. Clinical Research Fellow, Department of Infectious Diseases, University of Texas M.D. Anderson Cancer Center, Houston, Texas

Emilio Montserrat, M.D. Professor of Medicine, Department of Hematology, University of Barcelona Hospital Clinic, Barcelona, Spain

Lee M. Nadler, M.D. Associate Professor of Medicine, Division of Tumor Immunology, Dana-Farber Cancer Institute, Boston, Massachusetts

Kenneth Nilsson, M.D., Ph.D. Professor, Department of Pathology, University of Uppsala Hospital, Uppsala, Sweden

LoAnn Peterson, M.D. Director of Hematology, Department of Pathology, Northwestern University Medical School, Chicago, Illinois

William Plunkett, Ph.D. Hubert L. and Olive Stringer Professor, Department of Medical Oncology, The University of Texas M.D. Anderson Cancer Center, Houston, Texas

Milan Potmesil, M.D., Ph.D. Director, Laboratory of Experimental Therapy, and Professor, Department of Radiology, New York University Medical Center, New York, New York

Susan N. Rabinowe, M.D. Instructor in Medicine, Division of Tumor Immunology, Dana-Farber Cancer Institute, Boston, Massachusetts

Kanti R. Rai, M.B., F.A.C.P. Professor of Medicine, Albert Einstein College of Medicine, Bronx, New York, and Chief, Division of Hematology/Oncology, Long Island Jewish Medical Center, New Hyde Park, New York

Juan-Carlos Reverter, M.D. Department of Hemostasis and Blood Bank, University of Barcelona Hospital Clinic, Barcelona, Spain

Ciril Rozman, M.D. Professor of Medicine, Department of Hematology, University of Barcelona Hospital Clinic, Barcelona, Spain

Robert Silber, M.D. Professor, Department of Medicine, and Director, Division of Hematology, New York University Medical Center, New York, New York

Yoshihide Tsujimoto The Wistar Institute of Anatomy and Biology, Philadelphia, Pennsylvania

Nuria Viñolas, M.D. Department of Oncology, University of Barcelona Hospital Clinic, Barcelona, Spain

1

Immunologic Markers in B-Cell Chronic Lymphocytic Leukemia

Arnold S. Freedman and Lee M. Nadler
Dana-Farber Cancer Institute, Boston, Massachusetts

INTRODUCTION

Chronic lymphocytic leukemia (CLL) cells have been previously hypothe-sized to be the neoplastic counterparts of peripheral blood lymphocytes, based on their morphology and tendency to involve peripheral blood and bone marrow. Further support for this hypothesis was the demonstration that CLLs had surface characteristics of mature B or T cells. Specifically, the majority of CLLs weakly expressed monoclonal cell surface immuno-globulin (sIg) (1,2) and were therefore of B-cell lineage, whereas approxi-mately 5% of CLLs formed rosettes with sheep erythrocytes, demonstrating their T-cell origin (3). These observations were important since they demon-strated that the lineage derivation of the neoplastic cell could be correlated with clinical presentation and disease course. CLLs of B-cell derivation appeared to restrict their infiltration to the lymph node, bone marrow, and spleen and generally had an indolent course. In contrast, T-cell CLLs, which demonstrated a more malignant course, also invaded the skin and CNS, and frequently lacked lymphadenopathy.

The identification of cell surface structures expressed on B lymphocytes provided the opportunity to relate CLL cells with stages of normal B-cell ontogeny (see Fig. 1). CLL cells were examined for the expression of a number of B-cell-restricted and -associated markers, including the isotypes

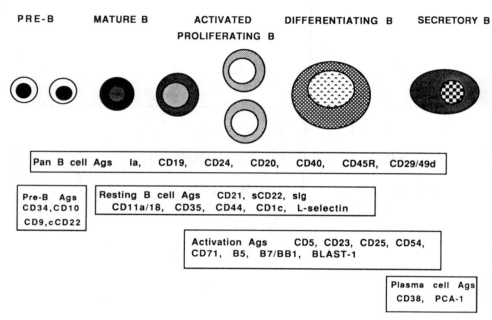

PRE-B   MATURE B   ACTIVATED   DIFFERENTIATING B   SECRETORY B
                                 PROLIFERATING B

| Pan B cell Ags | Ia, | CD19, | CD24, | CD20, | CD40, | CD45R, | CD29/49d |

| Pre-B Ags | Resting B cell Ags | CD21, sCD22, sIg |
| CD34,CD10 | CD11a/18, CD35, CD44, CD1c, L-selectin |
| CD9,cCD22 |

| Activation Ags | CD5, CD23, CD25, CD54, |
| CD71, B5, B7/BB1, BLAST-1 |

| Plasma cell Ags |
| CD38, PCA-1 |

Figure 1 Stages of normal B-cell differentiation. The expression of B-cell antigens defines stages of normal B-cell ontogeny. These include pan-B-cell antigens, which are expressed throughout differentiation; antigens expressed on pre-B cells; antigens on mature resting B cells; activation antigens induced on stimulated B cells; and antigens expressed on plasma cells.

of cell surface Ig, complement receptors, and mouse red blood cell rosette receptors (MRBC-R). Most B-CLLs expressed sIgM, often with sIgD (1,2,4–6), and the intensity of expression of sIg on B-cell CLLs (B-CLLs) was generally much weaker than that seen on peripheral blood B cells, suggesting a difference between these two cellular populations. Further evidence for the notion that B-CLLs were not derived from a major population of circulating B lymphocytes arose from their discordant expression of MRBC-R and complement receptors. Virtually every B-CLL forms MRBC rosettes (7–9). This marker has been classically considered to be the best diagnostic marker of B-CLL, since peripheral blood B cells have not been shown to form MRBC-R. Similarly, whereas nearly all peripheral blood B cells form rosettes with red blood cells coated with the C3b and C3d complement components, most B-CLLs form rosettes only with C3d (10,11).

These phenotypic differences between peripheral blood B cells and B-CLL cells provided compelling evidence that B-CLL might not be the neoplastic counterpart of the circulating peripheral blood B lymphocyte.

In this review, the immunology of B-CLL will be discussed, by relating the cell surface phenotype of B-CLL cells to normal B lymphocytes. The phenotype of B-CLL cells will be approached by defining the lineage and state of differentiation of the malignant cells. In addition, CLL cells will be related to normal B cell ontogeny through the identification of normal cellular counterparts of the neoplastic cells.

NORMAL B-CELL ONTOGENY

Normal B-Cell ontogeny has been operationally divided into stages, including pre-B cell, resting B cell, activated/proliferating B cell, differentiating B cell, and plasma cell. These stages can be defined by the expression of unique cytoplasmic and cell surface antigens (Ags). In this regard, human B-cell Ags can be subgrouped into broad categories including: Ags that span ontogeny, the so-called pan-B cell Ags; Ags that appear in the resting B-cell stage and that are lost with activation; Ags that are not expressed on the resting B cell but that appear following activation; and Ags that appear at the terminal stages of differentiation (see Table 1).

The earliest pre-B cells have been defined by their expression of cell surface Ags, including major histocompatibility complex (MHC) class II (Ia) and CD19, and rearrangements of immunoglobulin-μ heavy-chain genes (12–15). CD19 is a 95-kD glycoprotein and is a member of the Ig superfamily (16) consisting of two Ig-like extracellular domains with an extensive cytoplasmic region (17,18). Studies by several investigators suggested that CD19 may be a receptor involved in the regulation of B-cell proliferation (19,20). More recently, it has been shown that CD19 is a component of a multimolecular complex of cell surface membrane proteins (21). This complex can include the CD21 complement receptor CR2 and several other proteins. The CD19 complex is capable of signal transduction to the B cell via activation of protein kinase C. By virtue of its B lineage restriction, CD19 is the most reliable marker of B lineage at the pre-B-cell level.

The earliest pre-B cells also express CD34, a 115-kD type I transmembrane glycoprotein that is also present on immature myeloid cells and identifies a population of immature progenitor cells (22–25). CD34 has no known homology to other proteins. In addition to these cell surface Ags, a B-cell-restricted Ag, CD22, is present in the cytoplasm (cCD22) at the earliest stages of pre-B-cell differentiation but is not exported to the cell surface until the mature resting B-cell stage, when sIgD is first expressed (26).

Table 1   B-Cell Antigens

CD/Ag	Expression in normal B-cell ontogeny	Function/nature of Ag
Ia	Pan-B	MHC class II
CD19	Pan-B	Ig superfamily, signal transduction
CD22	Pan-B	NCAM-1-like, adhesion molecule
CD20	Pan-B	Ion channel
CD24	Pan-B	Unknown
CD29/49d	Pan-B	β1 integrin, adhesion molecule for VCAM-1, fibro-nectin
CD40	Pan-B	Nerve growth factor receptorlike, signal transduction
CD45	Pan-B	Leukocyte common antigen, tyrosine phosphatase
CD10	Pre-B	Enkephalinase
CD34	Pre-B	Identifies pluripotent stem cells
CD21	Mature B	C3d/EBV receptor
sIg	Mature B	Antigen receptor
CD44	Mature B	Adhesion molecule
L-selectin	Mature B	Adhesion to HEV
CD11a/18	Mature B	β2 integrin (LFA-1), cell-cell adhesion
CD35	Mature B	C3b receptor
CD1	Mature B	Ig superfamily
CD71	Activated B	Transferring receptor
4F2	Activated B	Unknown
B5	Activated B	Unknown
CD54	Activated B	Ig superfamily, adhesion molecule, LFA-1 ligand
B7/BB1	Activated B	Ig superfamily, ligand for CD28
CD23	Activated B	Low-affinity FcE receptor
CD25	Activated B	Low-affinity IL-2 receptor
CD5	Activated B	Signal transduction, ligand for CD72
CD38	Plasma cells	Unknown
PCA-1	Plasma cells	Unknown

CD22 has five Ig-like domains and significant homology to neural cellular adhesion molecule, NCAM, and myelin-associated glycoprotein (27). CD22 may be involved in signal transduction following activation of B cells through the Ag receptor, surface Ig (28). There is more recent evidence that CD22 is an adhesion molecule, which can mediate interaction with B cells, monocytes, and erythrocytes (27). CD22 may also be capable of homophilic interaction as well as heterophilic interaction with CD45 on a subset of T cells.

The stages of normal pre-B-cell differentiation have been examined by isolating pre-B cells from fetal hematopoietic tissues and adult bone marrow and then inducing them to differentiate in vitro (29–33). Following the appearance of CD19 and cytoplasmic CD22, cells express CD10 (CALLA) (34,35). CD10 is a zinc metalloprotease, which is identical to neutral endopeptidase 24.11 or enkephalinase (36,37). This enzyme is capable of inactivating a variety of peptide hormones, including glucagon, enkephalin, atrial natriuretic peptide, substance P, oxytocin, bradykinin, neurotensin, and angiotensins I and II, as well as f-met-leu-phe. Studies in murine systems suggest that CD10 is involved in stromal cell-dependent lymphopoeisis (38). Pre-B cells next express the pan-B-cell restricted Ag CD20 (39–43), which is a nonglycosylated phosphoprotein. In-vitro functional studies suggest that CD20 regulates B-cell activation (44–46), and there is evidence that CD20 is involved in transmembrane ion flux and may regulate intracellular Ca^{2+} levels (47).

The expression of these cell surface Ags define stages of pre-B-cell development including CD34 + Ia + CD19 + cCD22 + CD10 − CD20 − , CD34 + Ia + CD19 + cCD22 + CD10 + CD20 − , and CD34 + Ia + CD19 + cCD22 + CD10 + CD20 + . The last stage of pre-B-cell ontogeny appears with the expression of cytoplasmic μ (cμ) Ig heavy chain without the expression of light chains. The expression of cμ further divides the CD34 + Ia + CD19 + cCD22 + CD10 + CD20 + stage into cμ − and cμ + stages.

Several other Ags are expressed during pre-B-cell development, including CD29/49d, CD40, and CD45R (leukocyte common Ag/T200), CD9, and CD24. CD29/49d (also known as VLA-4 and $\alpha 4 \beta 1$) is a member of the $\beta 1$ integrin family of cell adhesion molecules (48–51). CD29/49d is involved in the adhesion of pre-B cells to bone marrow stromal cells through its ligand VCAM-1 (52). CD40 is a 50-kD phosphoprotein expressed on a subset of pre-B cells (46,53–57). CD40 is homologous to both the nerve and epidermal growth factor receptors. CD40 has been shown to be involved in growth regulation of B cells, since mAbs against CD40 prevent programmed cell death of B cells in vitro (58). It has been suggested that the natural ligand of CD40 is located in germinal centers but to date remains unknown. The leukocyte common Ag family of molecules, CD45, are widely expressed on hematopoietic cells (59,60). Monoclonal antibodies directed against CD45 precipitate four chains of 220, 205, 190, and 180 kD. The generation of these different polypeptide chains is through differential mRNA splicing of a single transcript (61). The 220- and 200-kD chains are preferentially expressed by B lymphocytes (termed CD45RA). Recent studies have shown that the cytoplasmic domain of CD45 has tyrosine phosphatase activity, suggesting a regulatory function of this cell surface molecule (62). Further evidence for this is recent studies which have shown that

CD45 can be associated with sIg, the B-cell antigen receptor (63). The tyrosine phosphatase activity of CD45 may regulate B-cell activation through dephosphorylation of proteins associated with the antigen receptor, which are involved in signal transduction. CD9 is a 26-kD glycoprotein present on thymocytes, activated B and T cells, and platelets (64,65). CD24 is a 45-kD sialoglycoprotein that is also expressed on granulocytes (66).

In adults, pre-B-cell development takes place in the bone marrow. In the fetus, in contrast, B-cell development begins in the liver, followed by bone marrow, spleen, and lymph node (67–70). Although fetal B-cell ontogeny in the liver and bone marrow follow the above-discussed sequence of Ag expression, B cells isolated from lymph node and spleen demonstrate a unique cell surface phenotype. At approximately 22–24 weeks of gestation, the major population of fetal B cells that are weakly sIgM+ and IgD+ coexpress the T-cell-associated Ag CD5. CD5, a 67-kD glycoprotein originally described to be present on mature T cells (71–74), functions as a receptor that transmits a costimulatory signal which leads to enhanced proliferation of T cells in association with ligation of the T-cell Ag receptor (75). It has been recently shown that the B-cell antigen CD72, which is present on pre-B and mature B cells, serves as a natural ligand for CD5 (76). To date, the function of CD5 on B cells is unknown, but it is likely that it is important in B-cell activation through a B-B cell interaction.

As pre-B cells mature, they are exported to the peripheral blood and migrate to secondary lymphoid tissues. The mature resting B cells continue to express Ia, CD19, CD20, CD24, CD22, CD40, and CD45R, but they no longer express CD9, CD10, and CD34. The localization of lymphocytes from peripheral blood to secondary lymphoid organs involves their binding to a specialized endothelium within small vessels in tonsil and lymph nodes known as high endothelial venules (77–79). Mature B cells express two molecules, CD44 (80–83) and L-selectin (also known as LAM-1, Leu 8, TQ1, Mel 14) (84–88), which has been shown to be involved in lymphocyte recirculation, homing, and the adhesion of lymphocytes to high endothelial venules. Within secondary lymphoid tissues, B and T lymphocytes are not randomly distributed, but inhabit highly organized tissues where there are areas in which B and T cells are largely segregated, and other areas in which different populations of cells can interact and differentiate (89). Specifically, T cells localize to the interfollicular areas, whereas B cells localize to follicles (89–92). Coincident with the maturation to the sIg+ stage, B cells express a number of antigens that mediate cell-cell and cell-extracellular matrix adhesive interactions within lymphoid follicles. These include CD11a/18 (LFA-1) (93,94) and CD29/49d (VLA-4). CD11a is noncovalently associated with CD18 and is a member of the integrin family of molecules, which are involved in a variety of cell-cell and cell-matrix interactions (95-97). Within secondary lymphoid tissues, CD11a/18 mediates B-cell binding to B cells, T cells, monocytes, and follicular dendritic cells through its ligand ICAM-1 (CD54) (98-105). CD29/49d mediates adhesion of activated B cells to follicular dendritic cells in germinal centers through binding to its ligand VCAM-1 (INCAM-110) (106-109). CD29/49d also mediates binding of B cells to an alternatively spliced fragment of fibronectin (termed FN-40 or CS-1) (110,111). In addition to these adhesion molecules, B cells utilize complement component receptors for binding to immune complexes localized in the B-cell zones of lymphoid tissues. These include CD21, which is the receptor for the C3d cleavage fragment of complement and for Epstein-Barr virus (EBV) (112-115); and CD35, which is the C3b complement receptor (116). The expression of CD21 is relatively restricted to B cells and follicular dendritic cells, whereas CD35 is present on granulocytes, monocytes, red blood cells, and dendritic cells.

A subset of mature B cells has been described that express the T-cell associated Ag CD1 (117). CD1 is a member of the immunoglobulin superfamily and shares homology to both MHC class I and class II. CD1 exists as these molecules, CD1a (49 kD), CD1b (45 kD), and CD1c (43 kD), which are noncovalently associated with beta-2 microglobulin. Approximately 50% of normal adult splenic B cells and a proportion of peripheral blood B cells are CD1c+, and following activation CD1c is upregulated (118,119).

Following exposure to Ag or various polyclonal mitogens, resting B cells are activated and subsequently proliferate (120). In vitro, DNA synthesis begins between 30 and 48 h and peaks at 72 h. From in-vitro, in-vivo, and in-situ studies, the activation of resting B cells is accompanied by a sequence of changes in cell surface Ags (121). Within 24 h of activation, resting B cells begin to lose sIgD, CD21, and CD22, and this process is complete by 72 to 96 h. As these Ags are lost, a number of B-cell-restricted and -associated Ags sequentially appear (122). These activation Ags are excellent candidates for growth factor receptors, molecules that regulate proliferation and differentiation, structures involved in cell-cell interaction, and molecules that play a role in the localization and binding of activated B cells in various microenvironments.

The activation Ags include those whose expression is not limited to B cells, including CD71 (123), 4F2 (124), CD54 (98), Blast-1 (125), CD25 (126,127), CD5 (70,128-131), B7/BB-1 (132,133), and CD23 (134); and those that are more restricted in their expression on B cells, including CD77 (135), B5 (136), and Bac-1 (137). The majority of these activation Ags demonstrate peak expression by 72 h and are no longer expressed on the cell surface at 120 h. The functions of several of these antigens have been identified. CD71 is the transferrin receptor and is expressed on all proliferating cells (138). CD25, the 55-kD Tac Ag, is a component of the IL-2 receptor (low affinity) and is present on activated B cells, T cells, and monocytes (126,127). CD23, a 45-kD glycoprotein, is the low-affinity receptor for IgE, and a soluble form is reported to have B-cell growth-promoting activity (139–142). CD23 is preferentially expressed on B cells following activation with EBV, phorbol esters, and IL-4, and is also present on monocytes, eosinophils, platelets, and activated T cells. Intracellular adhesion molecule-1 (ICAM-1) (CD54) is a 90-kD glycoprotein that is the ligand for LFA-1 and is involved in homotypic adhesion of activated B cells, as well as the binding of activated B cells to T cells, monocytes, and endothelial cells (100,102–104,143). T-cell proliferation is also upregulated by ligation of LFA-1 by its ligand ICAM-1. B7/BB-1 is a 50-kD glycoprotein (132,133) that has been identified as a member of the Ig gene superfamily (144). The B7/BB-1 molecule has been recently shown to be the natural ligand for the T-cell antigen CD28, also a member of the Ig gene superfamily (145). CD28, like CD5, transmits a constimulatory signal to T cells that have been activated through the T-cell receptor (146). This signal leads to augmented cytokine secretion, including IL-2, TNF-α, GM-CSF, and interferon-γ (145,147–150). Therefore, during the cognate interaction of activated B cells with T cells, the ligation of B7/BB-1 with CD28 may also regulate B-cell proliferation and differentiation into Ig secreting or memory B cells through enhanced lymphokine production by T lymphocytes.

Following activation, B cells are competent to proliferate in response to a variety of cytokines (151). There is evidence that IL-2, IL-4, low- and high-molecular-weight B-cell growth factor (BCGF), IFN-γ, and IL-1 can induce B-cell proliferation. Proliferating B cells then are induced to secrete Ig and undergo Ig heavy-chain class switching in response to various cytokines. IL-2 in high concentrations, IL-6, and IL-1 have been shown in various systems to induce IgG secretion, whereas IL-5 appears to specifically induce IgA secretion. IL-4 promotes isotype switching to IgE and IgG1, but inhibits IgM, IgG3, IgG2a, and IgG2b. In contrast, IFN-γ stimulates IgG2a isotype but inhibits IgG3, Ig2b, IgG1, and IgE production (152). Accompanying this differentiative stage is the gradual loss of the B-cell activation Ags as well as pan-B-cell Ags including Ia, CD19, CD20, CD24, CD40, and CD45R. This terminal differentiation stage is also characterized by the appearance of several other Ags, including CD38 and PCA-1, which are expressed on plasma cells (117,153,154).

CELL SURFACE PHENOTYPE OF B-CLL

In this section, the Ags that are on most B-CLLs will be discussed followed by those Ags whose expression is heterogeneous and may define subgroups of B-CLL.

Pan-B-Cell Antigens

Most B-CLLs, like most other B-cell leukemias and lymphomas, uniformly express pan-B cell Ags (70,155–157). B-CLLs are MHC class II+, and when the different loci of class II Ags have been examined, B-CLLs are DR+, DC+ but are heterogeneous for the expression of DQ (69%+) (158). B-CLLs are also CD19, CD20, CD24, CD40, and CD45RA+, although there is less intense expression of CD45RA than on normal B cells (159,160). Following stimulation of B-CLLs with phorbol esters, there is gradual decrease in expression of pan-B-cell antigens and expression of the lower-molecular-weight isoform of the leukocyte common antigen family, CD45RO.

Pre-B-Cell Antigens

CD10 (CALLA), which is expressed during normal pre-B-cell ontogeny, and on the B-cell NHLs including follicular small cleaved cell and small noncleaved cell (Burkitt's) NHL (161), has not been demonstrated on B-CLLs (162–164). CLLs do not express the antigen that is present on pluripotent stem cells, CD34. The CD9 Ag that is present on normal pre-B, a subpopulation of normal activated B cells, and a subset of pre-B-cell ALLs is detected on only 20% of B-CLLs (164).

Mature B-Cell Antigens

The expression of sIg defines the B-cell lineage derivation of B-CLL and its monoclonality. Although all B-CLLs express B-cell-restricted Ags and clonally rearranged Ig genes (165), sIg is detected on only 80–90% of B-CLLs examined (2,4–6,70). A recent study has shown that essentially all cases that lack sIg have monoclonal Ig present in the cytoplasm (166). Cells from almost all sIg-positive CLLs express sIgM or coexpress sIgM and sIgD. Occasional cases have been identified that are sIgG+ or combinations of IgG with IgM and IgD. It has been suggested that the sIgG in these cases is not of the same idiotype but is bound by Fc receptors to the cell surface (167). Rare cases of sIgA+ CLL have been reported. Several investigators have suggested that both Ig heavy-chain and light-chain isotypes correlate with clinical stage or survival, but these studies remain controversial (4,168,169).

The sIg expressed on B-CLL cells is of very low density, and is much less than that seen on normal B cells isolated from peripheral blood or lymphoid tissues. Similarly, the density of sIg is less than that observed on other B-cell-derived leukemias and lymphomas (170). However, several studies have suggested that the total cellular IgM of CLL cells is equivalent to most normal B cells. This discrepancy between the density of cell sIgM and the total cellular IgM is explained by the observation that B-CLL cells appear to have a higher density of cytoplasmic IgM (171). Therefore, B-CLL cells possess a low level of sIgM and a high level of cytoplasmic IgM, whereas normal cells express higher levels of sIgM and lower cytoplasmic IgM. The faint expression of sIgM might suggest that B-CLL cells may correspond to early B cells, after the cm+ pre-B-cell stage. However, the presence of sIgD on a significant number of CLLs supports the hypothesis that CLLs are counterparts of B cells that are later in normal ontogeny.

CLLs are heterogeneous for the expression of molecules involved in the adhesion with other cells or with extracellular matrix proteins. Unlike normal peripheral blood B lymphocytes, CLL cells have low to absent expression of LFA-1 (CD11a/CD18) (93,172–174). Moreover, CLLs generally have low to absent expression of ICAM-1 (CD54), the ligand for LFA-1 (175,176). This correlates with the low degree of homotypic adhesion seen when CLL cells are cultured in vitro (172). In contrast to normal peripheral blood B cells, CLLs express the other members of this glycoprotein family that are normally thought to be restricted to myeloid cells, including CD11b and CD11c noncovalently associated with CD18 (177–179). Similar to peripheral blood B cells, most CLLs express the lymphocyte homing receptors CD44 (76% of cases) (180,181) and L-selectin (55% of cases) (182). In-vitro studies have further demonstrated that L-selectin is functionally intact in mediating binding of CLL cells to high endothelial venules (182). The lack of the cell-cell adhesion molecules LFA-1, ICAM-1, but more importantly the expression of homing receptors L-selectin and CD44, may in part explain the capacity of B-CLLs to recirculate and widely disseminate.

Several other Ags on mature B cells have been investigated in B-CLL. The B-cell Ag-restricted CD22 is expressed on only 25% of B-CLLs (164). This observation again supports the notion that B-CLL is not the neoplastic counterpart of the "common" small resting B cell. Moreover, it has been suggested that the subset of B-CLLs that are CD22+ may have a more indolent course (183). Whereas 40–50% of peripheral blood B cells express CD1c, only a small proportion of B-CLLs are CD1c+ (20–40%) (118,184,185). This is in contrast to the majority of cases of B-PLL, HCL, and B-NHL, which have increased CD1c expression. The monoclonal antibody FMC7 reacts with 30–60% of sIg+ cells from peripheral blood and virtually all MRBC-R+ peripheral blood mononuclear cells (186). FMC7 has been reported to be unreactive with most B-CLLs (187), but some reports have observed reactivity with up to 50% of cases (163). A major difference between B-CLLs and virtually all B-cell prolymphocytic leukemias and hairy cell leukemias examined is that the PLLs and HCLs are FMC7+.

Complement Receptors

The receptors for the C3 fragments of complement are B-cell Ags with limited expression in ontogeny, which have heterogeneous expression on B-CLL. The majority of B-CLLs express CD21 (70), which is the C3d (C3dR) and EBV receptor, but B-CLLs express only 30% of the CD21 present on normal B cells (188). Although they express the receptor for EBV, it is controversial whether B-CLL cells proliferate in response to EBV (171). In contrast to the expression of C3dR, it is controversial whether CLLs express CD35, which is the C3b receptor.

B-Cell Activation Antigens

B-cell malignancies have been examined for the expression of B-cell activation Ags. These studies have demonstrated that virtually all B-cell NHLs express activation Ags, suggesting that B-cell malignancies do not correspond phenotypically to the small resting B cell that expresses Ia, CD19, CD20, CD21, CD22, CD24, CD40, CD44, CD45R, and sIgM/D and lacks activation Ags (189). This suggests that B-cell NHLs may be derived from neoplastic transformations of subpopulations of normal activated B cells. B-CLL have been similarly studied for the expression of activation Ags (70). Of the B-cell activation Ags examined, virtually all cases were B5+. Blast-1 and CD25 are expressed on approximately 50% of the cases and are generally present on the same cases. Other B-cell activation Ags, including B7/BB-1, B8.7, CD54, CD71, CD77, and 4F2, were less frequently expressed (190–192). The low-affinity Fcε receptor is reported to be present on a proportion of B-CLLs (184). Soluble CD23, which represents serum IgE-binding factor, is also elevated in B-CLL patients (57). Furthermore, the normal upregulation of CD23 by IL-4 that exists for normal B cells is also intact in B-CLL (193).

Studies from this laboratory have demonstrated by immunoprecipitation that the identical 55-kD protein, low-affinity IL-2 receptor (TAC Ag) (CD25), is present on B-CLLs, activated T cells, and activated B cells (70,127). Although not an activation Ag, normal B cells and B-CLLs also express low levels of the p75 IL-2 receptor (194). Other investigators have also confirmed the expression and release of soluble CD25 by B-CLLs (195), but it is controversial whether B-CLLs proliferate in response to exogenous recombinant IL-2 (70,196–203).

Terminal B-Cell Differentiation Antigens

B-CLLs uniformly lack Ags that are expressed on terminally differentiated B cells, including PCA-1 and CD38 (161). Therefore, B-CLL does not correspond to a terminally differentiated secretory B cell.

Antigens Expressed on Minor Subpopulations of B Cells

A number of Ags are present on minor subpopulations of normal B lymphocytes but are expressed on the majority of B-CLLs. These minor subpopulations of normal B cells do not represent the majority of B cells isolated from peripheral blood, lymph node, tonsil, and spleen.

Greater than 95% of B-CLLs express the MRBC-R (7–9). More important, within the B-cell malignancies this marker appears to be restricted to B-CLL, although some cases of hairy cell leukemia are MRBC-R +. The expression of MRBC-R is not restricted to malignant B cells, as a minor subpopulation of weakly sIg + normal B cells are MRBC-R positive. These cells have been observed to be present in fetal lymph node and liver, and in adult tonsil, but not in adult or fetal bone marrow (68,204). MRBC-R is therefore a useful marker for both B-CLL cells and a distinct minor subpopulation of normal B lymphocytes.

The CD5 Ag that is present on mature T cells and stage III thymocytes is also present on virtually all B-CLLs (70–73,156). As discussed previously, CD5 + B cells are observed in normal B-cell ontogeny, and the identification of addition sources of these cells will be discussed below.

COMMON B-CLL PHENOTYPE AND B-CLL HETEROGENEITY

A large study of the cell surface phenotype of cells isolated from patients with the clinical and morphologic features of B-CLL has been reported (70). Tumor cells in all cases were of B-cell derivation by the expression of CD19 and CD20. All but five cases expressed CD5, and 90 of 100 cases expressed the EBV/C3dR, CD21. Monoclonal sIg was not detectable on the tumor cells of 21 patients. C3b receptors (CD35) were detected on only 19 of the 100 cases. Therefore the overwhelming majority of B-CLLs coexpressed Ia, CD19, CD20, CD5, and CD21. Three major subgroups could be identified by the examination of expression of sIg and CD21: (a) sIg + CD21 − (n = 51); (b) sIg + CD21 + (n = 17); and (e) sIg − CD21 − (n = 15). When the intensity of Ag expression was examined, Ia and CD20 were strongly expressed on all tumor cells. The CD21 and CD19 Ags were less intensely expressed but were clearly positive on most tumor cells (60–80%) in the neoplastic population. Cell surface Ig, CD5, and CD35 were weakly expressed on the cell surface. When compared to small resting B cells isolated from peripheral blood or spleen, which are Ia +, CD19 +, CD20 +, CD21 +, sIg +, and CD35 +, the intensity of sIg and CD35 was significantly less intense on B-CLL cells. As stated above, most B-CLLs express B5, and approximately 50% express Blast-1 and CD25. Approximately a third were CD23 +, and only two cases expressed B7/BB-1. The transferrin receptor (CD71) was not detected on any of the cases examined.

More recently, further heterogeneity of B-CLLs has been demonstrated by the expression of the $\beta2$ integrin CD11c (178,179). Although CD11c is frequently present on HCL, a subset of CLLs that are CD11c+ have been studied. In contrast to typical CLLs, these CD11c+ cells were larger and had lower nuclear : cytoplasm ratios, but lacked nucleolar characteristics of PLL. Clinically, patients with CD11c+CD5+ leukemias presented with features of CLL and not HCL, with the characteristic splenomegaly and pancytopenia.

NORMAL CELLULAR COUNTERPARTS OF B-CLL

Identification of CD5+ B Cells in Normal Tissues

Normal B lymphocytes have been identified that resemble B-CLL cells by virtue of the coexpression of B-cell-restricted antigens and CD5 (see Fig. 2). As discussed previously, CD5+ B cells are a major population of fetal B cells present in lymph node and spleen, but not bone marrow or liver (67,69,70,204). Studies from our laboratory have isolated and demonstrated that CD5+CD20+ fetal splenocytes also express Ia, CD19, CD21, weak sIgM/D, but not CD35. This immunophenotype as well as the intensity of antigen expression on these cells was remarkably similar to that observed for the majority of B-CLLs. In-situ studies have identified CD5+ B cells in very small numbers at the periphery of the germinal center of normal adult lymph node (204). CD5+ B cells have also been observed in small numbers in adult peripheral blood and tonsil but not bone marrow (70). The more recent finding that B-CLLs express the $\beta2$ integrin CD11c has led to further studies of adult peripheral blood CD5+ B cell, and normal CD11c+CD5+CD20+ B cells have been identified (179). The CD5+ subpopulation of B cells have been noted in increased numbers in the peripheral blood of patients following allogeneic transplantation (205, 206) and the peripheral blood of patients with rheumatoid arthritis and systemic lupus erythematosis (207).

Studies of Normal Activated CD5+ B Cells

The initial observation that most B-CLLs express B-cell activation antigens led to studies of normal activated B cells for presence of CD5+. With the previous observations that some of the B-cell activation antigens can be variably induced by different stimuli, we examined splenic B cells following exposure to a variety of B-cell mitogens for the expression of CD5 (70,129). Of the various B-cell mitogens examined, only phobol myristic acetate (TPA) induced CD5 expression. Other B-cell stimuli that activate B cells via different receptors and pathways, including anti-Ig, EBV, or the anti-

B-CLL CELL

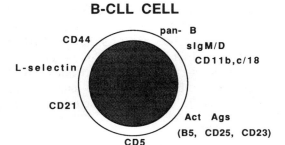

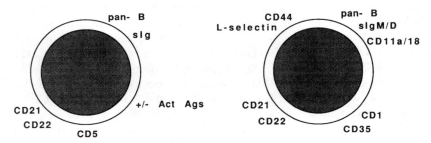

Figure 2 Cell surface phenotype of B-CLL cells; normal mature B cells; and in-vitro-activated, fetal, and a subset of normal adult peripheral blood and tonsillar B cells.

CD20 mAb 1F5, did not induce CD5. Similarly, culturing splenic B cells with IL-1, IL-2, IL-4, IFN-γ, and low-molecular-weight B-cell growth factor (LMW-BCGF), individually or in combination, failed to induce CD5. However, it has been reported that supernatants derived from the EL4 murine thymoma cell line can induce CD5 expression on normal B cells (131). The cell surface expression of CD5 was confirmed by immunoprecipitation studies demonstrating that resting B cells lack detectable CD5 protein whereas both ^{125}I- and ^{32}P-labeled CD5 could be identified from both activated B cells and T cells (130). Moreover, the CD5 protein immunoprecipitated from both activated B cells and normal mature T cells were structurally similar by limited peptide mapping.

The regulation of CD5 expression on normal activated B cells has been further studied by our laboratory. CD5 mRNA was not detected in resting splenic B cells, but following exposure to TPA, the mRNA was detected at 8 h, and maximally present at 48 h (130). Cell surface CD5 was detected at 48 h and declined after 96 h. With the observations that various cytokines regulated B-cell activation antigen expression, we examined the effect of a large number of cytokines for their effects on TPA-induced CD5 expression. We observed that both cell surface CD5 and CD5 mRNA were specifically inhibited by IL-4 but not by other cytokines examined. This effect was specific for CD5, as other B-cell activation Ags were generally unaffected by IL-4, except for induction of CD23. This suggested that a T-cell-derived lymphokine was involved in the expression of CD5 by activated B cells.

Further characterization of in-vitro-activated CD5+ B cells provided evidence that they are phenotypically similar to B-CLL cells. In-vitro-activated CD5+ B cells coexpressed other activation Ags found on B-CLLs, including B5, CD23, and CD25 (129). Other investigators have similarly examined normal CD5+ B cells isolated from peripheral blood for the expression of an activated cell surface phenotype. CD5+ B cells from cord blood coexpress CD23, CD25, and CD71, suggesting that they are preactivated (208). When these cells were cultured in the presence of only IL-1 and IL-2, without any other B-cell stimuli such as anti-Ig or TPA, the cells resembled a subset of activated B cells. The cells lost sIgD and CD5 and acquired CD10 and CD38 as well as the morphologic appearance of germinal center B cell blasts. It has also been noted that normal CD5+ tonsillar B cells express the B-cell-associated activation Ag 4F2 (209). In contrast to these reports, adult peripheral blood CD5+ B cells from normal individuals and patients with autoimmune diseases are reported not to express the activation Ags CD25, CD71, and Ba (210). Therefore, these studies suggest that normal CD5+ cells are a very heterogeneous population and include cells that are activated.

Functional studies of CD5+ cells have provided similar evidence that these cells are activated. In-vitro-activated CD5+ B cells proliferate in response to IL-2 but not BCGF (129). Similarly, cord blood CD5+ B cells proliferate spontaneously to IL-2 as well as LMW-BCGF. Finally, although both CD5− and CD5+ tonsillar B cells proliferate in response to LMW-BCGF (208), only the CD5+ respond to high-molecular-weight BCGF (209). Although the detection of CD5+ B cells in adult peripheral blood is reported to be quite variable, one study of normal CD5+ B cells from peripheral blood demonstrated that these cells do not proliferate spontaneously in the absence of other stimuli such as SAC or EBV.

In contrast to the CD5+ B cells from normals, it has been consistently observed that the CD5+ B cells present in association with autoimmune disorders are an activated cell population (211). Increased numbers of

CD5+ B cells are reported to be present in peripheral blood of both mice and humans with autoimmune disorders (211–213). These conditions are known to be associated with polyclonal B cell activation (214). CD5+ B cells isolated from patients with rheumatoid arthritis both spontaneously proliferate and secrete Ig of μ, γ, and α heavy-chain isotypes, in vitro. In addition, the size and internal complexity of the rheumatoid arthritis CD5+ B cells (forward angle and log 90° light scatter) is increased, suggesting that they are activated in vivo. Normal B cells as well as those from patients with rheumatoid arthritis are the population responsible for the secretion of rheumatoid factor, and anti-DNA antibodies belong to the CD5+ subset (210,215). Normal CD5+ B cells secrete rheumatoid factor as well as anti-DNA antibodies following mitogen stimulation. However, one study has observed that the CD5+ B cells from rheumatoid arthritis patients produced greater amounts of rheumatoid factor following stimulation with SAC than normal CD5+ B cells. These studies complement the phenotypic studies demonstrating heterogeneity of the activation state of CD5+ B cells.

Neoplastic CD5+ B cells (B-CLL) have been associated with autoimmune phenomena, including hemolytic anemia and IgM rheumatoid factor (216). Similarly, Waldenstroms macroglogulinemia is more frequently associated with monoclonal immunoglobulin autoantibodies. More recently it has been shown that B-CLL cells can frequently secrete autoantibodies (217,218). In rheumatoid arthritis, abnormal immune regulation would lead to production of rheumatoid factor and other autoantibodies. Neoplastic transformation of normal CD5+ B cells can therefore lead to malignant clones that are capable of producing autoantibodies.

SUMMARY

The majority of CLLs are of B-lineage derivation, with about 5% of cases of T lineage. Although morphologically resembling the small peripheral blood B cell, by virtue of the expression of B-cell-restricted and -associated cell surface antigens, B-CLLs are not the neoplastic counterparts of normal resting B cells. Similar to the peripheral blood B cell, B-CLLs express CD19, CD20, CD21, CD24, CD29/49d, CD40, CD44, CD45R, L-selectin, and sIgM/D. However, unlike peripheral blood B cells, B-CLLs generally do not express C3b complement receptor (CD35), LFA-1 (CD11a/18), or CD22, In addition, B-CLLs express the T-cell-associated antigen CD5, and a number of antigens induced on normal B cells following in-vitro activation. Normal CD5+ B cells, which phenotypically resemble B-CLL, are present in fetal lymphoid tissues and in small numbers in adults. Moreover, normal CD5+ B cells are present in increased numbers in patients with autoimmune diseases, and a subset of normal in-vitro-activated B cells phenotypically resemble B-CLL. These findings support the hypothesis that B-CLLs are the neoplastic counterparts of one or more unique subpopulations of normal B cells.

ACKNOWLEDGEMENTS

This work was supported by PHS grant number CA40216 and CA55207, awarded by the National Cancer Institute, DHHS.

REFERENCES

1. A. C. Aisenberg and K. J. Bloch, Immunoglobulins on the surface of neoplastic lymphocytes, *N. Engl. J. Med., 287*:272–276 (1972).
2. J. L. Preud'homme and M. Seligman, Surface bound immunoglobulins as a cell marker in human lymphoproliferative diseases, *Blood, 40,*:777–791 (1972).
3. J. C. Brouet, F. Flandrin, and M. Sasportes, Chronic lymphocytic leukemia of T cell origin. Immunologic and clinical evaluation in eleven patients, *Lancet, 2*:890–893 (1975).
4. L. Baldini, R. Mozzann, A. Cortelezzi, A. Neri, F. Radaelli, B. Cesana, A. T. Maiolo, and E. E. Polli, Prognostic significance of immunologic phenotype in B cell chronic lymphocytic leukemia, *Blood, 65*:340–344 (1985).
5. T. Han, N. Sadamori, H. Ozer, R. Gajera, G. A. Gomez, E. S. Henderson, A. Bhargava, J. Fitzpatrick, J. Minowada, M. L. Bloom, and A. A. Sandberg, Cytogenetic studies in 77 patients with chronic lymphocytic leukemia: Correlations with clinical, immunologic, and phenotypic data, *J. Clin. Oncol., 2*:1121–1132 (1984).
6. J. L. Preud'homme, J. C. Brouet, J. P. Clanvel, and M. Seligman, Surface IgD in immunoproliferative disorder, *Scand. J. Immunol., 3*:853–859 (1974).
7. D. Catovsky, M. Cherchi, A. Okos, U. Hedge, and D. A. G. Galton, Mouse red blood cell rosettes in B lymphoproliferative disorders, *Br. J. Haematol., 33*:173–177 (1976).
8. S. Gupta, R. A. Good, and F. P. Siegal, Rosette formation with mouse erythrocytes. II. A marker for human B and non-T lymphocytes, *Clin. Exp. Immunol., 25*:319–327 (1976).
9. G. Stathopoulos and E. V. Elliot, Formation of mouse or sheep red blood cell rosettes by lymphocytes from normal and leukemic individuals, *Lancet, 2*:600–602 (1974).
10. G. D. Ross, E. M. Rabellino, M. J. Polley, and H. M. Grey, Combined studies of complement receptor and surface immunoglobulin bearing cells and sheep erythrocyte rosette forming cells in normal and leukemic human lymphocytes, *J. Clin. Invest., 52*:377–385 (1973).

11. E. M. Shevach, R. Heberman, M. M. Frank, and I. Green, Receptors for complement and immunoglobulins on human leukemic cells and human lymphoblastoid cell lines, *51*:1933–1938.

12. J. C. Brouet, J. L. Preud'homme, C. Penit, F. Valensi, P. Rouget, and M. Seligmann, Acute lymphoblastic leukemia with pre-B cell characteristics, *Blood, 54*:269–273 (1979).

13. J. S. Korsemeyer, A. Arnold, A. Bakhshi, J. V. Ravetch, V. Siebenlist, P. A. Hieter, S. O. Sharrow, T. W. LeBien, J. H. Kersey, D. G. Poplack, P. Leder, and T. A. Waldman, Immunoglobulin gene rearrangement and cell surface antigen expression in acute lymphocytic leukemias of T cell and B cell precursor origins, *J. Clin. Invest., 71*:301–313 (1983).

14. L. M. Nadler, K. C. Anderson, G. Marti, M. Bates, E. Paark, J. F. Daley, and S. F. Schlossman, B4, a human B cell associated antigen expressed on normal, mitogen activated, and malignant B lymphocytes, *J. Immunol., 131*: 244–250 (1983).

15. L. M. Nadler, S. J. Korsmeyer, K. C. Anderson, A. W. Boyd, B. Slaughenhoupt, E. Park, J. Jensen, F. Coral, R. J. Mayer, S. E. Sallen, J. Ritz, and S. F. Schlossman, B cell origin of non-T cell acute lymphoblastic leukemia, *J. Clin. Invest., 74*:332–340 (1984).

16. A. F. Williams and A. N. Barclay, The immunoglobulin superfamily—Domains for cell surface recognition, *Ann. Rev. Immunol., 6*:381 (1988).

17. T. F. Tedder and C. Isaacs, Isolation of cDNAs encoding the CD19 antigen of human and mouse B lymphocytes. A new member of the immunoglobulin superfamily, *J. Immunol., 143*:712–717 (1989).

18. I. Stamenkovic and B. Seed, CD19, the earliest differentiation antigen of B cell lineage, bears three extracellular immunoglobulin-like domains and an Epstein-Barr virus related cytoplasmic tail, *J. Exp. Med., 168*:1205–1210 (1988).

19. A. Pezzutto, G. Dorken, P. S. Rabinovitch, P. Snow, E. Reinherz, and S. F. Schlossman, CD19 monoclonal antibody HD37 inhibits anti-immunoglobulin induced B cell activation and proliferation, *J. Immunol., 138*:2793–2799 (1986).

20. A. Pezzuto, G. L. Shu, T. B. Barrett, L. Ellingswoth, B. Dorken, and E. A. Clark, Downregulation of B cell activation by CD19 monoclonal antibodies vs inhibition by surface Ig Fc receptor cross-linking or TGF-beta, *Tissue Antigens, 33*:144 (1989).

21. R. Carter, D. Tuveson, D. Park, S. Rhee, and D. Fearon, The CD19 complex of lymphocytes. Activation of phospholipase C by a protein tyrosine kinase-dependent pathway that can be enhanced by the membrane IgM complex. *J. Immunol., 147*:3663–3671 (1991).

22. L. C. Strauss and C. I. Civin, MY10, a human progenitor cell surface antigen identified by a monoclonal antibody, *Exp. Hematol., 11 (suppl. 14)*:370a (1983).

23. L. C. Strauss, K. M. Skubitz, J. T. August, and C. I. Civin, Antigenic analysis of hematopoiesis: II. Expression of human neutrophil antigens on normal and leukemic marrow cells, *Blood, 63*:574–578 (1984).

24. C. A. Hurwitz, M. R. Loken, M. L. Graham, J. E. Kzarp, M. J. Borowitz, D. J. Pullen, and C. I. Civin, Asynchronous antigen expression in B lineage acute lymphoblastic leukemia, *Blood, 72*:299–307 (1988).

25. X. He, V. Antao, D. Basila, J. Marx, and B. Davis, Molecular characterization of the human CD34 gene, *Blood, 78*:371a (1991).

26. B. Dorken, G. Moldenhauer, A. Pezzutto, R. Schwartz, A. Feller, S. Kiesel, and L. M. Nadler, HD39 (B3), a B lineage-restricted antigen whose cell surface expression is limited to resting and activated human B lymphocytes, *J. Immunol., 136*:4470–4479 (1986).

27. I. Stamenkovic and B. Seed, The B-cell antigen CD22 mediates monocyte and erythrocyte adhesion, *Nature, 345*:74–77 (1990).

28. A. Pezzutto, B. Dorken, G. Moldenhauer, and E. A. Clark, Amplification of human B cell activation by a monoclonal antibody to the B cell-specific antigen CD22, Bp 130/140, *J. Immunol., 138*:98–103 (1987).

29. J. Cossman, L. M. Neckers, A. Arnold, and S. J. Korsmeyer, Induction of differentiation in a case of common acute lymphoblastic, *N. Engl. J. Med., 307*:1251–1254 (1982).

30. P. Hokland, P. Rosenthal, J. Griffin, L. M. Nadler, J. F. Daley, M. Hokland, S. F. Schlossman, and J. Ritz, Purification and characterization of fetal hematopoietic cells that express the common acute lymphoblastic leukemia antigen (CALLA), *J. Exp. Med., 157*:114–129 (1983).

31. P. Hokland, L. M. Nadler, J. D. Griffin, S. F. Schlossman, and J. Ritz, Purification of the common acute lymphoblastic leukemia antigen (CALLA) positive cells from normal bone marrow, *Blood, 64*:662–666 (1984).

32. P. Hokland, J. Ritz, S. F. Schlossman, and L. M. Nadler, Orderly expression of B cell antigens during the in vitro differentiation of non-malignant human pre-B cell, *J. Immunol., 135*:1746–1751 (1985).

33. L. M. Nadler, J. Ritz, M. P. Bates, E. K. Park, K. C. Anderson, S. E. Sallan, and S. F. Schlossman, Induction of human B cell antigen in non-T cell acute lymphoblastic leukemia, *J. Clin. Invest., 70*:433–442 (1982).

34. M. F. Greaves, G. Hariri, R. A. Newman, D. R. Sutherland, M. A. Ritter, and J. Ritz, Selective expression of the common acute lymphoblastic leukemia (gp100) antigen on immature lymphoid cells and their malignant counterparts, *Blood, 61*:628–639 (1983).

35. J. Ritz, M. Pesando, J. Notis-McConarty, H. Lazarus, and S. F. Schlossman, A monoclonal antibody to human acute lymphoblastic leukemia antigen, *Nature, 283*:583–585 (1980).

36. M. A. Shipp, N. E. Richardson, P. H. Sayre, N. R. Brown, E. L. Masteller, L. K. Clayton, J. Ritz, and E. L. Reinherz, Molecular cloning of the common acute lymphoblastic leukemia antigen (CALLA) identifies a type II integral membrane protein, *Proc. Natl. Acad. Sci. USA, 85*:4819–4823 (1988).

37. M. A. Shipp, J. Vijayaraghavan, E. V. Schmidt, E. L. Masteller, L. D'Adamio, L. B. Hersh, and E. L. Reinherz, Common acute lymphoblastic leukemia antigen (CALLA) is active neutral endopeptidase 24.11 ("enkephalinase") direct evidence by cDNA transfection analysis, *Proc. Natl. Acad. Sci. USA, 86*:297–301 (1989).

38. G. Salles, E. Reinherz, and M. Shipp, CD10/NEP inhibition potentiates stromal cell dependent lymphopoeisis, *Blood, 78*:158a (1991).

39. P. Stashenko, L. M. Nadler, R. Hardy, and S. F. Schlossman, Characterization of a new B lymphocyte specific antigen in man, *J. Immunol., 125*:1678–1685 (1980).

40. L. M. Nadler, P. Stashenko, J. Ritz, R. Hardy, J. M. Pesando, and S. F. Schlossman, A unique cell surface antigen identifying lymphoid malignancies of B cell origin, *J. Clin. Invest., 67*:134–140 (1981).

41. D. A. Einfeld, J. P. Brown, M. A. Valentine, E. A. Clark, and J. A. Ledbetter, Molecular cloning of the human B cell CD20 receptor predicts a hydrophobic protein with multiple transmembrane domains, *EMBO, 7*:711–717 (1988).

42. I. Stamenkovic and B. Seed, Analysis of two cDNA clones encoding the B lymphocyte antigen CD20 (B1,Bp35), a type III integral membrane protein, *J. Exp. Med., 167*:1975–1980 (1988).

43. T. F. Tedder, M. Streuli, S. F. Schlossman, and H. Saito, Isolation and structure of a cDNA encoding the B1 (CD20) cell surface antigen of human B lymphocytes, *Proc. Natl. Acad. Sci. USA, 85*:208–212 (1988).

44. T. F. Tedder, A. W. Boyd, A. S. Freedman, and L. M. Nadler, The B cell surface molecule B1 is functionally linked with B cell activation and differentiation, *J. Immunol., 135*:973–979 (1985).

45. E. A. Clark, G. Shu, and J. A. Ledbetter, Role of the Bp35 cell surface polypeptide on human B-cell activation, *Proc. Natl. Acad. Sci. USA, 82*:1766–1770 (1985).

46. K. Beiske, E. A. Clark, H. Holte, J. A. Ledbetter, E. B. Smeland, and T. Godal, Triggering of neoplastic B cells via surface IgM and the cell surface antigen CD20 and CDw40. Responses differ from normal blood B cells and are restricted to certain morphologic subsets, *Int. J. Cancer, 42*:521–528 (1988).

47. T. F. Tedder, P. D. Bell, R. A. Frizzell, and J. K. Bubien, CD20 directly regulates transmembrane ion flux in B lymphocytes, *Tissue Antigen, 33*:145 (1989).

48. C. Morimoto, N. L. Letvin, A. W. Boyd, M. Hagan, H. M. Brown, M. M. Kornacki, and S. F. Schlossman, The isolation and characterization of the human helper inducer T cell subset, *J. Immunol., 134*:3762–3769 (1985).

49. M. E. Hemler, C. Huang, and L. Schwarz, The VLA protein family: Characterization of five distinct cell surface heterodimers each with a common 130,000 molecular weight β subunit, *J. Biol. Chem., 262*:3300–3309 (1987).

50. M. E. Hemler, C. Huang, Y. Takada, L. Schwarz, J. L. Strominger, and M. L. Clabby, Characterization of the cell surface heterodimer VLA-4 and related peptides, *J. Biol. Chem., 262*:11478–11485 (1987).

51. M. E. Helmer, VLA proteins in the integrin family: Structure, functions, and their role on leukocytes, *Ann. Rev. Immunol., 8*:365–400 (1990).

52. D. Ryan, B. Nuccie, C. Abboud, and J. Winslow, Vascular cell adhesion molecule-1 and the integrin VLA-4 mediate adhesion of human B cell precursers to cultured bone marrow adherent cells, *J. Clin. Invest., 88*:995–1004 (1991).

53. E. A. Clark and J. A. Ledbetter, Structure, function, and genetics of human B cell-associated surface molecules, in *Advances in Cancer Research* (G. F. Vande Woude, ed.) Academic Press, Boca Raton, FL, pp. 81–149 (1989).

54. S. Braesch-Anderson, S. Paulie, P. Aspenstrom, H. Koho, and P. Perlmann, Biochemical characteristics of the human B-cell and carcinoma antigen Cdw40, *Tissue Antigens, 33*:129 (1989).

55. S. Inui, T. Kaisho, E. A. Clark, B. Seed, H. Kikutani, and T. Klshimoto, Expression of intact and mutant CDw40 on murine lymphocytes (cytoplasmic portion is essential for signal transduction through CDw40), *Tissue Antigens, 33*:133 (1989).

56. F. Uckun and J. A. Ledbetter, Expression and function of CDw40/Bp50 antigen in early human B-lymphocyte ontogeny, *Tissue Antigens, 33*:146 (1989).

57. J. Cairns, L. Flores-Romo, M. J. Millsum, G. R. Guy, S. Gillis, J. A. Ledbetter, and J. Gordon, Soluble CD23 is released by B lymphocytes cycling in response to interleukin 4 and anti-Bp50 (CD40), *Eur. J. Immunol., 18*: 349–353 (1988).

58. Y.-J. Liu, D. E. Joshua, G. T. Williams, C. A. Smith, J. Gordon, and I. C. M. MacLennan, Mechanism of antigen-driven selection in germinal centres, *Nature, 342*:929–931 (1989).

59. C. Morimoto, N. Letvin, J. Distaso, W. Aldrich, and S. Schlossman, The isolation and characterization of the human suppressor inducer T cell subset, *J. Immunol., 134*:1508–1515 (1985).

60. M. A. Ritter, C. A. Sauvage, S. M. Pegram, C. D. Myers, R. Dalchau, and J. W. Fabre, The human leukocyte-common (LC) molecule: dissection of leukemias using monoclonal antibodies directed against framework and restricted antigenic determinants, *Leuk. Res., 9*:1249–1254 (1985).

61. M. Streuli, L. R. Hall, Y. Saga, S. F. Schlossman, and H. Saito, Differential usage of three exons generates at least five different mRNAs encoding human leukocyte common antigens, *J. Exp. Med., 166*:1548–1566 (1987).

62. H. Charbonneau, N. K. Tonks, K. A. Walsh, and E. H. Fischer, The leukocyte common antigen (CD45): A putative receptor-linked protein tyrosine phosphatase, *Proc. Natl. Acad. Sci. USA, 85*:7182–7186 (1988).

63. L. Justement, K. Campbell, N. Chien, and J. Cambier, Regulation of B cell antigen receptor signal transduction and phosphorylation by CD45, *Science, 252*:1839–1842 (1991).

64. T. Hercend, L. M. Nadler, J. M. Pesando, E. L. Reinherz, S. F. Schlossman, and J. Ritz, Expression of a 26,000 dalton glycoprotein on activated human T cells. *Cell. Immunol., 64*:192–199 (1981).

65. J. H. Kersey, T. W. LeBien, C. S. Abramson, R. Newman, R. Sutherland, and M. Greaves, A human hemopoietic progenitor and acute lymphoblastic leukemia-associated cell surface structure identified with a monoclonal antibody, *153, 153*:726–731 (1981).

66. C. Abramson, J. R. Kersey, and T. W. LeBien, A monoclonal antibody (BA-1) primarily reactive with cells of human B lymphocyte lineage, *J. Immunol., 126*:83–88 (1981).

67. P. Rosenthal, I. J. Rimm, T. Umiel, J. D. Griffin, R. Osathanondh, S. F. Schlossman, and L. M. Nadler, Ontogeny of human hematopoietic cells: Analysis utilizing monoclonal antibodies, *J. Immunol., 31*:232–237 (1983).

68. M. Bofill, G. Janossy, M. Janossa, G. D. Burford, G. J. Seymor, P. Wernet, and E. Keleman, Human B cell development, II. Subpopulations in the human fetus. *J. Immunol., 134*:1531–1538 (1985).

69. J. H. Antin, S. G. Emerson, P. Martin, N. Gadol, and K. A. Ault, Leu-1+ (CD5+) B cells. A major lymphoid subpopulation in human fetal spleen: Phenotypic and functional studies, *J. Immunol., 136*:505–510 (1986).

70. A. S. Freedman, A. W. Boyd, F. Bieber, J. Daley, K. Rosen, J. Horowitz, D. Levy, and L. M. Nadler, Normal cellular counterparts of B cell chronic lymphocytic leukemia, *Blood, 70*:418–427 (1987).

71. L. Boumsell, H. Coppin, D. Pham, B. Raynal, J. Lemerle, J. Dausset, and A. Bernard, An antigen shared by a human T cell subset and B cell chronic lymphocytic leukemic cells, *J. Exp. Med., 152*:229–234 (1980).

72. M. Kamoun, M. F. Kadin, P. J. Martin, J. Nettleton, and J. A. Hansen, A novel human T cell antigen preferentially expressed on mature T cells and also on (B type) chronic lymphatic leukemic cells, *J. Immunol., 127*:987–996 (1981).

73. P. J. Martin, J. A. Hansen, A. W. Siadak, and R. C. Nowinski, Monoclonal antibodies recognizing normal human T lymphocytes and malignant B lymphocytes: A comparative study, *J. Immunol., 127*:1920–1923 (1981).

74. N. H. Jones, M. L. Clabby, D. P. Dialynast, H.-J. S. Huang, L. A. Herzenberg, and J. L. Strominger, Isolation of complementary DNA clones encoding the human lymphocyte glycoprotein T1/Leu-1, *Nature, 323*:346–349 (1986).

75. J. A. Ledbetter, P. J. Martin, C. E. Spooner, D. Wofsy, T. T. Tsu, P. G. Beatty, and P. Gladstone, Antibodies to Tp67 and Tp44 augment and sustain proliferative responses of activated T cell, *J. Immunol., 135*:2331–2336 (1985).

76. H. Van de Velde, I. von Hoegen, W. Luo, J. Parnes, and K. Thielemans, The B cell surface protein CD72/Lyb-2 is the ligand for CD5, *Nature, 351*: 662–665 (1991).

77. J. L. Gowans and E. J. Knight, The route of recirculation of lymphocytes in the rat, *Proc. Roy. Soc. London (Biol.), 159*:257 (1964).

78. H. B. Stamper and J. J. Woodruff, Lymphocyte homing into lymph nodes: In vitro demonstration of the selective affinity of recirculating lymphocytes for high endothelial venules, *J. Exp. Med., 144*:828–833 (1976).

79. E. C. Butcher, R. G. Scollay, and I. Weissman, Lymphocyte adherence to high endothelial venules: Characterization of a modified in vitro assay and examination of the binding of syngeneic and allogeneic lymphocyte populations, *J. Immunol., 123*:1996–2003 (1979).

80. W. M. Gallatin, I. L. Weissman, and E. C. Butcher, A cell-surface molecule involved in organ-specific homing of lymphocytes, *Nature, 304*:30–34 (1983).

81. L. A. Goldstein, D. F. H. Zhou, L. J. Picker, C. N. Minty, R. F. Bargatze, J. F. Ding, and E. C. Butcher, A human lymphocyte homing receptor the

Hermes antigen, is related to cartilage proteoglycan core and link proteins, *Cell, 56*:1063–1072 (1989).

82. T. St. John, J. Meyer, R. Idzerda, and W. M. Gallatin, Expression of CD44 confers a new adhesive phenotype on transfected cells, *Cell, 60*:45–52 (1990).

83. I. Stamemkovic, M. Amiot, J. M. Pesando, and B. Seed, A lymphocyte molecule implicated in lymph node homing is a member of the catilage link protein family, *Cell, 56*:1057–1062 (1989).

84. L. M. Stoolman, Adhesion molecules controlling lymphocyte migration, *Cell, 56*:907–910 (1989).

85. T. F. Tedder, C. M. Isaacs, T. J. Ernst, G. D. Demetri, D. A. Adler, and C. M. Disteche, Isolation and chromosomal localization of cDNAs encoding a novel human lymphocyte cell surface molecule, LAM-1. Homology with the mouse lymphocyte homing receptor and other human adhesion proteins, *J. Exp. Med., 170*:123–134 (1989).

86. D. Camerini, S. P. James, I. Stamenkovic, and B. Seed, Leu-8/TQ1 is the human equivalent of the Mel-14 lymph node homing receptor, *Nature, 342*: 78–82 (1989).

87. M. H. Siegelman, M. Van De Rijn, and I. L. Weissman, Mouse lymph node homing receptor cDNA clone encodes a glycoprotein revealing tandem interaction domains, *Science, 243*:1165–1172 (1989).

88. O. Spertini, G. Kansas, J. Munro, J. Griffin, and T. Tedder, Regulation of leukocyte migration by activation of the leukocyte adhesion molecule-1 (LAM-1) selectin, *Nature, 349*:691–694 (1991).

89. G. Gutman and I. Weissman, Lymphoid tissue architecture. Experimental analysis of the origin and distribution of T-cells and B-cells, *Immunology, 23*:465–471 (1972).

90. P. Nieuwenhuis and F. J. Keuning, Germinal centres and the origin of the B cell system II. Germainal centers in the rabbit spleen and popliteal lymph nodes, *Immunology, 26*:509–519 (1974).

91. P. Nieuwenhuis and W. L. Ford, Comparative migration of B and T lymphocytes in the rat spleen and lymph nodes, *Cell. Immunol., 23*:254–267 (1976).

92. R. F. Coico, S. Bhogal, and G. J. Thorbecke, Relationship of germinal centers in lymphoid tissue to immunologic memory. VI. Transfer of B cell memory with lymph node cells fractionated according to their receptors for peanut agglutinin, *J. Immunol. 131*:2254–2257 (1983).

93. F. Meidema, J. F. Tromp, M. B. Veer, S. Poppema, and C. J. M. Melief, Lymphocyte function-associated antigen 1 (LFA-1) is a marker of mature (immunocompetent) lymphoid cells. A survey of lymphoproliferative disease in man, *Leuk. Res., 9*:1099–1104 (1985).

94. D. Campana, B. Sheridan, N. Tidman, A. V. Hoffbrand, and G. Janossay, Human leukocyte function-associated antigens on lympho-hematopoetic precurser cells, *Eur. J. Immunol., 16*:537–542 (1986).

95. R. O. Hynes, Integrins: A family of cell surface receptors, *Cell, 48*:549–554 (1987).

96. T. A. Springer, Adhesion receptors of the immune system, *Nature, 346*:425–434 (1990).

97. S. M. Albelda and C. A. Buck, Integrins and other cell adhesion molecules, *FASEB J., 4*:2868–2880 (1990).
98. R. Rothlein, D. M. L., S. D. Marlin, and T. A. Springer, A human intracellular adhesion molecule (ICAM-1) distinct from LFA-1, *J. Immunol., 137*: 1270–1274 (1985).
99. R. Rothlein and T. A. Springer, The requirement for lymphocyte function associated antigen 1 in homotypic leukocyte adhesion stimulated by phorbol ester, *J. Exp. Med., 163*:1132–1149 (1986).
100. S. D. Marlin and T. A. Pringer, Purified intracellular adhesion molecule-1 (ICAM-1) is a ligand for lymphocyte-functional antigen 1 (LFA-1), *Cell, 51*: 813–819 (1987).
101. S. J. Mentzer, S. H. Gromkowski, A. M. Krensky, S. J.Burakoff, and E. Martz, LFA-1 membrane molecule in the regulation of Homotypic adhesion of human B lymphocytes, *J. Immunol., 135*:9–11 (1985).
102. M. Patarroyo, E. A. Clark, J. Prieto, C. Kantor, and C. G. Gahmberg, Identification of a novel adhesion molecule in human leukocytes by monoclonal antibody LB-2, *FEBS Lett., 210*:127–131 (1987).
103. M. Patarroyo, J. Prieto, P. G. Betty, E. A. Clark, and C. G. Gahmberg, Adhesion-mediating molecules of human monocytes, *Cell, Immunol., 113*: 278–289 (1988).
104. J. Prieto, P. G. Beatty, E. A. Clark, and M. Patarroyo, Molecules mediating adhesion of T and B cells, monocytes and granulocytes to vascular endothelial, *Cell, 63*:631–637 (1988).
105. G. Koopman, H. K. Parmentier, H.-K. Schuurman, W. Newman, C. J. L. M. Meijer, and S. Pals, Adhesion of human B cells to follicular dendritic cells involves both the lymphocyte function-associated antigen 1/intercellular adhesion molecule 1 and very late antigen 4/vascular cell adhesion molecule 1 pathways, *J. Exp. Med., 173*:1297–1304 (1991).
106. G. E. Rice and M. P. Bevilacqua, An inducible endothelial cell surface glycoprotein mediates melenoma adhesion, *Science, 246*:1303–1306 (1989).
107. A. S. Freedman, M. J. Munro, G. E. Rice, M. P. Bevilacqua, C. Morimoto, B. W. McIntyre, K. Rhynhart, J. S. Pober, and L. M. Nadler, Adhesion of human B cells to germinal centers in vitro involves VLA-4 and INCAM-110, *Science, 249*:1030–1033 (1990).
108. G. E. Rice, J. M. Munro, and M. P. Bevilacqua, Inducible cell adhesion molecule 110 (INCAM-110) is an endothelial receptor for lymphocytes, *J. Exp. Med., 171*:1369–1374 (1990).
109. G. E. Rice, J. M. Munro, C. Corless, and M. P. Bevilacqua, Vascular and nonvascular expression of INCAM-110, *Am. J. Pathol., 138*:385–393 (1991).
110. A. Garcia-Pardo, E. A. Wayner, W. G. Carter, and O. C. Ferreira, Human B lymphocytes define an alternative mechanism of adhesion to fibronectin, *J. Immunol., 144*:3361–3366 (1990).
111. J. L. Guan and R. O. Hynes, Lymphoid cells recognize an alternatively spliced segment of fibronectin via the integrin receptor $\alpha 4\beta 1$, *Cell, 60*:53–61 (1990).
112. L. M. Nadler, P. Stashenko, R. Hardy, A. van Agthoven, C. Terhorst, and

S. F. Schlossman, Characterization of a B cell specific (B2) distinct from B1, *J. Immunol., 126*:1941–1947 (1981).

113. K. Iida, L. M. Nadler, and V. Nussenzweig, The complement fragment C3d is a ligand for the human B lymphocyte membrane antigen B2, *J. Exp. Med., 158*:1021–1033 (1983).

114. J. D. Fingeroth, J. Weis, T. F. Tedder, J. L. Strominger, P. A. Biro, and D. T. Fearon, Epstein-Barr virus receptor of human B lymphocytes is the C3d receptor CR2, , *81*:4510–4514 (1984).

115. L. M. Nadler, A. W. Boyd, E. Park, K. C. Anderson, D. Fisher, B. Slaughenhoupt, D. A. Thorley-Lawson, and S. F. Schlossman, The B cell-restricted glycoprotein (B2) is the receptor for Epstein-Barr virus, in *Leukocyte Typing II* (E. L. Reinherz, B. F. Haynes, L. M. Nadler, and I. D. Bernstein, eds.), Springer-Verlag, Berlin, p. 509 (1986).

116. K. Iida, L. M. Nadler, and V. Nussenzweig, The identification of the membrane receptor for the complement fragment C3d by means of a monoclonal antibody, *J. Exp. Med., 158*:1021–1033 (1983).

117. C. Terhorst, A. van Agthoven, K. LeClair, J. A. Ledbetter, G. Moldenhauer, and E. A. Clark, Biochemical studies in the human thymocyte antigens T6, T9, and T10, *Cell, 23*:771–780 (1981).

118. D. Delia, G. Cattoretti, N. Polli, E. Fontanella, A. Aiello, R. Giardini, F. Rilke, and G. Della Porta, CD1c but neither CD1a nor CD1b molecules are expressed on normal, activated, and malignant human B cells: Identification of a new B-cell subset, *Blood, 72*:241–247 (1988).

119. T. N. Small, C. A. Keever, R. W. Knowles, R. J. O'Reilly, and N. Flomenberg, CD1c expression during normal B cell ontogeny, *Tissue Antigens, 33*: 71 (1989).

120. W. E. Paul, J. Mizuguchi, M. Brown, K. Nakanishi, P. Horbeck, E. Rabin, and J. Ohara, Regulation of B-lymphocyte activation, proliferation, and immunoglobulin secretion, *Cell. Immunol., 99*:7–13 (1986).

121. A. W. Boyd, K. C. Anderson, A. S. Freedman, D. C. Fisher, B. L. Slaughenhoupt, S. F. Schlossman, and L. M. Nadler, Studies of in vitro activation and differentiation of human B lymphocytes. I. Phenotypic and functional characterization of the B cell population responding to anti-Ig antibody, *J. Immunol., 134*:1516–1523 (1985).

122. J. H. Kehrl, A. Muraguchi, and A. S. Fauci, Differential expression of cell activation markers after stimulation of resting human B lymphocytes, *J. Immunol., 132*:2857–2861 (1984).

123. B. Haynes, B. F. Hemler, T. Cotner, D. L. Mann, G. S. Eisenberth, J. L. Strominger, and A. S. Fauci, Characterization of a monoclonal antibody (5E9) that defines a human cell surface antigen of cell activation, *J. Immunol., 127*:347–351 (1981).

124. B. F. Haynes, M. E. Hemler, D. L. Mann, G. S. Eisenberth, J. Shelhamer, H. S. Mostowski, C. A. Thomas, J. L. Strominger, and A. S. Fauci, Characterization of a monoclonal antibody (4F2) that binds to human monocytes and to a subset of activated lymphocytes, *J. Immunol., 126*:1409–1420 (1981).

125. D. A. Thorley-Lawson, R. T. Schooley, A. K. Bhan, and L. M. Nadler, Epstein-Barr virus superinduces a new human B cell differentiation antigen (B-LAST-1) expressed on transformed lymphoblasts, *Cell, 30*:415–425 (1982).

126. M. Tsudo, T. Uchiyama, and H. Uchino, Expression of TAC antigen on activated normal human B cells, *J. Exp. Med., 160*:612–617 (1984).

127. A. W. Boyd, D. C. Fisher, D. Fox, S. F. Schlossman, and L. M. Nadler, Structural and functional characterization of II-2 receptors on activated B cells, *J. Immunol., 134*:2387–2392 (1985).

128. R. A. Miller and J. Gralow, The induction of Leu-1 antigen expression in human malignant and normal B cells by Phorbol myristic acetate (PMA), *J. Immunol., 133*:3408–3414 (1984).

129. A. S. Freedman, G. Freeman, J. Whitman, J. Segil, J. Daley, and L. M. Nadler, Studies on in vitro activated CD5+ B cells, *Blood, 73*:202–208 (1989).

130. A. S. Freedman, G. Freeman, J. Whitman, J. Segil, J. Daley, H. Levine, and L. M. Nadler, Expression and regulation of CD5 on in vitro activated human B cells, *Eur. J. Immunol., 19*:849–855 (1989).

131. C. Werner-Favre, T. Vischer, D. Wohlwend, and R. Zubler, Cell surface CD5 is a marker for activated human B cells, *Eur. J. Immunol., 19*:1209–1213 (1989).

132. A. S. Freedman, G. Freeman, J. C. Horowitz, J. Daley, and L. M. Nadler, B7, a B cell restricted antigen which identifies pre-activated B cells, *J. Immunol., 137*:3260–3267 (1987).

133. T. Yokochi, R. D. Holly, and E. A. Clark, B lymphoblast antigen (BB1) expressed on Epstein-Barr virus-activated B cell blasts. B lymphoblastoid cell lines, and Burkitt's lymphomas, *J. Immunol., 128*:823–827 (1982).

134. D. A. Thorley-Lawson, L. M. Nadler, A. Bhan, and R. T. Schooley, Blast-2 (EBVCS): An early cell surface marker of human B cell activation is superinduced by Epstein-Barr virus, *J. Immunol., 134*:3007–3012 (1985).

135. L. J. Murray, J. A. Habeshaw, J. Wiels, and M. F. Greaves, Expression of Burkitt lymphoma-associated antigen (defined by the monoclonal antibody 38.13) on both normal and malignant germinal-centre B cells, *Int. J. Cancer, 36*:561–565 (1985).

136. A. S. Freedman, A. W. Boyd, K. C. Anderson, D. C. Fisher, S. F. Schlossman, and L. M. Nadler, B5, a new B cell restricted activation antigen, *J. Immunol., 134*:2228–2235 (1985).

137. T. Suzuki, S. K. Sanders, J. L. Butler, G. L. Gartland, K. Komiyama, and M. D. Cooper, Identification of an early activation antigen (Bac-1) on human B cells, *J. Immunol., 137*:1208–1213 (1986).

138. L. M. Neckers, G. Yenokida, and S. P. James, The role of the transferrin receptor in human B lymphocyte activation, *J. Immunol., 133*:2437–2441 (1984).

139. T. Defrance, J. P. Aubry, F. Rousset, B. Vanberulist, J. Y. Bonnefoy, N. Arai, Y. Takebe, T. Yokota, F. Lee, K. Aral, J. DeVries, and J. Banchereau, Human recombinant interleukin 4 induces FcE receptors (CD23) on normal human B lymphocytes, *J. Exp. Med., 165*:1459–1467 (1987).

140. J. Gordon, M. Rowe, L. Walker, and G. Guy, Ligation of the CD23 p45 antigen triggers cell-cycle progression of activated B lymphocytes, *J. Immunol., 16*:1075–1080 (1986).

141. K. Ikuta, M. Takami, C. W. Kim, T. Honjo, T. Miyoshi, Y. Tagaya, T. Kawabe, and J. Yodoi, Human lymphocyte Fc receptor for IgE: Sequence homology of its cloned cDNA with animal lectins, *Proc. Natl. Acad. Sci. USA, 84*:819–823 (1987).

142. H. Kikutani, S. Inui, R. Sato, L. E. Barsumain, H. Owaki, K. Yamaski, T. Kaisho, N. Uchibayshi, R. R. Hardy, T. Hirano, S. Tsunasawa, F. Sakiyama, M. Suemura, and T. Kishimato, Molecular structure of human lymphocyte receptor for immunoglobulin E, *Cell, 47*:657–665 (1986).

143. E. A. Clark and T. Yokochi, Human B cell and B cell blast-associated surface molecules defined with monoclonal antibodies, in *Leukocyte Typing I* (A. Bernard et al., eds.), Springer-Verlag, Berlin, pp. 339–346 (1984).

144. G. J. Freeman, A. S. Freedman, J. M. Segil, G. Lee, J. F. Whitman, and L. M. Nadler, B7, a new member of the Ig superfamily with unique expression on activated and neoplastic B cells, *J. Immunol., 143*:2714–2722 (1989).

145. P. S. Linsley, E. A. Clark, and J. A. Ledbetter, T-cell antigen CD28 mediates adhesion with B cells by interacting with activation antigen B7/BB-1, *Proc. Natl. Acad. Sci. USA, 87*:5031–5035 (1990).

146. C. H. June, J. A. Ledbetter, M. M. Gillespie, T. Lindsten, and C. B. Thompson, T-cell proliferation involving the CD28 pathway is associated with cyclosporin-resistant interleukin 2 gene expression, *Mol. Cell. Biol., 7*:4472–4481 (1987).

147. C. B. Thompson, T. Lindsten, J. A. Ledbetter, K. S. L., H. A. Young, S. G. Emerson, J. M. Leiden, and C. H. June, CD28 activation pathway regulates the production of multiple T-cell-derived lymphokines/cytokines, *Proc. Natl. Acad. Sci. USA, 86*:1333–1337 (1989).

148. C. H. June, J. A. Ledbetter, P. S. Linsley, and C. B. Thompson, Role of the CD28 receptor in T-cell activation, *Immunol. Today, 58*:271–276 (1990).

149. J. A. Ledbetter, J. B. Imboden, G. L. Schieven, L. S. Grosmaire, P. S. Rabinovitch, T. Lindsten, C. B. Thompson, and C. H. June, CD28 ligation in T-cell activation: Evidence for two signal transduction pathways, *Blood, 75*:1531–1539 (1990).

150. C. D. Gimmi, G. J. Freeman, J. G. Gribben, K. Sugita, A. S. Freedman, C. Morimoto, and L. M. Nadler, B7 provides a costimulatory signal which induces T cells to proliferate and secrete interleukin 2, *Proc. Natl. Acad. Sci. USA, 88*:6575–6579 (1991).

151. T. Kishimoto, Factors affecting B cell growth and differentiation, *Ann. Rev. Immunol., 3*:133–155 (1985).

152. C. M. Snapper and W. E. Paul, Interferon-γ and B cell stimulatory factor-1 reciprocally regulate Ig isotype production, *Science, 236*:944–947 (1987).

153. I. Stamenkovic and B. Seed, Molecular cloning of CD38, *Tissue Antigens, 33*:139 (1989).

154. K. C. Anderson, K. Park, M. Bates, R. C. F. Leonard, R. Hurdy, S. F. Schlossman, and L. M. Nadler, Antigens on human plasma cells identified by monoclonal antibodies, *J. Immunol., 130*:1132–1138 (1983).

155. R. O. Dillman, J. L. Beauregard, J. W. Lea, M. R. Green, R. E. Sobol, and I. Royston, Chronic lymphocytic leukemia and other chronic lymphoid proliferations: Surface marker phenotypes and clinical correlations, *J. Clin. Oncol., 3*:190–197 (1983).

156. R. T. Perri, I. Royston, T. LeBien, and N. E. Kay, Chronic lymphocytic leukemia progenitor cells carry the antigens T65, BA-1, and Ia, *Blood, 61*: 871–875 (1983).

157. L. Baldini, L. Cro, A. Cortelezzi, R. Calori, L. Nobili, A. Maiolo, and E. Polli, Immunophenotypes in "classical" B-cell chronic lymphocytic leukemia. Correlation with normal cellular counterpart and clinical findings, *Cancer, 66*:1738–1742 (1990).

158. J. P. Fermand, C. Schmitt, and J. C. Bronet, Distribution of class II DC antigens on normal and leukemic lymphoid cells, *Eur. J. Immunol., 15*:1183–1187 (1985).

159. V. Brown, S. Smith, E. Dewart, and A. Maddy, The correlation between surface immunoglobulin expression and the leucocyte-common antigen in B-cell chronic lymphocytic leukaemia, *Leuk. Res., 11*:903–910 (1987).

160. A. E. Roxburgh and I. A. Cooper, Expression of leukocytic-common antigen and large sialoglycoprotein on leukemic cells in B cell chronic lymphocytic leukemia and non-Hodgkin's lymphoma, *Leuk. Res., 1987*:891–901 (1987).

161. K. C. Anderson, M. P. Bates, B. L. Slaughenhoupt, G. S. Pinkus, C. O'Hara, S. F. Schlossman, and L. M. Nadler, Expression of human B cell associated antigens on leukemias and lymphomas: A model of B cell differentiation, *Blood, 63*:1424–1431 (1984).

162. J. Cossman, L. M. Neckers, T. Jones, S. M. Hsu, and E. S. Jaffe, Low grade lymphomas: Expression of developmentally regulated B cell antigens, *Am. J. Pathol., 115*:117–124 (1984).

163. M. Menon, H. G. Drexler, and J. Minowada, Heterogeneity of marker expression on B-cell leukemias and its diagnostic significance, *Leuk. Res., 10*: 25–28 (1986).

164. L. M. Nadler, B cell/leukemia panel workshop: Summary and comments in human B lymphocytes, in *Leukocyte Typing II* (E. L. Reinherz, B. F. Haynes, L. M. Nadler, and I. Bernstein, eds.), Springer-Verlag, Berlin, pp. 1–43 (1986).

165. A. Arnold, J. Cossman, A. Bakhshi, E. S. Jaffa, T. A. Waldmann, and S. J. Korsmeyer, Immunoglobulin-gene rearrangement as unique clonal markers in human lymphoid neoplasms, *N. Engl. J. Med., 309*:1593–1599 (1983).

166. G. Pianezze, I. Gentilini, M. Casini, P. Fabris, and P. Coser, Cytoplasmic immunoglobulins in chronic lymphocytic leukemia B cells, *Blood, 69*:1011–1014 (1987).

167. F. K. Stevenson, T. J. Hamblin, and G. T. Stevenson, The nature of the immunogloublin G on the surface of B lymphocytes in chronic lymphocytic leukemia, *J. Exp. Med. 154*:1965–1969 (1981).

168. T. J. Hamblin, D. G. Oscier, J. R. Stevens, and J. L. Smith, Long term survival in B-CLL correlates with surface IgM k phenotype, *Br. J. Haematol., 66*:21–26 (1987).

169. F. S. Ligler, J. R. Kettemen, R. G. Smith, and E. P. Frenkel, The nature of the immunoglobulin G on the surface of B lymphocytes in chronic lymphocytic leukemia, *Blood, 62*:256–263 (1983).

170. Y. H. Chen and P. Heller, Lymphocyte surface immunoglobulin density and immunoglobulin secretion in vitro in chronic lymphocytic leukemia (CLL), *Blood, 52*:601–608 (1978).

171. A. P. Johnstone, Chronic lymphocytic leukemia and its relationship to normal B lymphopoiesis, *Immunol. Today, 3*:342–348 (1982).

172. G. Inghirami, R. Wieczorek, B. Zhu, R. Silber, R. Dalla-Favera, and D. M. Knowles, Differential expression of LFA-1 molecules in non-Hodgkins's lymphoma and lymphoid leukemia, *Blood, 72*:1431–1434 (1988).

173. F. Morabito, E. F. Prasthofer, N. E. Dunlap, C. E. Grossi, and A. B. Tilden, Expression of myelomonocytic antigen on chronic lymphocytic leukemia B cells correlates with their ability to produce Interleukin 1, *Blood, 70*:1750–1757 (1987).

174. L. J. Medeiros, L. M. Weiss, L. J. Picker, C. Clayberger, S. J. Horning, A. M. Krensky, and R. A. Warnke, Expression of LFA-1 in non-Hodgkin's lymphoma, *Cancer, 63*:255–259 (1989).

175. R. Strauder, R. Greil, T. F. Schulz, J. Thaler, C. Gattringer, T. Radaskie-wicz, M. P. Dierich, and H. Huber, Expression of leukocyte function-associated antigen-1 and 7F7-antigen, an adhesion molecule related to intercellular adhesion molecule-1 (ICAM-1) in non-Hodgkin's lymphomas and leukemias: Possible influence on growth patterns and leukemic behavior, *Clin. Exp. Immunol., 77*:234–238 (1989).

176. M. Maio, A. Pinto, A. Carbone, V. Zagonel, A. Gloghini, G. Marotta, D. Cirillo, A. Colombatti, F. Ferrara, L. Del Vecchio, and S. Ferrone, Differential expression of CD54/intercellular adhesion molecule-1 in myeloid leukemias and in lymphoprolioferative disorders, *Blood, 76*:783–790 (1990).

177. A. De la Hera, M. Alvarez-Mon, F. Sanchez-Madrid, C. Marinez-A, and A. Durantez, Co-expression of Mac-1 and p150,95 on CD5+ B cells. Structural and functional characterization in a human chronic lymphocytic leukemia, *Eur. J. Immunol., 18*:1131–1134 (1988).

178. C. Hanson, T. Gribbin, B. Schnitzer, J. Schlegelmilch, B. Mitchell, and L. Stoolman, CD11c (LEU-M5) expression characterizes a B-cell chronic lymphoproliferative disorder with features of both chronic lymphocytic leukemia and hairy cell leukemia, *Blood, 76*:2360–2367 (1990).

179. S. Wormsley, S. Baird, N. Gadol, K. Rai, and R. Sobol, Characteristics of CD11c+CD5+ chronic B-cell leukemias and the identification of novel peripheral blood B-cell subsets with chronic lymphoid leukemia immunophenotypes, *Blood, 76*:123–130 (1990).

180. S. T. Pals, E. Horst, G. J. Ossekoppels, C. G. Figdor, R. J. Scheper, and C. J. L. M. Meijer, Expression of lymphocyte homing receptor as a mechanism of dissemination in non-Hodgkin's lymphoma, *Blood, 73*:885–888 (1989).

181. L. J. Picker, L. J. Medeiros, L. M. Weiss, R. A. Warnke, and E. C. Butcher, Expression of lymphocyte homing receptor antigen in non-Hodgkin's lymphoma, *Am. J. Pathol., 130*:496–504 (1988).

182. O. Spertini, A. S. Freedman, M. P. Belvin, A. C. Penta, T. A. Yednock, S. D. Rosen, J. D. Griffin, and T. F. Tedder, Regulation of leukocyte adhesion molecule-1 (TQ1, Leu-8) expression and shedding by normal and malignant cells, *Leukemia*.

183. F. Caligaris-Cappio, M. Gobbi, L. Bergui, D. Campand, F. Lauria, M. T. Fierro, and R. Foa, B-chronic lymphocytic leukemia patients with stable benign disease show a distinctive membrane phenotype, *Br. J. Haematol., 56*:655–660 (1984).

184. A. Orazi, G. Cattoretti, N. Polli, and F. Rike, CD1c and CD23 expression distinguish chronic B-lymphoctic leukemias from other chronic leukemias and leukemic lymphomas, *Tissue Antigens, 33*:68 (1989).

185. R. A. Jones, P. S. Master, J. A. Child, B. E. Roberts, and C. S. Scott, Diagnostic differentiation of chronic B malignancies using monoclonal antibody L161 (CD1c), *Br. J. Haematol., 71*:43–46 (1989).

186. D. A. Brooks, I. G. R. Beckman, J. Bradley, P. J. McNamara, M. E. Thomas, and H. Zola, Human lymphocyte markers defined by antibodies derived from somatic cell hybrids. IV. A monoclonal antibody reacting specifically with a subpopulation of human B lymphocytes, *J. Immunol., 126*: 1373–1377 (1981).

187. D. Catovsky, M. Cherchi, D. Brooks, J. Bradley, and H. Zola, Heterogeneity of B-cell leukemias demonstrated by the monoclonal antibody FMC7, *Blood, 33*:173–177 (1981).

188. J. Tooze and D. Bevan, Decreased expression of complement receptor type 2 (CR2) on neoplastic B cells of chronic lymphocytic leukaemia, *Clin. Exp. Immunol., 83*:423–429 (1991).

189. A. S. Freedman, A. W. Boyd, A. Berrebi, J. C. Horowitz, K. J. Rosen, B. Slaughenhoupt, D. Levy, J. Daley, H. Levine, and L. M. Nadler, Expression of B cell activation antigens on normal and malignant B cells, *Leukemia, 1*: 9–15 (1987).

190. J. Gordon, H. Mellstedt, P. Aman, P. Biberfield, M. Bjorkkholm, and G. Klein, Phenotypes in chronic B-lymphocytic leukemia probed by monoclonal antibodies and immunoglobulin secretion studies: Identification of stages of maturation arrest and the relation to clinical findings, *Blood, 62*:910–917 (1983).

191. K. Lewandrowski, L. Medeiros, and N. Harris, Expression of the activation antigen, 4F2, by non-Hodgkin's lymphomas of B-cell phenotype, *Cancer, 66*: 1158–1164 (1990).

192. S. Karray, C. Leprince, H. Merle-Beral, P. Debre, Y. Richard, and P. Galanaud, B8.7 antigen expression on B-CLL cells and its relationship to the LMW-BCGF responsiveness, *Leuk. Res., 14*:809–814 (1990).

193. M. Sarfati, S. Fournier, M. Christoffersen, and G. Biron, Expression of CD23 antigen and its regulation by IL-4 in chronic lymphocytic leukemia, *Leuk. Res., 14*:47–55 (1990).

194. C. Begley, J. Burton, M. Tsudo, B. Brownstein, J. Ambrus, and T. Waldmann, Human B lymphocytes express the p75 component of the interleukin 2 receptor, *Leuk. Res., 14*:263–271 (1990).

195. G. Semenzato, R. Foa, C. Agostini, R. Zambello, L. Trentin, F. Vinante, F.

Benedetti, M. Chilosi, and G. Pizzolo, High serum levels of soluble interleukin 2 receptor in patients with B chronic lymphocytic leukemia, *Blood, 70*: 396–400 (1987).

196. D. Kabelitz, K. Pfeffer, D. Von Steldern, P. Bartman, O. Brudler, C. Nerl, and H. Wagner, In vitro maturation B cells in chronic lymphocytic leukemia. I. Synergistic action of phorbol ester and interleukin-2 in the induction of Tac antigen expression and interleukin-2 responsiveness in leukemic B cells, *J. Immunol., 135*:2876–2881 (1985).

197. O. Lantz, C. Grillot-Courvalin, C. Schmitt, J.-P. Ferman, and J.-C. Brouet, Interleukin-2 induced proliferation of leukemic human B cells, *J. Exp. Med., 161*:1225–1230 (1985).

198. B. W. Grant, J. L. Platt, H. S. Jacob, and N. E. Kay, Lymphocyte populations and Tac-antigen in diffuse B-cell lymphomas, *Leuk. Res., 10*:1271–1278 (1986).

199. C. Hivroz, C. Grillot-Courvalin, J.-C. Brouet, and M. Seligmann, Heterogeneity of responsiveness of chronic lymphocytic leukemic B cells to B cell growth factor or interleukin 2, *Eur. J. Immunol., 16*:1001–1004 (1986).

200. R. T. Perri and N. E. Kay, Malignant chronic lymphocytic leukemia B cells express interleukin 2 receptors but fail to respond to interleukin 2's proliferative signal, *Leukemia, 1*:127–130 (1987).

201. I. Touw, L. Dorssers, and B. Lowenberg, The proliferative response of B cell chronic lymphocytic leukemia to interleukin 2: Functional characterization of the interleukin 2 membrane receptors, *Blood, 69*:1667–1673 (1987).

202. J. J. Murphy, V. Malkovska, L. Hudson, and R. E. Millard, Expression of functional interleukin 2 receptors on chronic lymphocytic leukemia B lymphocytes is modulated by recombinant interleukin 2, *Clin. Exp. Immunol., 70*:182–191 (1987).

203. N. E. Kay, J. Burton, D. Wagner, and D. L. Nelson, The malignant B cells from B-chronic lymphocytic leukemia patients release TAC-soluble interleukin-2 receptors, *Blood, 72*:447–450 (1988).

204. F. Caligaris-Cappio, M. Gobbi, M. Bofill, and G. Janossy, Infrequent normal B lymphocytes express features of B chronic lymphoxyic leukemia, *J. Exp. Med., 155*:623–627 (1982).

205. J. H. Antin, K. A. Ault, J. M. Rappeport, and B. R. Smith, B lymphocyte reconstitution after human bone marrow transplantation, *J. Clin. Invest., 80*:325–332 (1987).

206. K. A. Ault, J. H. Antin, D. Ginssburg, S. H. Orkin, J. M. Rappeport, M. L. Keohan, P. Martin, and B. R. Smith, Phenotype of recovering lymphoid cell populations after marrow transplantation, *J. Exp. Med., 161*: 1483–1502 (1985).

207. C. Plater-Zyberk, R. N. Maini, K. Lam, T. D. Kennedy, and G. Janossy, A rheumatoid arthritis B cell subset expresses a phenotype similar to that in chronic lymphocytic leukemia, *Arthritis Rheum., 28*:971–976 (1985).

208. F. Caligaris-Cappio, M. Riva, L. Tesio, M. Schena, G. Gaidano, and L. Bergui, Human normal CD5[+] B lymphocytes can be induced to differentiated to CD5[−] B lymphocytes with germinal center cell features, *Blood, 73*:1403–1408 (1989).

209. Y. Richard, C. Leprince, B. Dugas, D. Treton, and P. Galanaud, Reactivity of Leu-1 tonsillar B cells to a high molecular weight B cell growth factor, *J. Immunol. 139*:1563–1567 (1987).

210. R. R. Hardy, K. Hayakawa, M. Shimizu, K. Yamasaki, and T. Kishimoto, Rheumatoid factor secretion from human Leu-1+ B cells, *Science, 236*:81–83 (1987).

211. S. E. Burastero, P. Casali, R. L. Wilder, and A. L. Notkins, Monoreactive high affinity and polyreactive low affinity rheumatoid factors are produced by CD5+ B cells from patients with rheumatoid arthritis, *J. Exp. Med., 168*:1979–1992 (1988).

212. K. Hayakawa, R. R. Hardy, M. Hondo, L. A. Herzenberg, A. D. Steinberg, and L. A. Herzenberg, Ly-1 B cells: Functionally distinct lymphocytes that secrete IgM autoantibodies, *Proc. Natl. Acad. Sci. USA, 81*:2494–2498 (1984).

213. K. Hayakawa, R. R. Hardy, and L. A. Herzenberg, Progenitors for Ly-1 B cells are different from progenitors for other B cells, *J. Exp. Med., 161*:1554–1568 (1985).

214. D. M. Klinman and S. A. D., Systemic antoimmune disease arises from polyclonal B cell activation, *J. Exp. Med., 165*:1755–1761 (1987).

215. P. Casali, S. E. Burastero, M. Nakamura, G. Inghirami, and A. L. Notkins, Human lymphocytes making rheumatoid factor and antibody to ssDNA belong to Leu-1+ B-cells subset, *Science, 236*:77–80 (1987).

216. J. Michaeli, G. Lugassy, I. Raz, and A. Polliack, Chronic lymphocytic leukemia, lymphoma and autoimmunity in *Chronic Lymphocytic Leukemia* (A. Polliak and D. Catovsky, eds.), Harwood Academic Publishers, pp. 353–368 (1988).

217. L. Borche, A. Lim, J. Binet, and G. Dighiero, Evidence that chronic lymphocytic leukemia B lymphocytes are frequently committed to production of natural autoantibodies, *Blood, 76*:562–569 (1990).

218. T. Kipps, B. Robbins, A. Tefferi, G. Meisenholder, P. Banks, and D. Carson, CD5-positive B-cell malignancies frequently express cross-reactive idiotypes associated with IgM autoantibodies, *Am. J. Pathol., 136*:809–816 (1990).

2

The Control of Growth and Differentiation in Chronic Lymphocytic Leukemia (B-CLL) Cells

Kenneth Nilsson
University of Uppsala Hospital, Uppsala, Sweden

INTRODUCTION

Chronic lymphocytic leukemia (CLL) is a heterogeneous disease with respect to both its clinical behavior and its cellular biology in vitro (1,2). CLL has a variable clinical course and is characterized by the accumulation of clonal tumor cells with the morphology of small blood lymphocytes. Patients with CLL may have polyreactive autoantibodies, produced by the leukemic cells, in the serum. They frequently suffer from infections, probably related to not fully defined immune deficiencies, including hypogammaglobulemia, deficient granulocyte motility, and T-cell abnormalities, which may have developed as a consequence of suppressive immunoregulatory functions of the CLL cells (1–3). Since CLL cells are easily accessible and survive comparatively well in vitro, they have been examined extensively during recent years with respect to genotypic and phenotypic properties.

During the early 1970s it became clear that most CLL cells express low levels of immunoglobulin (Ig) M, or coexpress IgM and IgD (4), while a minority (5%) form rosettes with sheep red blood cells (5). With the introduction of the method for production of mouse monoclonal antibodies (moab), the flow cytometer, various molecular biology techniques, and new methods for cell separation, it has been possible to further define the surface Ig-expressing CLL cells as CD5+ B cells and to identify some features of B-CLL cells possibly associated with their malignant state. During the 1980s cellular immunologists and molecular biologists have extensively characterized the various stages of B-cell differentiation in the bone marrow and the peripheral lymphoid organs (6), and have defined various compartments of the normal immune system with respect to cellular genotypes and phenotypes, cell-cell interactions, and cellular recirculation (7). A picture of the normal hematopoietic and immune systems as cellular network systems has emerged from these studies. The growth and differentiation of the various cell types appear to be regulated by complex homeostatic mechanisms, including interactions between cells by signals provided by specific cell-cell contacts and soluble hormonelike factors, the cytokines. This new knowledge is of fundamental importance for the understanding of the neoplastic process in B-CLL.

This review will show that B-CLL cells should no longer be regarded as autonomous resting cells, irreversibly arrested in their differentiation at a stage of B-cell development roughly corresponding to that of normal peripheral blood B cells. In-vitro experiments over the last decade have rather convincingly demonstrated that fresh B-CLL cells interact, although frequently less well than normal B cells, and with extensive variability, with cytokines and T cells in their microenvironment. B-CLL cells in vivo may be thus subjected to most if not all of the growth and differentiation control mechanisms that tightly control the expansion and function of normal B cells. This fact gives hope that it should be possible to correct the genetically determined malignant growth behavior of B-CLL cells in the future by manipulating the microenvironment in which the tumor clone expands, and to prolong the life of the patient. Such therapeutic interventions should aim at controlling the growth of the B-CLL cells directly by cytokines, or indirectly by stimulating nonneoplastic cells with capacity to restrict the proliferation of the B-CLL cells within the immunologic cellular network, e.g., T cells and monocytes.

GENERAL ASPECTS OF THE CONTROL OF GROWTH AND DIFFERENTIATION OF NORMAL AND MALIGNANT HEMATOPOIETIC CELLS

Mature cells of the hematopoietic system are the progeny of the pluripotent stem cell (PSC) population in the bone marrow. The hematopoiesis seems to have a hiarchic structure. According to common models the PSC, which has the capacity for self-renewal through asymmetric division, restricts its potency by a process of commitment and develops into either a lymphoid or a myeloid precursor cell (8). Such cells evolve into unipotent precursor cells from which the various specific cell lineages develop. The commitment of the PSC may be a stochastic process (8), which, however, is influenced not only by signals (cell-cell contacts and cytokines) from cells of the microenvironment (particularly stromal cells), but also by hormones and cytokines produced at a distance, e.g., inflammatory cells and kidney epithelium (9). Figure 1 presents schematically the complex control of the growth and differentiation of hematopoietic cells by stimulatory and inhibitory cellular interactions via adhesion molecules and paracrine cytokines, autocrine loops, and hormones.

The expansion of the progeny of a unipotent precursor cells within each cell lineage by proliferation occurs in parallel with functional specialization (maturation). The capacity for proliferation thus diminishes as maturation proceeds, and the terminally differentiated end cells become irreversely arrested in the G_0/G_1 of the cell cycle. Proliferation and maturation are thus inversely related processes that seem to be controlled by separate, but coupled, gene programs.

In leukemia/lymphoma the gene programs for growth and differentiation are frequently uncoupled as a consequence of genetic changes (10). In agreement with the concept of "frozen" differentiation, lymphocytic leukemias, including B-CLL, have been found to represent clonal expansions of neoplastic cells with a phenotype representing a particular, discrete stage of lymphoid differentiation (11).

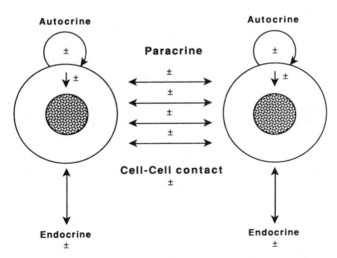

Figure 1 General scheme of the complex signaling that controls the growth and differentiation of any two cells within the hematopoietic and immune systems.

NORMAL HUMAN B-CELL DEVELOPMENT

The description of the control and growth and differentiation of B-CLL cells to follow requires, as a background, a short summary of the complex regulatory mechanisms that control normal B cells at various stages of the B-cell differentiation lineage and the extensive differences in the architecture of the organ-specific B-cell microenvironment that exist. Since B-CLL cells express the CD5 antigen, the distinguishing features of normal CD5 + B cells will be described.

The Development of B Cells in the Bone Marrow

Putative lymphoid stem cells in the bone marrow appear to develop independently of antigenic stimulation through successive, functionally and morphologically definable stages of differentiation into virgin B cells. By analyses of the expression of surface antigens, terminal deoxynucleotidyl transferase, and the rearrangement of Ig heavy and light chains of leukemia and lymphoma cell clones, representing frozen stages of B-cell differentiation (6,11,12), and by studies of B-cell development in in-vitro bone marrow cultures (13,14), several discrete stages of normal B-cell development have been defined (6). The earliest recognizable cells within the B lineage are the pro-B cells. Once pro-B cells have rearranged the μ-Ig chain genes, they produce cytoplasmic μ chains and are termed pre-B cells. After successful rearrangement of one of the Ig light chains, early virgin B cells, expressing low levels of surface IgM, develop. Such cells migrate from the bone marrow to the peripheral lymphoid tissue, during which time they gradually evolve into functionally mature virgin B cells by initiating the expression of surface IgD and by increasing the density of surface IgM. The sequential expression of several B-cell antigens (6) allows the definition of developing B cells by moabs. The differentiation-specific expression of several surface antigens on the various categories of developing B cells suggests that the stepwise process of differentiation is controlled to a large extent by signals in the microenvironment (Fig. 1). Most surface antigens are not yet defined functionally. However, existing information shows that they may represent receptors for growth regulatory signals, molecules involved in the transduction of external signals, and adhesion molecules necessary for the interaction of the cells with their microenvironment, particularly with stromal cells and T cells (6,15).

The introduction of in-vitro methods for short-term culture of bone marrow cells has recently made it possible to study the regulatory role of stromal cells and paracrine cytokines in B-cell development (13,14). The results so far demonstrate that stimulation of pre-B cells with IL-3, Il-7, low-molecular-weight BCGF (LMW-BCGF), and the interaction of such cells with stromal cells by adhesion proteins and with matrix proteins, e.g., laminin and fibronectin, resulting in induction of proliferation and differentiation (6,16,17). The importance of stromal cells in the regulation of developing B cells has further been suggested by studies showing that glycosaminoglycans of such cells accumulate and present growth factors to hematopoietic cells (18,19).

CD5 + B cells are not detectable in adult bone marrow but are found as a large subpopulation after bone marrow transplantation (39). There are no data to support that bone marrow CD5 + B cells should be regulated differently from CD5 − B cells during development.

B-Cell Development in the Peripheral Lymphoid Organs

In the peripheral lymphoid organs the process by which further differentiation of the virgin B cells occurs is only partly known but seems to depend on antigenic stimulation in addition to the signals provided by cell-cell contacts and cytokines (20). The lymphoid organs, e.g., lymph nodes, are highly structured tissues in which the virgin B cells encounter antigens and receive the necessary activation-, growth-, and differentiation-inducing signals from antigen-specific T cells and cells of monocytic derivation. The responding cells may develop during an extrafollicular, paracortical (primary) response into short-lived plasma cells, or they may become part of the pool of recirculating follicular B cells. Virgin B cells not selected by antigen appear to die during their recirculation in the blood. Later, in a T-cell-dependent antigenic response, the follicle is the major B-cell area. In the primary follicle, the network of follicular dendritic cells (FDC) is filled with recirculating B cells, which become activated by the interaction with antigen-presenting FDC to become proliferating B blasts. The follicles will later transform into secondary follicles with germinal centers, following the development of the B blasts into highly proliferating, surface Ig-negative centroblasts, which undergo the process of sIg V-region hypermutation. The Ig isotype class switch also occurs in the germinal centers. The progeny of the centroblasts, the centrocytes, reexpress surface Ig and become growth arrested in the G_0 phase of the cell cycle. Centrocytes expressing high-affinity Ig will be selected to become follicular B blasts, which subsequently develop into either memory B cells or long-lived plasma cells. Unselected centrocytes die by apoptosis, as suggested by the presence of apoptotic bodies in the germinal centers and by in-vitro experiments (21). The mechanism by which centrocytes may be rescued from apoptotic death by FDCs is poorly understood. Indirect evidence from in-vitro experiments suggests that FDCs interact with centrocytes by presenting antigen, by cell-cell contacts, and by the production of cytokines (IL-1α, LMW-BCGF, CD23), thereby preventing apoptosis (21,22).

Cytokines and Adhesion Molecules Involved in the Regulation of Mature B Cells

B-cell proliferation thus occurs both in the bone marrow, as the result of antigen-independent stimulation of precursor B cells that develop into short-lived virgin B cells, and in the periphery, following antigen-dependent activation of virgin B cells and memory B cells. However, most peripheral blood B cells seem to have a long life span as resting G_0 cells. Many B cells recirculate and are in constant flux between the various lymphoid tissues via the blood and lymph.

It is obvious that the regulation of growth and differentiation of mature B cells is complex. Usually more than one signal is required to induce a mitogenic response. Distinct signals seem to activate the resting B cell to undergo G_0-to-G_1 transition with concomitant RNA and protein synthesis, leading to a morphological blast transformation. The activation is associated with an increased expression of several adhesion proteins and receptors for growth and differentiation factors. Interactions with the adhesion molecules during the cell-cell contacts with T cells, monocytes, and other immunoregulatory cells, and the interaction of cytokines with their receptors, transmit signals that regulate the gene transcription necessary for entry into the S phase. In the proper environment, cells will thus traverse the S and G_2 phases of the cell cycle and undergo mitosis.

B cells express different types of adhesion proteins. Both the stage of differentiation and the state of activation influence the type of adhesion proteins expressed and their quantity. Of special interest is the expression of integrin adhesion proteins of the $\beta 1$ and $\beta 2$ groups (23,24), which may mediate interaction of B cells with extracellular matrix proteins and with T cells and monocytes, and several surface structures of importance for the homing of circulating B cells in the peripheral lymphoid organs (25,26).

Depending on the stage of differentiation and the activation status peripheral B cells in vitro respond differently to various cytokines. This observation is expected since, as mentioned above, the expression of cytokine receptors, and other surface structures transmitting noncytokine external signals, appear to be dynamic and associated with the differentiation stage and activation status. Nevertheless, this makes the critical assessment of the data on cytokine effects on B cells in vitro difficult. The species studied, the source of B cells used, the method for B-cell purification, contamination with non-B cells, the source of serum used, the cell density, the method for activation, and the methods used to determine induced proliferation and differentiation will all affect the results from studies on the effect of a given cytokine on the growth and differentiation of B cells. The following cytokines, however, appear to have documented stimulatory effect on DNA synthesis and differentiation on normal B cells: IL-1α, IL-1β (27), IL-2 (28), IL-6 (29), LMW-BCGF (30), IFN-γ (31), and TNF-α (32). Differentiation only has been induced by IL-5 (33) and IFN-α and -γ (34), while TNF-α and IL-10 seem to preferentially induce proliferation and minimal differentiation (35,36). Depending on the costimulatory activation signal(s), IL-4 has been reported either to stimulate or inhibit DNA synthesis and differentiation (37). TGF-β (38) and IFN-α (34), in contrast, have been found to inhibit DNA synthesis.

CD5 + B cells recirculate in the peripheral blood and constitute about 10% of the splenic and 30% of lymph nodes and tonsils (39). They differ from CD5 − B cells in antigen expression (see also below) and may have immunoregulatory functions (40). These features and the fact that the CD5 surface molecule might be involved in the transmission of cytokine signals, either as a receptor or as a molecule associating with other cytokine receptors, e.g., the IL-1R (39), suggest that the presence of CD5 on B-CLL cells may be decisive for their impaired response to growth-regulating signals as compared to CD5 − normal B cells.

THE PHENOTYPE OF B-CLL CELLS

The extensive studies on various aspects of the phenotype of B-CLL cells have recently been summarized in several excellent reviews (1,2,11,39,41). The reader is referred to these articles for detailed information, particularly about antigenic expression, which will be summarized only briefly in the following.

Taken together, the phenotypic studies of B-CLL cells seem to show that the well-known clinical heterogeneity of B-CLL is a reflection of considerable heterogeneity present between different B-CLL clones at the cellular level. Nevertheless, most B-CLL clones appear to have a morphology roughly corresponding to that of recirculating small B cells resting in the G_0 phase of the cell cycle, as illustrated by Fig. 2. The following summary will focus on the description of this "common" type of B-CLL. The aspects of heterogeneity will be stressed whenever relevant.

Surface Antigen Expression

B-CLL cells express most of the surface antigens typical of mature or slightly immature B cells (Fig. 2). Thus, associated with the common

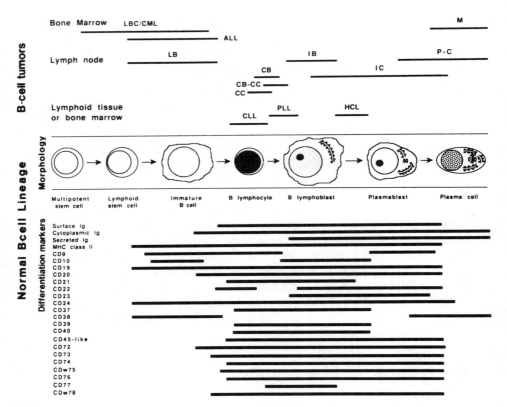

Figure 2   The relationship of human B-cell tumors to normal B-cell development. Data on the expression of Ig and surface markers on normal and malignant B cells are from Refs. 6, 11, and 12. Tumors are classified according to the Kiel classification. Abbreviations: LBC/CML, lymphoid blast crisis of chronic myeloid leukemia; M, multiple myeloma; ALL, acute lymphoblastic leukemia; LB, lymphoblastic lymphoma; IB, immunoblastic lymphoma; P-C, plasmacytoma; CB, centroblastic lymphoma; IC, immunocytoma; CB-CC, centroblastic-centrocytic lymphoma; CC, centrocytic lymphoma; PLL, prolymphocytic leukemia; HCL, hairy cell leukemia; B-CLL, chronic lymphocytic leukemia.

B-CLL immunophenotype is the expression of MHC class II antigen, CD5 (see below), CD19, CD20, CD21 (C3d receptor), CD24, CD40, CD44, CD45R, and B5 (2). Less frequently expressed are CD11c, CD9, CD22, CD35 (C3b receptor), and FMC7 (2), illustrating that B-CLL is heterogeneous with respect to the stage of normal B-cell differentiation.

The heterogeneity is also apparent from the expression of some antigens not expressed on normal mature B cells (1,2,41). Thus, CD11a/CD18 (LFA-1, mediating homotypic adhesion) is absent on B-CLL cells or expressed at a low level (42,43), and several antigens, usually assumed to represent antigens of myelomonocytic cells, i.e., CD11b/CD18, CD11c/CD18, CD14, and CD15, are variably expressed (39,44). As discussed below, these antigens may not exemplify lineage infidelity but rather reflect that B-CLL cells are derived from CD5 + normal cells, which express myelomonocytic antigens as part of their lineage-specific antigen repertoire.

Also antigens, normally associated with an activated normal B-cell phenotype, are detectable on B-CLL cells with variable frequency, with CD5 (see below), B5, Blast-1, CD23, and CD25 most frequently expressed. Less prevalent and/or weakly expressed are BB-1/B7, CD54, CD71, and CD77 (2,45).

Cytokine Receptor Expression

Comparatively little is known about the expression of cytokine receptors on B-CLL cells. From the biologic effects noted in the studies on cytokine-induced proliferation and/or differentiation of B-CLL cells in vitro (see below), it is, however, clear that IL-2, IL-4, TNF-α, IFN-α, IFN-γ, LW-BGGF, and HMW-BCGF stimulate such cells. It can therefore be assumed that B-CLL cells express receptors for at least these cytokines. However, only in the case of the receptors for IL-2 (IL-2R), TNF-α, IL-6, LMW-BCGF, and HMW-BCGF have direct assays on the receptor expression been reported.

The IL-2R is, as described above, expressed on a variable fraction of B-CLL clones (46–49). The IL-2Rs are functional, since IL-2 stimulation can be blocked by anti-IL-2R moabs (47,48). Characterization of the IL-2R expression on B-CLL cells by radiolabeled IL-2 binding assay demonstrated the presence of both high- and low-affinity receptors (49). The expression of the IL-2R is upregulated after stimulation with phorbolester, SAC, or by IL-2 (48,50). IL-4 seems to inhibit the formation of a functional, high-affinity IL-2R on anti-μ antibody and SAC-activated cells, but not the expression of the synthesis of the α- and β-IL-2R chains (50).

The TNF-αR is described by Hoffbrand in this volume. Suffice it to say that, although this receptor mediates a growth stimulatory signal in vitro, freshly isolated cells seem to be TNF-αR negative (51).

The expression and/or function of a few cytokine receptors may be abnormal in B-CLL cells. The HMW-BCGFR has been reported to be contitutively expressed in B-CLL cells but not in normal resting B cells (52). The expression of LMW-BCGF may be impaired (53). Finally, recent data show no activation-associated increase in IL6R expression in one

B-CLL clone, and, in contrast to activated normal B cells, the B-CLL cells do not respond to IL-6 (54).

Cytokine Production

Like normal B cells, B-CLL cells produce several cytokines as determined by assays for cytokine protein and/or mRNA. In the interpretation of these data, one is confronted with several problems. One is that highly purified B-CLL cells were usually not studied. It is therefore difficult to exclude that non-B-CLL cells among the peripheral blood mononuclear cells were the main source of the cytokines detected. The reports on production of IL-2 and IFN-γ in B-CLL cells are for this reason controversial. Another difficulty is how to interpret the cytokine studies at the mRNA level. Although cytokine mRNAs are commonly translated and secreted, one cannot conclude from such studies that the cytokines examined indeed are synthesized and exported. A third problem is the heterogeneity of B-CLL clones. It is likely that synthesis of cytokines is associated with the level of differentiation, the type of activating agent, and the state of activation. Due to the heterogeneity with respect to maturation and the variability in response to different activation signals among B-CLL clones, the cytokine profile is therefore expected to be variable.

With these reservations, the studies demonstrate that B-CLL clones may produce IL-1α (55), IL-1β (55), IL-6 (54–57), TNF-α (57–59), TNF-β (54), TGF-β (57), and release the soluble form of CD 23 (60). Of these cytokines, only TNF-α, TGF-β, and IL-1β were regularly found (55,57,58). The role of any of these cytokines as autocrine growth factors is controversial and not yet convincingly proven. The mere finding of the production of a cytokine, and that the producer cell may respond to the same exogenous cytokine, only suggest the possibility of an autocine loop. In B-CLL this problem is best exemplified by the studies on TNF-α (see Hoffbrand, this volume). Since B-CLL cells are expected to interact with the environment by paracrine loops according to Fig. 1, it is interesting to note that IL-6 production is constitutive (56,57) and inducible (54) in B-CLL clones, but that the B-CLL cells do not express functional IL-6R, neither spontaneously nor after induction. IL-6 may thus exemplify a paracrine cytokine produced by B-CLL cells to communicate with nonneoplastic cells in its microenvironment.

IL-2 and IL-4 do not seem to be produced by B-CLL cells (57).

Immunoglobulin Synthesis and Secretion

A few studies on the biosynthesis of Ig in vitro illustrate that the phenotype of B-CLL cells is heterogeneous (61,62), as expected from early studies on the expression of surface Ig and by the fact that a fraction of B-CLL patients have monoclonal Ig in their sera (1,2,4). B-CLL cells were analyzed for spontaneous and inducible Ig synthesis at the transcriptional level by northern blot analysis of Ig mRNA and at the translational level by protein synthesis studies. The results demonstrated that B-CLL clones of the common type spontaneously expressed membrane and secretory μ-chain mRNA. However, only membrane IgM was further processed and expressed at the cell surface. The secretory μ chains were degraded intracellularly (61,62). Another type of B-CLL clone had spontaneous secretion of IgM (61). A third type of B-CLL was at an intermediate stage of functional differentiation. The studies thus support the concept of frozen differentiation in B-CLL and agree with the studies of antigen expression that B-CLL is a heterogeneous B-cell neoplasia in which individual clones represent distinct, discrete stages of B-cell differentiation.

Similarities and Differences Between B-CLL Cells and Normal CD5+ B Cells

It is still a controversial issue whether CD5+ B cells constitute a separate B-cell subset or whether CD5 is an activation antigen on circulating, regular B cells. Since CD5 positivity is a hallmark of B-CLL cells, the issue is important. As recently reviewed by Freedman (2) and Kipps (39), B-CLL cells have many features in common with CD5+ normal B cells. However, some aspects of the phenotype differ between the two cells types, and the presence of the assumed, malignancy-associated abnormalities in B-CLL cells, have not been examined in CD5+ B cells.

The similarities between B-CLL and normal CD5+ cells seem to be: expression of surface Ig at a low level; expression of CD5, MRBC receptors and myelomonocytic antigens (e.g., CD14) (39); inability of surface Ig capping (63); absence of stimulatory function in MLC (64); poor response to mitogens (63,64); response to cytokines and TPA without the need for a second costimulatory signal (39,65); capacity of production of polyreactive antibodies encoded by V genes without hypermutation (39); an immunosuppressive function (64); and an unexplained long survival in vitro (39).

Some differences have been reported: B-CLL cells can cap CD5 (66), and only they express some activation antigens (67).

Finally, the knowledge about the presence or absence of most of the typical "B-CLL abnormalities," e.g., the high expression of activation antigens, the low density of LFA-1, and their susceptibility to transformation by EBV, in CD5+ normal B cells is incomplete.

Conclusions

Several facts make it difficult to discuss the nature of the normal counterpart of B-CLL cells. First, as pointed out before, the heterogeneity of

B-CLL clones and the many different methodological approaches used to study the phenotypic properties of B-CLL make it difficult to integrate existing data into a definition of the B-CLL phenotype(s). Second, we do not know the phenotypic consequences of the alternative genetic aberrations typical of B-CLL and therefore cannot interpret with certainty whether a marker is malignancy-associated or not. Third, the nature of the normal CD5+ cells is not yet characterized enough, making any comparisons of the B-CLL and CD5+ normal B-cell phenotype uncertain. However, at least three different possibilities seem to exist. The first is that B-CLL is derived from a subtype of normal, activated B cells, in which case the expression of CD5 is typical of its particular activation stage. The second possibility is that B-CLL is derived from a CD5+ B cell that is part of a unique B-cell subset. Both these hypotheses imply that the phenotype of B-CLL cells faithfully reflects the phenotype of the normal cell of origin, as has been shown for acute lymphocytic leukemia (11). The first hypothesis predicts that it should be possible to identify a new, unique subpopulation of normal B cells with features of B-CLL cells, and the second hypothesis that CD5+ normal B cells will be proven to represent a unique subset of B cells that will be able to express the antigens typical of B-CLL cells.

The third possibility is that B-CLL is derived from a normal B cell in which CD5 expression has been induced as a consequence of some early genetic events in the neoplastic transformation. the aberrant CD5 expression on the preneoplastic B cell may lead to an alteration of its interaction with the microenvironment. Cytokine signaling and cell-cell contacts, stimulating clonal expansion of the preneoplastic cells, together with further genetic changes, will then lead to the transformation of the pre-B-CLL cell to a typical B-CLL cell. Following the philosophy of Ockam, I favor one of the first two, simpler hypotheses.

INDUCTION OF GROWTH AND DIFFERENTIATION OF B-CLL CELLS

Several early studies on the kinetics of peripheral blood B-CLL cells showed that the leukemic cells were essentially nonproliferative (68). It was therefore assumed the majority of the tumor cells in B-CLL were long-lived and incapable of further proliferation. Putative precursor cells in the bone marrow, or the peripheral lymphoid organs, were supposed to represent the proliferative compartment.

As reviewed in detail (68), the attempts to stimulate blood B-CLL cells by mitogens during the early 1970s were largely unsuccessful. In 1974, when Fu and collaborators (69) used cells from B-CLL patients with a monoclonal serum IgM and stimulated them with PWM and allogeneic T cells, it was for the first time possible to reproducibly induce DNA synthesis and plasmacytoid differentiation in B-CLL cells in vitro. Later, Robért et al. (70) employed a large panel of T-cell-dependent and -independent polyclonal B-cell mitogens (PHA, PPD, PWM, EBV, LPS, and dextran sulfate) and were able to induce variable, minimal DNA synthesis and Ig secretion also in non-Ig secretory B-CLL clones. Studies in several other laboratories failed, however, to critically exclude that the small increase in ^{3}H-thymidine uptake recorded in mitogen, anti-μ antibodies, staphylococcal protein A, and calcium ionophore A23187 stimulated B-CLL cell cultures was indeed a reflection of DNA synthesis induced in the B-CLL cells and not in contaminating T cells. Taken together, these early studies demonstrated that at least Ig secretory B-CLL cells were not irreversibly arrested in differentiation and suggested that also in the common type of B-CLL clones the putative differentiation block was not absolute. Importantly, they also showed the T-cell dependency of mitogen-induced proliferation and differentiation of B-CLL cells and established that B-CLL cells generally responded poorly to mitogens and some other stimuli even during optimal tissue culture conditions with the presence of T cells.

In 1980, Tötterman et al. (71) demonstrated that the phorbol ester 12-0-tetradecanoylphorbol-13-acetate (TPA) induced efficient plasmacytoid differentiation in more than 50% of the B-CLL clones tested. As will be described, TPA-induced differentiation occurs in the absence of DNA synthesis and proliferation and is T-cell dependent. TPA induction of B-CLL cells has been found to be a reproducible method in many laboratories during the 1980s and has allowed studies on various aspects of B-CLL differentiation even under serum-free conditions (68). TPA can also be used to provide activation signals in studies aimed at studying the effect of proliferation inducing signals, e.g., cytokines.

With the introduction of refined methods for cell separation, the possibilities to define the vast majority of circulating leukocytes by moabs, and the availability of recombinant cytokines, it has recently been possible to study critically how the growth and differentiation in B-CLL cells are controlled by para- and autocrine cytokine signaling and cell-cell contacts. The results of these studies will be summarized below. In most of the studies by our own group during the last few years, only two B-CLL clones (I73 and I83), obtained at one bleeding of the patients, have been employed to avoid the problem of heterogeneity and intraindividual variability that was encountered during the early work with B-CLL cells in culture. Both clones had the common B-CLL cell morphology and cell surface phenotype and were resting G_0 cells. They had been selected on the basis of their capacity to undergo differentiation without proliferation in response to TPA, to differentiate with concomitant proliferation in response to thioredoxin and

TPA, *Staphylococcus* Cowan I (SAC) or anti-m antibodies, as activation signals, and to IL-2 or IL-4, as a second (progression) signal. Cells were harvested by leukapheresis, purified by density gradient centrifugation, and stored in liquid nitrogen. Upon revival they could be reproducibly induced to proliferation and/or differentiation according to various protocols of stimulation as depicted in Fig. 3.

Induction of Differentiation by TPA

About 50–60% of investigated B-CLL clones respond well to TPA by induction of differentiation (68). Different laboratories, using TPA as an inducer of differentiation of B-CLL cells, have reported very similar phenotypic changes, which will be summarized in the following. (For a detailed review, see Refs. 68 and 72.)

Changes in Morphology and Adhesion Properties

Most of the cells (80–90%) in a responsive clone will undergo a morphological blast transformation (Fig. 4) and subsequently develop into lymphoblastoid-plasmacytoid cells and, infrequently, into plasma cells, as judged by light and electron microscopy (71–78). The ultrastructure of the majority of the TPA-induced B-CLL cells was similar to that of EBV-transformed cells (73,78). Strong morphological and cytochemical (TRAP expression) similarities with hairy cell leukemia cells were also demonstrated (72,74,75). Recent studies on normal B cells and B-CLL cells, using other markers

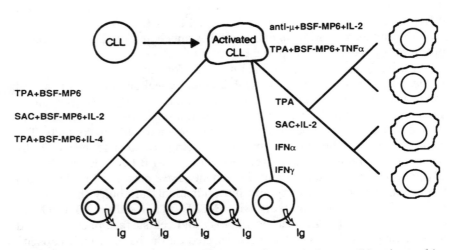

Figure 3 A summary of the various protocols used to induce proliferation and/or differentiation in the I73 and I83 B-CLL clones in vitro.

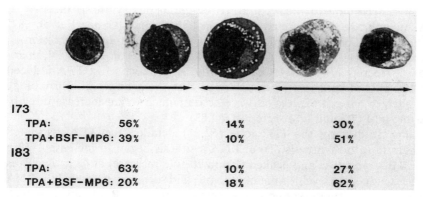

I73
     TPA: 56%   14%   30%
     TPA+BSF−MP6: 39%   10%   51%
I83
     TPA: 63%   10%   27%
     TPA+BSF−MP6: 20%   18%   62%

Figure 4   The stepwise morphological differentiation of the I73 and I83 B-CLL clones during TPA + TRx- and TPA-induced proliferation and/or differentiation (93).

including the hairy cell leukemia-specific B-Ly 7 moab, have, however, failed to confirm the suggested close relationship between TPA-induced B-CLL cells and hairy cell leukemia cells (79,80).

Following TPA induction, B-CLL cells form clumps and acquire new properties for substrate adhesion that differ from those of normal B cells (74,81).

Alterations of the Cell Surface

The cell surface changes (as described in Refs. 68 and 71–84) include a decrease in the expression of IgM, IgD, and the receptors for MRBC, Fc, and C3, an increased expression of MHC class II antigen, and an increase in the capacity to present antigens and to stimulate in conventional mixed lymphocyte reaction (MLR) and in autologous MLR.

Altered expression of B-cell activation and differentiation-associated surface antigens were also found (74,85,86). The changes include an increased BB-1 and LB-1 expression and decreased expression of B1 and B2. Carlsson et al. (81) examined I83 cells during TPA induction by the B-cell antigen panel of the Fourth International Conference on Leukocyte Differentiation Antigens and found a decrease in CD20, CD21, CD37, and CD45R expression and an increase in CD25, CD23, and CD54 expression.

Functional Changes

Functional changes include increased expression of activation-associated cytokine receptors, e.g., the IL-2R (81), as described above, and differentiation-associated alterations of the Ig gene expression.

As described above, and in Refs. 85 and 87, B-CLL clones can be subgrouped according to their pattern of spontaneous synthesis in vitro of IgM (membrane and secreted IgM) and light chains. Gauazzi et al. (87) distinguished four groups of B-CLL clones: I, membrane − /secretion −; II, membrane + /secretion −; III, membrane + /secretion +; and IV, membrane − /secretion +. Early studies on the Ig production in TPA-induced B-CLL cells of category I demonstrated that the changes in morphology and surface antigen expression were accompanied by an increase in cytoplasmic IgM (71) and IgM secretion (68,83).

Later studies on the I73 clone (62,88) detailed the TPA-associated changes in Ig biosynthesis. Total RNA synthesis began to increase 4–12 h after TPA induction and peaked (10- to 20-fold increase) at 48 h. Analyses of the steady-state levels of membrane (m) and secretory (s) μ-chain mRNA demonstrated a rapid (within 4 h) decrease in total μmRNA, during which time the relative expression of μs and μm mRNA shifted from 1 : 1 to 4 : 1. Total μ mRNA then increased and reached a maximum (5- to 20-fold increase) at 24 h. The switch from μm to μs RNA is very rapid and even precedes the increase in total RNA and protein synthesis, which suggests an early regulation of Ig gene expression at the level of mRNA processing. The Ig genes do not appear to be selectively controlled by TPA, since no relative increase of μ mRNA to the control actin mRNA was found.

The studies on μ-heavy- and κ-light-chain synthesis showed a rapid increase in the production of both proteins, but secretion of pentameric IgM, at a rate of 1–2 μg/10^6 cells/24 h, was detectable only after transition of the cells from the G_0 to the G_1 phase of the cell cycle, at 24 h. The results of these studies show that Ig gene expression during the TPA-induced differentiation is regulated at the transcriptional level. Further, they demonstrate that regulatory events must occur also at the translational level, since the high rate of secretion of IgM is disproportionate to the small increase in μs mRNA. Finally, the presence of intracellular μ chains in the absence of IgM secretion shows that, in addition, posttranslational control mechanisms of Ig synthesis operate in differentiating B-CLL cells. Recently, Guazzi et al. (87) showed that B-CLL cells of categories I, II, and III, but not IV, were inducible to IgM secretion. Interestingly, their study also suggests that the Ig synthesis was regulated differently in B-CLL cells than in normal B cells, since μs mRNA was upregulated rather than downregulated after TPA induction. This conclusion is, however, controversial, since a rapid, although transient, decrease in μ-chain expression was found in the I73 B-CLL cells (88) and since a recent study demonstrated transcriptional downregulation of the IgM mRNA in one B-CLL cell line (89).

Cell Cycle Changes

Cell cycle studies have been performed by flow cytometric analysis of acridine orange-stained cells (48,90) and DNA synthesis measurements by ^{3}H-thymidine incorporation assays (48,85). The studies all agree that when a common B-CLL clone is induced by TPA, most cells will gradually traverse in the cell cycle from the G_0 to the G_1 phase of the cell cycle. No B-CLL cells entered S phase. In the study by Carlsson et al. (48), 10% of the cells were found in G_{1A} at 24 h. At day 5, about 60% of the total B-CLL population were found to be arrested in G_{1A} while 10% positioned in G_{1B}. Thirty percent of the cells thus remained in G_0. The small fraction of cells (3%) detected in the $G_2 + S$ phases were identified as T cells (48).

Normal B cells responded to TPA by a similar G_0-to-G_1 transition, but, in contrast to the B-CLL cells, they continued to traverse into S phase and further through the cell cycle to divide (90).

Conclusions

TPA induces B-CLL cells to undergo morphological, antigenic, and functional changes similar, if not identical, to those observed for normal B cells undergoing differentiation in vitro, but without concomitant proliferation. The differentiation leads to the development of lymphoblasts-plasmablasts and is terminal only in a small fraction of cells.

The nature of the hairy cell-like phenotype, which develops after TPA stimulation, is controversial. The recent data on antigen expression suggest that, contrary to a widely held view, hairy cells and B-CLL cells are not closely related.

However, some of the responses of B-CLL cells to TPA may be abnormal as compared to peripheral blood B cells—e.g., the absence of proliferation, the failure to upregulate the Bly-7 antigen expression, and perhaps also the upregulation of IgM transcription.

As will be discussed, B-CLL clones may be induced to proliferate by thioredoxin in combination with T-cell-derived cytokines. This shows that B-CLL cells are not refractory to proliferation-inducing signals. The poor response to TPA may therefore not necessarily signify an abnormality restricted to the B-CLL cells but also a subnormal function of cytokine producing nonneoplastic cells, e.g., T cells, which in normal blood B-cell cultures provide necessary progression signals to TPA-activated B cells and make them proliferate.

Induction of Growth and Differentiation by Physiologic Inducers

Recently, the effects of recombinant cytokines (IL-1, IL-2, IL-4, IL-5, IL-6, IL-10, TNF-α) and partially purified HW- and LMW-BCGF on B-CLL cells have been tested in several laboratories. The results show that the responses, as expected from previous studies with mitogens, "conditioned media," and TPA, were very heterogeneous. However, a few general conclusions may be drawn from these studies. (a) DNA synthesis and cell division may indeed be induced in common, resting B-CLL cells, although the frequency is uncertain. As pointed out by Drexler (91), a critical demonstration of cytokine-induced growth, and not only DNA synthesis, has only been made by Carlsson et al. (92). (b) Cytokines usually stimulate resting, nonactivated B-CLL cells poorly as compared to normal peripheral blood B cells. (c) Activation by a proper, alternative activation signal (anti-u antibodies, SAC, TPA) is a prerequisite for efficient cytokine stimulation of B-CLL cells. (d) Cytokines often act synergistically on B-CLL cells in inducing growth and differentiation. (e) Autocrine loops have been suggested but not proven. (f) Once initiated, growth and differentiation occur similarly to what has been described for normal B cells. (g) The most efficient inducers with an unequivocal DNA synthesis-inducing effect in B-CLL cells are IL-2, IL-4, TNF-α, and thioredoxin (see below).

Due to the pronounced heterogeneity among B-CLL clones, and the intraclonal variability during the course of the disease in single B-CLL patients, it has been difficult to detail the response to various cytokines using a panel of fresh B-CLL clones. The summary below on the effect of different cytokines on B-CLL cells will therefore emphasize to some extent the studies of our group, using the previously mentioned I73 and I83 clones in which these and other problems associated with contamination of nonmalignant cells are controlled (Fig. 3).

The Costimulatory Effect of Thioredoxin

In a screening for T-cell-derived factors, which might assist TPA in activating B-CLL cells also to proliferation, Carlsson et al. (93) found that a B-cell-stimulatory factor (BSF), distinct from known cytokines and produced by a T-cell hybridoma (MP6), had the desired property. BSF-MP6 strongly enhanced TPA-induced differentiation, as indicated by an increase in the fraction of developed plasma cells (Fig. 4), by an altered profile of surface marker expression, and by an increased rate of induced Ig secretion. Most important, however, proliferation was induced, as evidenced by studies on DNA synthesis and by cell cycle parameter analysis by flow cytometry. BSF-MP6 seemed to act directly on the B-CLL cells, since depletion of T cells and monocytes did not alter its effect.

Recently, Rosén et al. (94) have shown that BSF-MP6 is an extracellular isoform of a potent redox-regulating and thiol-disulfide exchange enzyme, thioredoxin (Trx). Trx was shown to act in synergy with IL-2, IL-4, TNF-α, LMW-BCGF, and anti-CD40 to stimulate proliferation of SAC- and TPA-activated normal B and B-CLL cells (94). Screening studies on the inducibility of growth and differentiation, according to the protocols for stimulation depicted in Fig. 3, have recently shown that about 50% of B-CLL clones respond, demonstrating that the I73 and I83 clones are not unique. The mechanism by which Trx facilitates growth and differentiation of normal and leukemic B cells is not yet known. It is, however, tempting to speculate that malignancy-associated deficient production of Trx or decreased sensitivity to this enzyme in B-CLL cells explains why these cells, in contrast to normal B cells, do not respond by proliferation to TPA and cytokine induction.

Effects of IL-2

DNA synthesis in B-CLL cultures treated with IL-2 was first described by Lantz et al. (46). The question whether IL-2 can stimulate B-CLL cells directly is controversial (91,95). As in normal peripheral B cells, DNA synthesis, and sometimes increased Ig secretion, have been noted in several laboratories after IL-2 stimulation of anti-m antibodies, SAC, or TPA-preactivated B-CLL cells (46,47,96–98). The synergism with BCGF, IFN-α, and IFN-γ to induce DNA synthesis (98–101) is also a characteristic feature of IL-2-induced proliferation of normal B cells.

In the I83 B-CLL clone, Carlsson et al. (92) documented induced differentiation and cell growth by IL-2. IL-2 was active only when cells were costimulated with SAC and Trx, and a synergistic effect between these factors was found (Fig. 3). The SAC activation was followed by an increase in IL-2R. Anti-CD25 antibodies inhibited the response in a dose-dependent manner. Flow cytometric analysis of acridine orange and BrdU-stained cells showed that the induced B-CLL cells underwent a complete transition through the cell cycle, divided, and eventually became arrested in G_1. The induced proliferation was dependent on the presence of serum but independent of contaminating T cells and monocytes.

Effects of IL-4

IL-4 has no direct effects on B-CLL cells in the absence of costimulatory activation signals and progression factors. In normal B cells, IL-4 is known either to inhibit or stimulate proliferation depending on the nature of the costimuli used (102,103).

In the I83 clone, IL-4 was found to enhance TPA + Trx-induced proliferation and differentiation strongly (104). Morphological and antigenic changes were indicative of advanced B-cell differentiation. As compared with TPA stimulation, the Ig secretion was increased sevenfold to a rate of secretion similar to that reported for human myeloma cells. Studies of Ig production at the single cell level by the ELISPOT technique showed that about 70% of the TPA + TrX + IL-4-stimulated cells were Ig secretory. This value corresponded to a frequency of plasma cells in the induced cultures of about 15%. Also, the induction of proliferation by TPA + Trx was enhanced by the costimulation with IL-4.

As is the case for normal B cells, the effect on B-CLL cells was dependent on the costimulatory activation and progression signals. Thus IL-4 inhibited the SAC + Trx + IL-2 stimulation completely (104). Cell cycle analyses demonstrated that IL-4 inhibited the G_0-to-G_1 and the G_1-to-S-phase transition of the B-CLL cells. Neither the stimulatory nor inhibitory effect of IL-4 seemed to be indirect via T cells or monocytes, as shown by depletion experiments. The mechanism by which IL-4 inhibits the SAC + Trx + IL-2 response is not fully understood, but it does not seem to inhibit the expression of the two IL-2R chains but may, as mentioned, inhibit to formation of a functional IL-2R (50,54).

Effects of Other Factors

TNF-α is a good inducer of optimally activated B-CLL cells (Fig. 3) and has been suggested to be involved in the control of B-CLL growth as an autocrine growth factor (detailed by Hoffbrand in this volume).

The effects of some other cytokines (LMW-BCGF, IL-1, IL-6), as measured by DNA synthesis assays and by cell cycle studies and quantitation of induced Ig secretion in our I73 and I83 B-CLL clones, if present, have generally been found to be minimal (91). Anti-CD40 antibodies induced proliferation in SAC + Trx-stimulated I83 cells (94), but its effect in general on B-CLL is unknown.

Uckun (52) reported on clonogenic growth of B-CLL cells in response to HW-BGCF and found that the receptors for this cytokine were constitutively expressed on noninduced B-CLL cells. If these findings can be reproduced independently, they might indicate a role of this factor in the growth control of B-CLL cells.

Conclusions

With Trx as a costimulator, TPA induction is followed not only by the characteristic differentiation but also by proliferation, demonstrating that B-CLL cells, although poor responders, are not refractory to proliferation-inducing signals.

B-CLL cells may be induced to growth and differentiation by physiologic inducers.

The initiation of a complete proliferation/differentiation response in B-CLL cells usually requires stimulation by an alternative activation inducer, Trx, and an alternative cytokine signal.

IL-2 seems to be the most potent inducer of proliferation.

The effects of IL-4 illustrate that a cytokine signal can either stimulate or inhibit induced growth/differentiation response in B-CLL cells, depending on the costimulatory activation and progression signals.

TNF-α, LMW-BCGF, and anti-CD40 may induce proliferation.

HMW-BCGF may stimulate clocogenic growth of B-CLL cells. Since HMW-BCGF receptors are constitutively expressed in B-CLL cells, this response may be abnormal and of pathogenetic significance.

GENERAL SUMMARY

B-CLL cells have heterogeneous phenotypic properties. Nevertheless, the common-type B-CLL cell is resting in the G_0 phase of the cell cycle and has morphological, antigenic, and functional properties similar to that of an activated B cell.

The normal counterparts of B-CLL clones are elusive and controversial. Obvious possibilities, depending on whether CD5+ B cells constitute a separate subpopulation of B cells or not, are (a) that the normal counterparts are subpopulations of activated normal B cells, expressing CD5 as one of its activation antigens, or (b) CD5+ B lineage cells. It is also possible, although less likely, that (c) the CD5 positivity of B-CLL cells represents a malignancy-associated, aberrant gene expression.

B-CLL seems not to be irreversibly arrested in differentiation. At least 50% of the clones are inducible to proliferation and/or differentiation by TPA and physiological inducers, e.g., SAC, anti-IgM, IL-2, IL-4, and TNF-α.

B-CLL cells survive better in vitro than normal B cells, the mechanism for which is unknown. They respond poorly to growth and differentiation stimuli. However, growth and differentiation, when successfully induced, seem to be essentially normal, as evidenced by several detailed studies on cell cycle parameters and functional markers of these processes.

The subnormal response to mitogens and cytokines may either reflect characteristics of the normal counterpart B cell(s) or may be a malignancy-associated feature. The recent finding of comparatively high levels of bcl-2 protein in B-CLL cells is interesting in this regard, since the expression of this gene appears to prolong the survival of cells in the G_0 phase of the cell cycle. However, since B-CLL clones have several genetic alterations, other genetic changes than a deregulated bcl-2 expression may be responsible for, or contribute to, the relative anergy of B-CLL cells when stimulated by cytokines and other physiologic and nonphysiologic stimuli. Intriguing in this regard is their dependence on the Trx enzyme for a normal response to cytokines, which may be the manifestation of one of the genetic aberrations.

It is also possible that the subnormal responsiveness of the B-CLL cells depends on an autologous T-cell compartment, which functions subnormally in providing the necessary help for activated B-CLL cells to traverse the cell cycle, differentiate, and divide.

Taken together, the recent studies on growth and differentiation control of B-CLL cell clones in vitro suggest that they are not autonomous but can respond to the cytokine and cell-cell contact-induced signals in their microenvironment, although less well than normal B cells. It should therefore be possible to regulate B-CLL cells directly, by inhibitory cytokines (until now best exemplified by IL-4), or indirectly via nonneoplastic cells of the cellular network of the hematopoietic and immune systems. It remains as a challenge for the future to exploit the new knowledge on the cellular biology of B-CLL cells in the clinical management of B-CLL patients.

ACKNOWLEDGMENTS

I thank M. Carlsson for valuable discussions during the preparation of this paper and E. Harryson for excellent secretarial work. The work performed by the author and his collaborators and reviewed in this chapter was supported by the Swedish Cancer Society.

REFERENCES

1. K. A. Foon, K. R. Rai, and R. P. Gale, Chronic lymphocytic leukemia: New insights into biology and therapy, *Ann. Int. Med., 113*:525 (1990).
2. A. S. Freedman, Immunobiology of chronic lymphocytic leukemia, *Hematol./Oncol. Clin. N. Am., 4*:405 (1990).
3. A. Siegbahn, P. Venge, K. Nilsson, and B. Simonsson, Identification of a chemokinetic inhibitor in serum from patients with chronic lymphocytic leukemia, *Scand. J. Haematol., 28*:122 (1982).
4. A. C. Aisenberg and K. J. Block, Immunoglobulins on the surface of neoplastic lymphocytes, *N. Engl. J. Med., 287*:272 (1972).
5. J. C. Brouet, F. Flandrin, and M. Sasportes, Chronic lymphocytic leukemia of T cell origin. Immunologic and clinical evaluation in eleven patients, *Lancet, 2*:890 (1975).
6. F. M. Uckun, Regulation of human B-cell ontogeny, *Blood, 76*:1908 (1990).
7. I. C. M. MacLennan, Y. J. Liu, S. Oldenfield, J. Zhang, and P. J. L. Lane, The evolution of B-cell clones, *Curr. Top. Microbiol. Immunol., 159*:37 (1990).
8. M. Ogawa, P. N. Porter, and T. Nakahata, Renewal and commitment to differentiation of hemopoietic stem cells (an interpretive review), *Blood, 61*: 823 (1983).
9. D. Metcalf, The molecular control of cell division, differentiation commitment and maturation in haemopoietic cells, *Nature* (Lond.), *339*:27 (1989).
10. L. Sachs, Constitutive uncoupling of pathways of gene expression that control growth and differentiation in myeloid leukemia: A model for the origin and progression of malignancy, *Proc. Natl. Acad. Sci. USA, 77*:6153 (1980).
11. M. F. Greaves, Differentiation-linked leukaemogenesis in lymphocytes, *Science, 234*:697 (1986).
12. K. Nilsson, L. C. Andersson, C. G. Gahmberg, and K. Forsbeck, Differentiation in vitro of human leukemia and lymphoma cell lines. International symposium on new trends in human immunology and cancer immunotherapy, in *International Symposium on New Trends in Human Immunology and Cancer*

Immunotherapy (B. Serrou and C. Rosenfeld, eds.), Doin Editeurs, Paris, p. 271 (1980).

13. F. M. Uckun and J. A. Ledbetter, Immunobiologic differences between normal and leukemic human B-cell precursors. *Proc. Natl. Acad. Sci. USA, 85*: 8603 (1988).

14. P. W. Kincade, G. Lee, C. E. Pietrangeli, S. Hayashi, and J. Gimble, Cells and molecules that regulate B lymphopoiesis in bone marrow, *Ann. Rev. Immunol., 7*:111 (1989).

15. E. A. Clark and P. J. L. Lane, Regulation of human B-cell activation and adhesion, *Ann. Rev. Immunol., 9*:97 (1991).

16. F. M. Uckun, I. Dibirdik, R. Smith, L. Tuel-Ahlgren, M. Chandan-Langlie, G. L. Schieven, K. G. Waddick, M. Hanson, and J. A. Ledbetter, Interleukin 7 receptor ligation stimulates tyrosine phosphorylation, inositol phospholipid turnover, and clonal proliferation of human B-cell precursors, *Proc. Natl. Acad. Sci. USA, 89*:3589 (1991).

17. J. G. Villablanca, J. M. Anderson, M. Moseley, C.-L. Law, R. L. Elstrom, and T. W. LeBien, Differentiation of normal human pre-B cells in vitro, *J. Exp. Med., 172*:325 (1990).

18. M. Y. Gordon, G. P. Riley, S. M. Watt, and M. F. Greaves, Compartmentalization of a haematopoietic growth factor (GM-CSF) by glycosaminoglycans in the bone marrow microenvironment, *Nature, 326*:403 (1987).

19. R. Roberts, J. Gallagher, E. Spooncer, T. D. Allen, F. Bloomfield, and T. M. Dexter, Heparan sulphate bound growth factors: A mechanism for stromal cell mediated haemopoiesis, *Nature, 332*:376 (1988).

20. I. C. M. MacLennan, Y. J. Liu, S. Oldfield, J. Zhang, and P. J. L. Lane, The evolution of B-cell clones, *Curr. Top. Microbiol. Immunol., 159*:37 (1990).

21. Y.-J. Liu, D. E. Joshua, G. T. Williams, C. A. Smith, J. Gordon, and I. C. M. MacLennan, The mechanism of antigen-driven selection in germinal centres, *Nature, 342*:929 (1989).

22. R. B. Gallagher and D. G. Osmond, To B or not to B: That is the question, *Immunol. Today, 12*:1 (1991).

23. M. E. Hemler, Adhesive protein receptors on hematopoietic cells, *Immunol. Today, 9*:109 (1988).

24. T. A. Springer, M. L. Dustin, T. K. Kishimoto, and S. D. Marlin, The lymphocyte function-associated LFA-1, CD2, and LFA-3 molecules: Cell adhesion receptors of the immune system, *Ann. Rev. Immunol., 5*:223 (1987).

25. T. A. Yednock and S. D. Rosén, Lymphocyte homing, *Adv. Immunol., 44*: 313 (1989).

26. E. L. Berg, L. A. Goldstein, M. A. Jutila, M. Nakache, L. J. Picker, P. R. Streeter, N. W. Wu, D. Zhou, and E. C. Butcher, Homing receptors and vascular addressins: Cell adhesion molecules that direct lymphocyte traffic, *Immunol. Rev., 108*:5 (1989).

27. C. J. March, B. Mosley, A. Larsen, D. P. Cerretti, G. Braedt, V. Price, S. Gillis, C. S. Henney, S. R. Kronheim, K. Grabstein, P. J. Conlon, T. P.

Hopp, and D. Cossman, Cloning, sequence and expression of two distinct human interleukin-1 complementary DNAs, *Nature, 315*:641 (1985).

28. T. Taniguchi, H. Matsui, T. Fujita, C. Takaoka, N. Kashima, R. Yoshimoto, and J. Hamuro, Structure and expression of a cloned cDNA for human interleukin-2, *Nature, 302*:305 (1983).

29. T. Hirano, K. Yasukawa, H. Harada, T. Taga, Y. Watanabe, H. Matsuda, S.-I. Kashiwamura, T. Hakajiama, K. Koyama, A. Iwamatsu, S. Tsunasawa, F. Sakiyama, H. Matsui, Y. Takahara, T. Taniguchi, and T. Kishimoto, Complementary DNA for a novel interleukin (BSF-2) that induces B lymphocytes to produce immunoglobulin, *Nature, 324*:73 (1986).

30. S. Sharma, S. Mehta, J. Morgan, and A. Maizel, Molecular cloning and expression of a human B-cell growth factor gene in *Escherichia coli, Science, 235*:1489 (1987).

31. P. W. Gray, D. W. Leung, D. Pennica, E. Yelverton, R. Najarian, C. C. Simonsen, R. Derynck, P. J. Sherwood, D. M. Wallace, S. L. Berger, A. D. Levinson, and D. V. Goedel, Expression of human immune interferon cDNA in *E. coli* and monkey cells, *Nature, 295*:503 (1982).

32. T. Shirai, H. Yamaguchi, H. Ito, C. W. Todd, and B. Wallace, Cloning and expression in *Escherichia coli* of the gene for human tumour necrosis factor, *Nature, 313*:803 (1985).

33. C. Azuma, T. Tanabe, M. Konishi, T. Noma, F. Matsuda, Y. Yaoita, K. Takatsu, L. Hammarström, C. I. E. Smith, E. Severinson, and T. Honjo, Cloning of cDNA for human T-cell replacing factor (interleukin-5) and comparison with the murine homologue, *Nucleic Acid Res., 14*:149 (1986).

34. D. V. Goeddel, E. Yelverton, A. Ullrich, H. L. Heyneker, G. Moizzari, W. Holmes, P. H. Seeburg, T. Dull, L. May, N. Stebbing, R. Crea, S. Maeda, R. McCandliss, A. Sloma, J. M. Tabor, M. Gross, P. C. Familletti, and S. Pestka, Human leukocyte interferon produced by *E. coli* is biologically active, *Nature, 287*:411 (1980).

35. D. F. Jelinek and P. E. Lipsky, Enhancement of human B cell proliferation and differentiation by tumor necrosis factor-α and interleukin 1, *J. Immunol., 138*:2970 (1987).

36. J. Banchereau, in *Mechanisms of B cell Neoplasia* (F. Melchers, and M. Potter, eds.), Editiones Roche, Basel, p. 129 (1991).

37. D. F. Jelinek, Inhibitory influence of IL-4 on human B cell responsiveness, *J. Immunol., 141*:164 (1988).

38. J. H. Kehrl, L. M. Wakefield, A. B. Roberts, S. Jakowlew, M. Alvarez-Mon, R. Derynck, M. B. Sporn, and A. S. Fauci, The production of TGF-β by human T lymphocytes and its potential role in the regulation of T cell growth, *J. Exp. Med., 163*:1037 (1986).

39. T. J. Kipps, The CD5 B cell, *Adv. Immunol., 47*:117 (1989).

40. T. Paglieroni and M. R. MacKenzie, Studies on the pathogenesis of an immune defect in multiple myeloma, *J. Clin. Invest., 59*:1120 (1977).

41. S. P. Mulligan, Human B cells: Differentiation and neoplasia, *Leuk. Lymph., 1*:275 (1990).

42. M. Kamoun, M. F. Kadin, P. J. Martin, J. Nettleton, and J. A. Hansen, A

novel human T cell antigen preferentially expressed on mature T cells and also on (B type) chronic lymphatic leukemic cells, *J. Immunol., 127*:987 (1981).

43. F. Morabito, E. F. Prasthofer, N. E. Dunlap, C. E. Grossi, and A. B. Tilden, Expression of myelomonocytic antigens on chronic lymphocytic leukemia B cells correlates with their ability to produce Interleukin 1, *Blood, 70*:1750 (1987).

44. A. De la Hera, M. Alvarez-Mon, F. Sanches-Madrid, C. Martinez, and A. Durantez, Co-expression of Mac-1 and p150,95 on CD5 + B cells. Structural and functional characterization in a human chronic lymphocytic leukemia, *Eur. J. Immunol., 18*:1131 (1988).

45. J. Gordon, H. Hellstedt, P. Åman, P. Biberfeld, M. Björkholm, and G. Klein, Phenotypes in chronic B-lymphocytic leukemia probed by monoclonal antibodies and immunoglobulin secretion studies: Identification of states of maturation arrest and the relation to clinical findings, *Blood, 62*:910 (1983).

46. O. Lantz, C. Grillot-Courvalin, C. Schmitt, J.-P. Fermand, and J.-C. Brouet, Interleukin-2 induced proliferation of leukemic human B cells, *J. Exp. Med., 161*:1225 (1985).

47. I. Touw, L. Dorssers, and B. Löwenberg, The proliferative response of B cell chronic lymphocytic leukemia to interleukin 2: Functional characterization of the interleukin 2 membrane receptors, *Blood, 69*:1667 (1987).

48. M. Carlsson, T. H. Tötterman, P. Matsson, and K. Nilsson, Cell cycle progression of B-chronic lymphocytic leukemia cells induced to differentiate by TPA, *Blood, 71*:415 (1988).

49. H. Yagura, T. Tamaki, T. Furitsu, Y. Tomiyama, T. Nishiura, N. Tominaga, S. Katagiri, T. Yonezawa, and S. Tarui, Demonstration of high-affinity interleukin-2 receptors on B-chronic lymphocytic leukemia cells: Functional and structural characterization, *Blut, 60*:181 (1990).

50. S. Karray, A. Dautry-Varsat, M. Tsudo, H. Merle-Beral, P. Debre, and P. Galanaud, IL-4 inhibits the expression of high affinity IL-2 receptors on monoclonal human B cells, *J. Immunol., 145*:1152 (1990).

51. W. Digel, W. Schöniger, M. Stefanic, H. Janssen, C. Buck, M. Schmid, A. Raghavachar, and F. Porzsolt, Receptors for tumor necrosis factor on neoplastic B cells from chronic lymphocytic leukemia are expressed in vitro but not in vivo, *Blood, 76*:1607 (1990).

52. F. M. Uckun, A. S. Fauci, M. Chandan-Langlie, D. E. Myers, and J. L. Ambrus, Detection and characterization of human high molecular weight B cell growth factor receptors on leukemic B cells in chronic lymphocytic leukemia, *J. Clin. Invest., 84*:1595 (1989).

53. R. T. Perri, Impaired expression of cell surface receptors for B cell growth factor by chronic lymphocytic leukemia B cells, *Blood, 67*:943 (1986).

54. M. Carlsson, unpublished data.

55. M. Aguilar-Santelises, R. Magnusson, S. B. Svenson, A. Loftenius, B. Andersson, H. Mellstedt, and M. Jondal, Expression of interleukin-1α interleukin-1β and interleukin-6 in chronic B lymphocytic leukaemia (B-CLL) cells from patients at different stages of disease progression, *Clin. Exp. Immunol., 84*:422 (1991).

56. A. Biondi, V. Rossi, R. Bassan, T. Barbui, S. Bettoni, M. Sironi, A. Manto-
     vani, and A. Rambaldi, Constitutive expression of the interleukin-6 gene in
     chronic lymphocytic leukemia, *Blood, 73*:1279 (1989).
57. M. Schena, G. Gaidano, D. Gottardi, F. Malavasi, L.-G. Larsson, K. Nils-
     son, and F. Caligaris-Cappio, Molecular investigation of the cytokines pro-
     duced by normal and malignant B lymphocytes, *Leukemia,* in press.
58. F. T. Cordingley, A. V. Hoffbrand, H. E. Heslop, M. Turner, A. Bianchi,
     J. E. Reittie, A. Vyakarnam, and A. Meager, Tumour necrosis factor as an
     autocrine tumour growth factor for chronic B-cell malignancies, *Lancet, 1*:
     969 (1988).
59. R. Foa, M. Massaia, S. Cardona, A. Gillio Tos, A. Bianchi, C. Attisano, A.
     Guarini, P. Francia di Celle, and M. T. Fierro, Production of tumor necrosis
     factor-alpha by B-cell chronic lymphocytic leukemia cells: A possible regula-
     tory role of TNF in the progression of the disease, *Blood, 76*:393 (1990).
60. M. Sarfati, D. Bron, L. Lagneaux, C. Fonteyn, H. Frost, and G. Delespesse,
     Elevation of IgE-binding factors in serum of patients with B cell-derived
     chronic lymphocytic leukemia, *Blood, 71*:94 (1988).
61. A. Rubartelli, R. Sitia, C. E. Grossi, and M. Ferrarini, Maturation of chronic
     lymphocytic leukemia B cells: Correlation between the capacity of responding
     to T-cell factors in vitro and the stage of maturation reached in vivo, *Clin.
     Immunol. Immunopathol., 34*:296 (1985).
62. K. Forsbeck, L. Hellman, A. Danersund, T. H. Tötterman, U. Pettersson,
     and K. Nilsson, TPA-induced differentiation of chronic lymphocytic leuke-
     mia cells: Studies on μ-chain expression, *Leukemia, 1*:38 (1987).
63. J. H. Antin, S. G. Emerson, P. Martin, N. Gadol, and K. A. Ault, Leu-1+
     (CD5+) B cells: A major lymphoid subpopulation in human fetal spleen:
     Phenotypic and functional studies, *J. Immunol., 136*:505 (1986).
64. M. R. MacKenzie, T. G. Paglieroni, and N. L. Warner, Multiple myeloma:
     A immunologic profile. IV. The EA rosette-forming cell is a Leu-1 positive
     immunoregulatory B cell, *J. Immunol., 139*:24 (1987).
65. Y. Richard, C. Leprince, B. Dugas, D. Treton, and P. Galanaud, Reactivity
     of Leu-1+ tonsillar B cells to a high molecular weight B cell growth factor,
     J. Immunol., 138:1563 (1987).
66. L. Bergui, L. Tesio, M. Schena, M. M. Riva, T. Schultz, P. C. Marchisio,
     and F. Caligaris-Cappio, CD5 and CD21 molecules are a functional unit in
     the cell/substrate adhesion of B-chronic lymphocytic leukemia cells, *Eur. J.
     Immunol., 18*:89 (1988).
67. R. R. Hardy, K. Hayakawa, M. Shimizu, K. Yamasaki, and T. Kishimoto,
     Rheumatoid factor secretion from human Leu-1+ B cells, *Science, 236*:81
     (1987).
68. T. H. Tötterman and K. Nilsson, Differentiation of B-chronic lymphocytic
     leukemia cells in vitro, in *Chronic Lymphocytic Leukemia*, (A. Polliack and
     D. Catovsky, eds.), Harwood Acad. Publ., Chur, Switzerland, pp. 353–368
     (1988).
69. S. M. Fu, R. J. Winchester, T. Feizi, P. D. Walzer, and H. G. Kunkel,
     Idiotypic specificity of surface immunoglobulin and the maturation of leuke-

mic bone-marrow-derived lymphocytes, *Proc. Natl. Acad. Sci. USA, 71*:4487 (1974).

70. K.-H. Robért, E. Möller, G. Garthon, H. Eriksson, and B. Nilsson, B-cell activation of peripheral blood lymphocytes from patients with chronic lymphatic leukemia, *Clin. Exp. Immunol., 33*:302 (1978).

71. T. H. Tötterman, K. Nilsson, and C. Sundström, Phorbol ester-induced differentiation of chronic lymphocytic leukaemia cells, *Nature, 288*:176 (1980).

72. A. Polliack, 12-0-tetradecanoyl phorbol-13-acetate (TPA) and its effect on leukaemic cells, in vitro — A review, *Leuk. Lymph., 3*:173 (1990).

73. K. Guy, V. Van Heyningen, E. Dewar, and C. M. Steel, Enhanced expression of human Ia antigens by chronic lymphocytic leukemia cells following treatment with 12-0-tetradenoylphorbol-13-acetate, *Eur. J. Immunol., 13*:156 (1983).

74. F. Caligaris-Cappio, G. Janossy, D. Campana, M. Chilosi, L. Bergui, R. Foa, D. Delia, M. C. Giubellino, P. Preda, and M. Giobbi, Lineage relationship of chronic lymphocytic leukemia and hairy cell leukemia: Studies with TPA, *Leukemia Res., 8*:567 (1984).

75. H. D. Drexler, M. Klein, N. Bhoopalam, G. Gaedicke, and Minowada, Morphological and isoenzymatic differentiation of B-chronic lymphocytic leukaemia cells induced by phorbolester, *Br. J. Cancer, 53*:181 (1986).

76. L. J. Forbes, P. D. Zalewski, L. Valente. and A. W. Murray, Loss of receptor activity for mouse erythrocytes precedes tumour promoter-induced maturation of chronic lymphocytic leukaemia cells, *Cancer Lett., 14*:187 (1981).

77. A. Rubartelli, R. Sitia, A. Zicca, C. E. Grossi, and M. Ferrarini, Differentiation of chronic lymphocytic leukemia cells: Correlation between the synthesis and secretion of immunoglobulins and the ultrastructure of the malignant cells, *Blood, 62*:495 (1983).

78. T. H. Tötterman, K. Nilsson, C. Sundström, and J. Sällström, Differentiation of chronic lymphocytic leukaemia cells in vitro II. Phorbol ester-induced changes in surface marker profile and ultrastructure, *Hum. Lymphocyte Diff., 1*:83 (1981).

79. L. Visser, and S. Poppema, Induction of B-cell chronic lymphocytic leukaemia and hairy cell leukaemia lika phenotypes by phorbol ester treatment of normal peripheral blood B-cells, *Br. J. Haematol., 75*:359 (1990).

80. M. Carlsson, I. Bashir Hassan, G. Paul, C. Sundström, K. Nilsson, and T. Tötterman, Hairy cell leukemia (HCL) associated antigen B-ly7 is an activation/differentiation-associated antigen on HCL and normal B cells but not on B-type chronic lymphocytic leukemia (B-CLL) cells, *Leuk. Lymph., 6*: 133 (1992).

81. M. Carlsson and K. Nilsson, Reactivity of workshop B-cell antibodies with B-CLL cells induced differentiation with or without concomitant proliferation, Proc. 4th Int. Conf. on Human Leucocyte Differentiation Antigens, Vienna, pp. 206–208 (1989).

82. D. Kabelitz, T. H. Tötterman, K. Nilsson, and M. Gidlund, Phorbol ester treated chronic B lymphocytic leukaemia cells induce autologous T cell prolif-

eration without generation of cytotoxic T cells, *Clin. Exp. Med., 57*:461 (1984).

83. J. Okamura, M. Letarte, L. D. Stein, N. H. Sigal, and E. W. Gelfand, Modulation of chronic lymphocytic stimulatory capacity, *J. Immunol., 128*: 2276 (1982).

84. M. Yasukawa, T. Shiroguchi, A. Inatsuki, and Y. Kobayashi, Antigen presentation in a HLA-DR-restricted fashion by B-cell chronic lymphocytic leukemia cells, *Blood, 72*:102 (1988).

85. J. Gordon, H. Mellstedt, P. Åman, P. Biberfeld, and G. Klein, Phenotypic modulation of chronic lymphocytic leukemia cells by phorbol ester: Induction of IgM secretion and changes in the expression of B cell-associated surface antigens, *J. Immunol., 132*:541 (1984).

86. A. P. Efremides, H. Haubenstock, J. F. Holland, and J. George Bekesi, TPA-induced maturation in secretory human B-leukemic cells in vitro: DNA synthesis, antigenic changes, and immunoglobulin secretion, *Blood, 66*:953 (1985).

87. S. Guazzi, R. Sitia, and A. Rubartelli, Regulation of IgM biosynthesis in human chronic lymphocytic leukemia. Normal and neoplastic B cells respond differently to TPA, *Leuk. Res., 13*:1105 (1989).

88. L.-G. Larsson, H. E. Gray, T. Tötterman, U. Pettersson, and K. Nilsson, Drastically increased expression of *MYC* and *FOS* protooncogenes during *in vitro* differentiation of chronic lymphocytic leukemia cells, *Proc. Natl. Acad. Sci. USA, 84*:223 (1987).

89. I.-I. Mårtensson, K. Nilsson, and T. Leanderson, Transcriptional regulation of immunoglobulin expression in a chronic lymphocytic leukemia cell line, *Eur. J. Immunol., 19*:1625 (1989).

90. R. Munker, J. Ellwart, and H. W. Löms Ziegler-Heitbrock, Flow cytometry of TPA-induced changes in cells of chronic B-cell leukaemias, *Folia Haematol., 114*: 177 (1987).

91. H. G. Drexler, Differential responses of B-CLL clones to in vitro stimulation with cytokines, *Leukemia, 4*:238 (1990).

92. M. Carlsson, T. H. Tötterman, A. Rosén, and K. Nilsson, IL-2 and a T cell hybridoma (MP6) derived B cell stimulatory factor act synergistically to induce proliferation and differentiation of human B-chronic lymphocytic leukemia cells, *Leukemia, 3*:593 (1989).

93. M. Carlsson, P. Matsson, A. Rosén, C. Sundström, T. H. Tötterman, and K. Nilsson, Phorbol ester and B cell-stimulatory factor synergize to induce B-chronic lymphocytic leukemia cells to simultaneous immunoglobulin secretion and DNA synthesis, *Leukemia, 2*:734 (1988).

94. A. Rosén, P. Lundman, M. Carlsson, K. Bhavani, B. R. Srinivasa, G. Kjellström, K. Nilsson, and A. Holmgren, Redox-controlled signal pathway in B lymphocytes involves a unique isoform of thioredoxin, to be published.

95. R. T. Perri, and K. E. Kay, Malignant chronic lymphocytic leukemia B cells express interleukin 2 receptors but fail to respond to interleukin 2's proliferative signal, *Leukemia, 1*:127 (1987).

96. P. Engel, J. Ingles, O. Delacalle, and T. Gallart, Cellular activation without

proliferation to B-cell growth factor and interleukin-2 in chronic lymphocytic leukaemia B-cells stimulated with phorbol ester plus calcium ionophore, *Clin. Exp. Immunol., 76*:61 (1989).

97. D. Kabelitz, K. Pfeffer, D. Von Steldern, P. Bartmann, O. Bruder, C. Nerl, and H. Wagner, *In vitro* maturation of B cells in chronic lymphocytic leukemia. I. Synergistic action of phorbol ester and interleukin 2 in the induction of tac antigen expression and interleukin 2 responsiveness in leukemic B cells, *J. Immunol., 135*:2876 (1985).

98. C. Hivroz, C. Grillot-Courvalin, J.-C. Brouet, and M. Seligmann, Heterogeneity of responsiveness of chronic lymphocytic leukemic B cells to B cell growth factor or interleukin 2, *Eur. J. Immunol., 16*:1001 (1986).

99. A. A. Ghaderi, P. Richardson, C. Cardona, M. J. Milssum, N. Ling, S. Gillis, J. Ledbetter, and J. Gordon, Stimulation of B-chronic lymphocytic leukemia populations by recombinant interleukin-4 and other defined growth promoting agents, *Leukemia, 2*:165 (1988).

100. S. Karray, A. Vasquez, H. Merle-Beral, D. Olive, P. Debre, and P. Galanaud, Synergistic effect of recombinant IL-2 and interferon-gamma on the proliferation of human monoclonal lymphocytes, *J. Immunol., 138*:3824 (1987).

101. S. Karray, J.-F. Delfraissy, H. Merle-Beral, C. Wallon, P. Debre, and P. Galanaud, Positive effects of interferon-α on B cell-type chronic lymphocytic leukemia proliferative response, *J. Immunol., 140*:774 (1988).

102. S. Karray, T. De France, H. Merle-Béral, J. Banchereau, and P. Galanaud, Interleukin 4 counteracts the interleukin 2-induced proliferation of monoclonal B cells, *J. Exp. Med., 168*:85 (1988).

103. A. Vallé, C. E. Zuber, T. Defrance, O. Djossou, M. De Rie, and J. Banchereau, Activation of human B lymphocytes through CD40 and interleukin 4, *Eur. J. Immunol., 19*:1463 (1989).

104. M. Carlsson, C. Sundström, M. Bengtsson, T. H. Tötterman, A. Rosén, and K. Nilsson, IL 4 strongly augments or inhibits DNA synthesis and differentiation of B-chronic lymphocytic leukemia cells depending on the co-stimulatory activation and progression signals, *Eur. J. Immunol., 19*:913 (1989).

3

Tumor Necrosis Factor and Autocrine Growth Loops: Implications for Therapy

A. V. Hoffbrand
Royal Free Hospital School of Medicine, London, England

H. E. Heslop and M. K. Brenner
St. Jude Children's Research Hospital, Memphis, Tennessee

In the last few years, data from a number of converging lines of research have established tumor necrosis factor (TNF) as an autocrine growth factor for normal B lymphocytes and some types of malignant B cells. This has led to further experiments, which suggest that interferon-α (IFN-α) is effective therapy in some B-cell tumors, particularly hairy cell leukemia and early-stage B-chronic lymphocytic leukemia, by interfering with an autocrine growth loop for TNF and possibly for other cytokines. The evidence supporting these concepts is reviewed here, and the implications of this new information for future research are discussed.

TUMOR NECROSIS FACTOR-α

Tumor necrosis factor-α (TNF) was discovered in mouse serum after injection of bacterial endotoxin and is now known to cause necrosis of some tumors in vivo and in vitro. TNF is a polypeptide cytokine of molecular weight 17,000, made up of 157 amino acids. It is involved in inflammatory and immune responses and in tumor cell growth (1–3). The single-copy gene is within the cluster of the major histocompatibility complex on the short arm of chromosome 6. It belongs to a class of hormone-like molecules called cytokines, including the hemopoietic growth factors, interferons, and interleukins, which form a complex network regulating their own produc-

63

tion and the growth, differentiation, and function of virtually all the cells of the body. TNF is produced by macrocytes/macrophages and by T and B lymphocytes and has a wide range of biologic activities because: (a) TNF receptors are present on virtually all cells; (b) TNF leads to activation of multiple signal transduction pathways, kinases, and transcription factors; and (c) TNF action activates a large number of cell genes (Table 1).

TNF has opposing effects on the early and late stages of hemopoiesis. It stimulates stromal cells (e.g., fibroblasts and endothelial cells) to produce the hemopoietic growth factors GM-CSF, G-CSF, and M-CSF, but inhibits proliferation of later hemopoietic progenitor cells. It is also involved in endotoxin shock and in bone resorption. A structurally and functionally related protein with a closely linked gene is called TNF-β or lymphotoxin, and is secreted mainly by lymphocytes.

TNF transmits its signal to target cells after binding to specific cell surface receptors. These appear to be two separate molecules, a high-affinity binder of apparent molecular weight 75,000 and a lower-affinity binder of molecular weight 55,000 (3). They differ in their intracellular domains and are likely to activate different intracellular signaling pathways. In some

Table 1 Examples of Genes Induced by TNF[a]

Cytokines	IL-1
	IL-6
	IL-8
	TNF
Growth factors	GM-CSF
	M-CSF
	PDGF
Receptors	IL-2
	EGF
Transcription factors	c-jun
	c-fos
	NF kappa B
	NF-IL6
Cell adhesion molecules	CAM-1
Inflammatory mediators and acute-phase proteins	Collagenase
	Serum ferritin
	Haptoglobin
Major histocompatibility molecules	Class 1
	Class 2

[a]Abbreviations: PDGF = platelet-derived GF; EGF = epidermal GF; for others, see text.

cells they are constitutively expressed, while in other TNF receptors are reversibly induced. Protein kinase C (PKC) activation leads to downregulation of TNF receptors but to secretion of TNF, whereas protein kinase A (PKA) activation upregulates TNF receptors but downregulates TNF production.

SIGNAL TRANSDUCTION

Following binding of TNF to its receptor, there is calcium influx from the exterior to the cytoplasm, followed by the activation of several cellular kinases. There is activation of phospholipase A_2, with release of arachidonic acid and prostaglandin E_2, enhanced cyclic AMP levels, and protein kinase A (PKA) activity. It is likely that these effects are mediated by a G protein. The exact spectrum of kinases activated is uncertain, but it probably includes PKC and PKA. Full activation of inositol lipid breakdown has not been observed. A series of cytoplasmic proteins are then activated, the signal being transmitted to the nucleus. Activated oxygen species also appear to be involved in the signal transduction (4).

TRANSCRIPTION FACTORS

Cytokine induction of genes involved in control of the cell cycle and in differentiation is thought to be mediated through transacting proteins called transcription factors. These bind to cis-acting DNA sequences including enhancers and promoters and determine transcriptional activity for both constitutive and inducible genes. A number of transcription factors can be activated by TNF, including AP-1, nuclear factor (NF) kappa B, and interferon-regulatory factors. A novel transcription factor, NF-GMa, has been described that is induced by TNF and binds to a common enhancer element CK-1 in a number of hemopoietic growth factor genes (5). More than one pathway or transcription factor may mediate activation of a single gene by TNF. Thus, induction of interleukin-6 (IL-6) requires three different cis-acting elements, and both NFKB and NF-IL-6 sites are required for IL-8 induction by TNF. Activation of the promoters for certain genes by TNF may occur through NF kappa B activation, and it is likely that these effects occur in normal B cells as well as in HCL and B-CLL cells. Gignac et al. (6) found that TNF induced the transcription of the protooncogenes c-fos and c-jun (which together make up the transcription factor AP-1) and c-myc in B-CLL cells. Induction by TNF was delayed compared to induction by the phorbol esters. This correlates with delayed induction of DNA synthesis by TNF in B-CLL cells compared with normal B cells (see later).

TNF-RESPONSIVE GENES

TNF (and IL-1) have the largest number of target genes of any known natural substances (Table 1). TNF induces a large number of genes, including those coding for certain transcription factors, cytokines (PDGF, GM-CSF, G-CSF, M-CSF), ferritin and other acute-phase proteins, and prostaglandin E_2, and in the context of the present chapter, TNF itself. TNF has been shown to increase its own synthesis (7). The TNF-responsive element in the TNF gene appears to be within a 5' region -125 to -82 in the TNF promoter region and to consist of a palindromic sequence similar but not identical to the consensus binding sequence for the transcription factor AP-1 and other transcription factors (8). As mentioned earlier, TNF also increases the synthesis of IL-6 and IL-8.

TNF may up- or downregulate expression of some genes depending on cell type. Thus, TNF induces c-myc in fibroblasts, which are stimulated to proliferate, whereas in cell types in which growth is inhibited, it may inhibit c-myc expression. It enhances the expression on the cell surface of certain adhesion molecules and the constitutively expressed genes encoding HLA class I and II antigens but inhibits expression of genes involved in lipogenesis, collagen synthesis, and muscle differentiation (for references see Ref. 8).

EVIDENCE FOR TNF AS A GROWTH FACTOR
FOR B LYMPHOCYTES

TNF is known to be a growth factor for fibroblasts, T cells, and thymocytes. Williamson et al. (9) first showed that the B lymphocyte may be a source of TNF. Kehrl et al. (10) then showed that TNF can enhance the proliferation of activated but not of resting normal B lymphocytes. They also found that B lymphocytes have receptors for TNF on the cell surface, increased by activation to about 6000 sites per cell. Sung et al. (11) showed that tonsillar lymphocytes could be induced by mitogens to express TNF messenger (m)RNA and to secrete TNF. This production of TNF correlated with their proliferation in response to mitogens. They also found that 9 of 15 B-cell leukemia lines tested and EBV-transformed normal B cells express TNF mRNA and protein. The phorbol ester, PMA (phorbol myristate acetate), could induce TNF mRNA in all these cell types. They postulated that TNF may be important for normal B-cell activation, growth, and differentiation. More recently, autocrine production of TNF by activated B cells has been shown to play an important role in maintenance of cell survival and production of immunoglobulin (12).

Cordingley et al. (13) first showed that TNF is an autocrine growth promoting factor in the B-cell diseases hairy cell leukemia (HCL) and B-chronic lymphocytic leukemia (B-CLL), inducing proliferation of the cells in vitro without terminal differentiation. In the case of HCL, the cells could be stimulated to undergo cell division and further proliferation. They also showed TNF receptors to be present on the surface of the malignant cells in both diseases. Cordingley et al. (13) and Bianchi et al. (14) found that the cell levels of TNF mRNA and TNF protein were increased when the cells were cultured with TNF itself. They suggested that endogenous TNF production may be important for growth and survival of these B-cell tumors, i.e., that an autocrine growth loop for TNF existed. Digel et al. (15) have confirmed that TNF causes proliferation in vitro in a dose-dependent fashion of the tumor cells in most cases of B-CLL. Interestingly, they found that low concentrations of TNF (e.g., 1 ng/mL of rTNF) reduced proliferation of these cells. The same group showed that the cells of 5 of 8 patients with HCL proliferated in response to TNF (16). Lymphotoxin (TNF-β) was inactive in this system. High-affinity TNF receptors were present on the cells whether or not they were responsive to TNF. More recently, this group have suggested that, unlike HCL cells, B-CLL cells in vivo do not express TNF receptors but gain them only after incubating the cells in vitro (17). Gignac et al. (6) have confirmed that TNF causes proliferation of B-CLL cells and showed that this was associated with induction of the protooncogenes c-jun and c-fos, which together form the transcription factor AP-1. On the other hand, Foa et al. (18) found that they could stimulate proliferation of B-CLL cells with TNF in only 4 of 24 cases at varying stages of the disease tested.

HEMOPOIETIC FAILURE

Pancytopenia is a feature of advanced disease in both HCL and B-CLL. In many cases this is out of proportion to the degree of marrow infiltration or of enlargement of the spleen. Taniguchi et al. (19) found that conditioned medium from hairy cells inhibited the growth of normal bone marrow myeloid progenitors (CFU-C) and erythroid progenitors (CFU-E). Conditioned medium from normal controls and from B-CLL patients did not have this effect. Lindemann et al. (20) found high levels of TNF in bone marrow serum of patients with HCL and showed that anti-TNF-neutralizing antibodies were able to increase the growth of hemopoietic progenitors (CFU-GM) from HCL marrow in vitro. TNF is known to suppress bone marrow hemopoietic progenitors from normal subjects. The improved growth of myeloid progenitors with anti-TNF antibodies has been confirmed for both peripheral blood and bone marrow progenitors (21). They showed that the addition of neutralizing anti-TNF antibodies increased the numbers of myeloid colonies in 11 of 15 patients with B-CLL, the effect being most marked on CFU-mix and BFU-E. They also showed high levels of TNF in conditioned medium from purified B-CLL cells.

SERUM LEVELS OF TNF

Lindemann et al. (20) first reported high levels of TNF in the peripheral blood and bone marrow plasma in HCL. Hahn et al. (22) studied supernatants prepared by incubating mononuclear cells or purified leukemic cells from the peripheral blood of patients with Rai stage 0 and stage 4 CLL. They showed spontaneous TNF production by both the peripheral blood mononuclear cells and the purified malignant cells. This was more marked in stage 0 than in stage 4 cases. This contrasts with an earlier study by the same group, which described reduced TNF secretion by peripheral blood mononuclear cells in HCL increased by IFN.

Foa et al. (18) found raised levels of TNF in the serum of 20 of 24 patients with HCL or B-CLL that they tested and confirmed that purified B-CLL or HCL cells constitutively release variable quantities of TNF. These quantities could be increased by incubating the cells with interferon-γ or phytohemagglutinin (PHA) plus PMA. They confirmed the results of Hahn that TNF release was higher per cell in stage 0-1 than in stage 2-3 B-CLL. On the other hand, Weiss et al. (23) could not detect TNF in serum in 14 of 20 patients with HCL or CLL. The differences may be due to the assay used, since we have observed raised levels using a Medgenix assay but undetectable levels using an Elisa assay (Reittie et al., unpublished).

EFFECTS OF ANTI-TNF ANTIBODY IN VIVO

If TNF production has a central role in the pathophysiology of HCL, then infusion of antibody to the cytokine might be expected to reverse many of the abnormalities seen. In a small pilot study of three patients with HCL, we gave 0.5–2 mg/kg of Celltech anti-TNF murine monoclonal antibody (Mab) (73). In lower doses the Mab was well tolerated, but at higher doses one patient developed features of serum sickness. In one patient there was a reduction in splenomegaly and in marrow infiltrate with HCL cells, and two patients showed a marked rise in circulating B cells associated with a rise in serum IL-6 levels. These limited clinical data further support the concept that TNF production contributes to the multiplicity of clinical abnormalities seen in HCL.

OTHER GROWTH FACTORS

IL-6 and IL-1 are additional further growth factors for normal and malignant B cells such as B-CLL and HCL (24). IL-6 and IL-1 are also produced by CLL and hairy cells (25–27), again raising the possibility of autocrine growth loops for these cytokines.

INTERLEUKIN-6

Normal B cells can synthesize IL-6, and anti-IL-6 antibody can reduce the Ig production response of normal B cells to pokeweed mitogen (PWM). Anti-IL6 also inhibits spontaneous IgG production by B cells from patients with diseases characterized by hypergammaglobulinemia, suggesting an autocrine IL-6 growth loop in B-cell differentiation in these diseases (28). Production of IL-6 may be stimulated by TNF, since anti-TNF reduces IL-6 production by stimulated normal B cells (12). This is consistent with the observation that TNF is synthesized earlier than IL-6 in activated normal B cells in vitro (12). B-CLL cells constitutively express the IL-6 gene and secrete IL-6 (25). A recent report (29) suggests that TNF may stimulate B-CLL cells by first inducing IL-6 synthesis, but this requires confirmation. HCL cells also produce IL-6 (26,27).

   In the context of a possible autocrine role of IL-6 in growth of B-CLL and HCL, it is relevant to review briefly the possible role of IL-6 in the autocrine or paracrine growth of another B-cell malignancy, multiple myeloma, particularly as this disease also has been reported to respond to interferon therapy. IL-6 was first established as a growth factor for multiple myeloma by Kawano et al. (30). Some workers, however, have failed to find IL-6 mRNA in fresh myeloma cells from patients and from myeloma cell lines and therefore suggest that growth of myeloma depends on paracrine rather than autocrine production of IL-6 (31). On the basis of studies with established human myeloma cell lines, Jernberg et al. (32) suggest heterogeneity—some lines being dependent on IL-6 for growth and survival, others being dependent on IL-6 for growth but not survival, and finally others being independent of IL-6. IL-6 dependence of the cell lines in general was lower than reported for fresh myeloma samples, implying that IL-6 independence may result from repeated passage in vitro. IL-6 mRNA has been detected in a proportion of fresh marrow cells isolated from patients with myeloma by some (30,33) but not other workers (31). Transfection of the IL-6 gene into IL-6 receptor-expressing, IL-6-dependent mouse plasmacytoma can result in autocrine growth stimulation in vitro and increased tumorgenicity in vivo (34). Whether human myeloma cells themselves produce IL-6 or whether this comes from macrophages and other cells in the marrow in myeloma thus remains unclear. Although responses to interferon are described in myeloma (see later), there is no published data on whether or not this can be attributed to interruption of autocrine or paracrine growth loops. At a clinical level, serum levels of IL-6 have been found to reflect disease severity in myeloma (35) and to be of prognostic significance (36).

INTERLEUKIN-1

Normal and malignant B lymphocytes including HCL cells produce IL-1 (27,37). Two main forms exist, IL-1α (associated with the cell membrane) and IL-1β, which is predominantly secreted. IL-1α and -β are produced by B-CLL cells (38,39), and there is evidence that production by individual cells is less in late compared to early-stage disease (40,41). IL-1β is frequently secreted but IL-1α is not, although all B-CLL cells also contain IL-1α. Secretion of IL-1 correlates with the cell expression of myelomonocytic antigens (e.g., CD14, CD16, CD15) (39).

The evidence that IL-1 acts as a growth factor for B-CLL cell is less complete. Although IL-1 is known to synergize with other growth factors in promoting growth of normal resting and activated B cells and of established B-cell lines, evidence that it directly stimulates B-CLL cells is lacking (42).

IL-1 levels are raised in HCL more than in any other hematologic malignancy (43). In this study IL-1 levels correlated with tumor bulk assessed by degree of bone marrow infiltration (hairy cell index) and by serum IL-2 receptor levels. No direct evidence was obtained that the tumor cells themselves synthesized IL-1. Ruco et al. (44) could not detect IL-1 produced by hairy cells in vitro, and Griffiths and Cawley (45) could not show that IL-1 enhanced the proliferation of hairy cells in vitro. Nevertheless, IL-1 can act as a growth factor for some B-cell neoplastic diseases, including myeloma (46) and possibly B-ALL (47). Hairy cells do express IL-1 mRNA when exposed to TNF, and this mRNA is reduced by interferon-α (27). Thus, an autocrine growth loop for IL-1 in HCL that can be interrupted by interferon cannot be entirely excluded.

RESULTS OF INTERFERON-α THERAPY IN B-CELL MALIGNANCIES

Interferon-α (IFN) was first established to be of value in therapy of HCL by Quesada et al. (48). Of seven patients treated, three achieved a complete response (CR) and four a partial response (PR). Many subsequent studies have shown up to a 90% response rate. It is unusual for hairy cells to disappear completely, but there is a gradual normalization of the blood counts in the vast majority of patients. Patients with the rare hairy cell variant are usually resistant. Improvement occurs over the first 12 months of therapy, and relapse occurs on average 2 years after stopping therapy (49). The dose of IFN usually used is 3 mU subcutaneously, 3–7 times weekly. Resistance may be associated with the development of neutralizing antibodies, although the exact significance of these is uncertain since they can be detected in many patients responding satisfactorily and also they may occur transiently despite continuation of IFN therapy (50).

Responses to IFN therapy have also been described in B-CLL, myeloma, and non-Hodgkin's lymphoma. In B-CLL, favorable responses have occurred in early-stage disease in one of four patients studied by O'Connell et al. (51), in five of seven patients studied by Ziegler-Heitbrook et al. (52), in all 10 studied by Rozman et al. (53), and in five of 10 patients treated by Pangalis and Griva (54). In late-stage disease, both partial and complete responses are unusual (55).

In myeloma, a number of studies have now shown some action in untreated cases, with less activity in late-stage disease. More recently, Mandelli et al. (56) have shown that IFN therapy may prolong the plateau phase and survival of patients who have already been treated with cytotoxic chemotherapy. The use of IFN in combination with chemotherapy for initial treatment of myeloma is now the subject of a randomized trial in Sweden (57). Initial results suggest that the addition of IFN to induction chemotherapy may improve survival for patients with stage 2 disease. Oken et al. (58), reporting for the ECOG group, also found that IFN improved response rate to VBMCP therapy compared to historical controls. It is of interest to speculate whether this clinical effect of IFN in myeloma is due to interruption of an autocrine or paracrine growth loop, e.g., for IL-6 by analogy with its suggested mode of action in B-CLL and HCL.

In lymphomas, the best responses have been described in low-grade B-cell disease, with fewer responses in intermediate or high-grade tumors. Prolongation of disease-free remission when IFN is used in combination with chemotherapy both in induction and maintenance has been shown (59). It is not yet clear if this will be translated into survival advantage. There have been no studies as yet of the action of IFN on cytokine growth loops in the lymphomas.

MECHANISM OF RESPONSE BY B-CELL MALIGNANCIES TO INTERFERON-α THERAPY

Earlier studies had suggested a number of possible mechanisms by which IFN is effective in therapy. These include enhanced natural killer activity against the tumor cells or breakdown of paracrine control mechanisms. Although IFN does enhance cytotoxic activity in vivo, there is no evidence in the case of the B-cell malignancies B-CLL or HCL that these cells are capable of killing the tumor cells, nor is there any relation between the degree of enhanced cytotoxic activity and the clinical response (60,61).

IFN can inhibit the proliferation of B-CLL and HCL cells induced by BCGF (IL-6) (62,63). Cordingley et al. (13) and Buck et al. (16) showed that IFN inhibits the increased thymidine uptake in HCL and B-CLL cells stimulated by TNF. IFN induces the synthesis of two enzyme systems capable of inhibiting B-cell proliferation. The first is 2-5′ oligo adenylate synthetase (2-5′ oligo AS). The product of the enzyme, 2-5′ oligo A stimulates the activity of a latent ribonuclease. This occurs in the malignant cells in both HCL and CLL (64,65). Favorable response in chronic myeloid leukemia (CML) correlates with the degree of 2-5′ oligo AS induction, and this may also be so in CLL (65), while resistance in CML is associated with a failure of induction (66). 2-5′ Oligo AS mRNA occurs in four different species. As yet, there is no information on whether different species are induced in different hemopoietic or lymphoid lineages or diseases or whether any other particular species of 2-5′ oligo AS relates to IFN action.

Increased cellular RNAase induced by IFN may lead to degradation of certain species of cellular RNA. This has been shown for the messenger RNA's encoding TNF, IL-1, and IL-6 in both HCL and B-CLL (27). The mRNA's for TNF, IL-6, and IL-1 normally induced by incubation with TNF protein were reduced or absent in the presence of IFN (Fig. 1). In addition, the half-life of mRNA for TNF in B-CLL and HCL upon incubation with IFN in vitro was reduced compared to control cells (Fig. 2). Moreover, time-course studies showed that 2-5′ oligo AS mRNA was increased in response to exposure to IFN shortly before levels of mRNA for these cytokines fall (Fig. 3).

If IFN achieves a therapeutic effect in HCL and B-CLL by interrupting autocrine (or paracrine) growth loops, the relative importance of the various cytokines downregulated by IFN remains uncertain. TNF, IL-6, and IL-1 are all downregulated (27). They are capable, separately or together, of inducing growth and/or differentiation of B-CLL/HCL cells, so the overall therapeutic benefit of IFN may be due to interruption of several growth factor loops.

The second enzyme system induced by interferon is a protein kinase that phosphorylates two proteins, the ribosome-associated protein PI and the peptide eukaryotic initiation factor ELF-2α. This system is capable of inhibiting protein synthesis; IFN is also able to downregulate expression of a variety of genes, including those involved in the cell entering the cell cycle including c-myc (67).

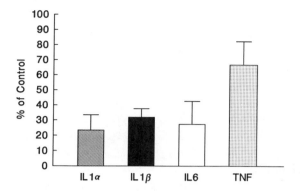

Figure 1   Effect of IFN-α on TNF, IL-1α, IL-1β, and IL-6 mRNA, accumulating at 24 h in the tumor cells of five patients with HCL or B-CLL. Cells were incubated with TNF with or without IFN. For each cytokine, bars represent the mean percent $\pm$ SD of cytokine mRNA in the presence of TNF and IFN-α, compared with that in the presence of TNF alone. Paired t test shows highly significant effect for IFN-α on all cytokine mRNA levels ($p < 0.01$). (*Source:* Reproduced with permission of the Rockefeller University Press.)

Not all cellular mRNAs are degraded by the RNAase activity stimulated by IFN. In the studies of Heslop et al. (27), it was shown that mRNA levels for structural proteins such as tubulin were unaffected. The explanation for this difference may be in the structure of different mRNA species. One of the major factors on which the stability of different mRNAs depends is the structure of 3' untranslated region (68,69), and cytokine mRNA contains a conserved AU sequence in this region that mediates instability (70).

Finally, Buck et al. (16) found that incubation with IFN downregulated receptors for TNF on HCL cells in vitro. The relevance of this to IFN action in vivo is unclear.

IMPLICATIONS

The response of IFN therapy in patients with various malignancies can now be examined in the light of the theory that IFN exerts its action in HCL and B-CLL and possibly in other B-cell malignancies by interrupting autocrine or paracrine growth loops for cytokines, particularly for TNF, IL-6, and possibly IL-1. The best responses occur in HCL, and it is in this disease that the highest TNF levels have been found in serum (18) and the highest levels of TNF are produced per cell in vitro. Moreover, the most consistent stimulation of DNA synthesis with TNF occurs in HCL, and only in this

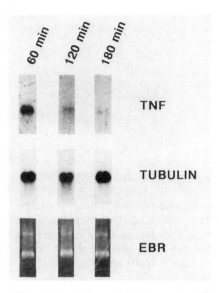

Figure 2 Effect of IFN-α on half-life of cytokine mRNA. B-CLL cells were cultured for 24 h in the presence of TNF or TNF and IFN-α. Actinomycin D was added to cultures, and mRNA was harvested at intervals for 4 h and run on a Northern blot. Ethidium bromide (EBR) staining shows equal loading at all time points. The figure shows that TNF mRNA degrades rapidly over this time course while tubulin mRNA is unaffected. (*Source:* Reproduced from Ref. 27, with permission of the Rockefeller University Press.)

disease and not in CLL can the cells be stimulated to undergo mitosis by TNF (13). It seems, therefore, that in HCL an autocrine growth loop for TNF is most marked, and this may make the cells particularly susceptible to IFN therapy. To a lesser degree, the same may be true of early compared to late-stage CLL. Although no clear-cut relation between stage of CLL and serum TNF levels has been shown (18), this may relate to total mass of disease rather than amount secreted by individual cells. Cytokine levels in plasma in B-cell non-Hodgkin's lymphoma has not yet been studied, nor has the dependence of these cells on autocrine or paracrine growth loop been reported, although responses to IFN are now well documented, particularly in early-stage disease.

The response to IFN therapy in individual patients with any one disease could depend on a variety of factors. These include presence of IFN receptors on the cells, degree of induction of 2-5′ oligo AS, degree of dependence of the tumor on cytokine stimulation, number and type of cytokine recep-

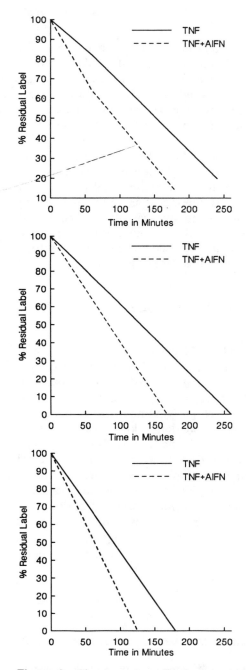

Figure 3 Time-course studies in three patients (one HCL, two B-CLL) showing that the half-life of cytokine mRNA is reduced still further in the presence of IFN-α. (*Source:* Reproduced from Ref. 27, with permission of the Rockefeller University Press.)

tors, and possibly other actions of IFN on tumor growth independent of a cytokine growth loop, of 2-5' oligo AS induction, and of cytokine mRNA degradation. Whether cytotoxic drugs, e.g., Fludarabine, deoxycoformycin, or chlorodeoxydenosine, active in HCL and B-CLL, specifically affect the cytokine growth loops in these diseases is unknown, although there is some preliminary evidence in the case of deoxycoformycin that this may be relevant to its action in HCL (71).

As mentioned earlier, it has been suggested that the hemopoietic failure in these B-cell malignancies may be due to inhibition of myelopoiesis by circulating TNF as well as to marrow infiltration by tumor cells. Interferon therapy by reducing TNF synthesis by the tumor cells as well as by reducing the number of tumor cells might be expected to lower circulating TNF levels. This would allow improved marrow hemopoiesis. Lauria et al. (72) found that the inhibiting effect of serum for hairy cell leukemia patients on normal myeloid progenitors disappeared after prolonged interferon therapy.

WHY DOES IFN SELECTIVELY CYTO-REDUCE HCL/B-CLL CELLS?

One major outstanding question is why IFN exerts a selective antitumor effect at all. Normal B cells produce and respond to the same growth factors as the malignant cells in B-CLL and HCL. If IFN exerts its therapeutic activity by interrupting autocrine growth loops, then it should downregulate both normal and malignant B-cell growth and differentiation and produce profound B lymphopenia. As yet, we do not know the mechanism by which selectivity occurs. One possibility is that normal B cells are sheltered from the consequences of IFN action because the environmental niches in which they grow can continue to supply necessary growth factors by direct cellular contact. Malignant cells, in their apparent independence of such niches, may be more vulnerable to interruption of endogenous growth factor loops. Other plausible explanations exist, and the issue will be resolved only when we have an improved understanding of normal and malignant B-cell physiology and when more is known about the lymphopoietic microenvironment.

REFERENCES

1. M. K. Brenner, Tumor necrosis factor (Annotation), *Br. J. Haematol., 69*: 149–152 (1988).
2. G. Semenzato, Tumor necrosis factor: A cytokine with multiple biological activities, *Br. J. Cancer, 61*:354–361 (1990).

3. J. Vilcek and T. H. Lee, Tumor necrosis factor: New insights into the molecular mechanisms of its multiple actions, *J. Biol. Chem.*, *266*:7313–7316 (1991).

4. R. Schreck, P. Rieber, and P. A. Baeuerle, Reactive oxygen intermediates as apparently widely used messengers in the activation of the NF-KB transcription factor and HIV-1, *EMBO J.*, *10*:2247–2258 (1991).

5. M. F. Shannon, L. M. Pell, M. J. Lenardo, E. S. Kuczek, F. S. Occhiodoro, S. M. Dunn, and M. A. Vadas, A novel tumor necrosis factor-responsive transcription factor which recognises a regulatory element in hemopoietic growth factor genes, *Mol. Cell. Biol.*, *10*:2950–2959 (1990).

6. S. M. Gignac, M. Buschle, H. E. Heslop, M. K. Brenner, A. V. Hoffbrand, and H. G. Drexler, Delayed induction of proto-onocogene expression in B-CLL cells in response to tumor necrosis factor, *Leuk. Lymph.*, *3*:37–43 (1990).

7. M. Kronke, S. Schutze, P. Scheurich, and K. Pfizenmaier, in *Tumor Necrosis Factor, Structure, Function and Mechanism of Action* (B. B. Aggarwal and J. Vilcek, eds.), Marcel Dekker, New York, pp. 189–216 (1991).

8. D. C. Leitman, R. C. J. Ribeiro, E. R. Mackow, J. D. Baxter, and B. L. West, Identification of a tumor necrosis factor-responsive element in the tumor necrosis factor α gene, *J. Biol. Chem.*, *266*:9343–9346 (1991).

9. B. D. Williamson, E. A. Carswell, B. J. Rubin, J. S. Predegast, and L. J. Old, Human tumor necrosis factor produced by human B-cell lines: Synergistic cytotoxic interaction with human interferon, *Proc. Natl. Acad. Sci. USA, 80*: 5397 (1983).

10. J. H. Kehrl, A. Miller, and A. S. Fauci, Effect of tumor necrosis factor α on mitogen-activated human B cells, *J. Exp. Med.*, *166*:786 (1987).

11. S. S. J. Sung, L. K. L. Jung, J. A. Walters, K. Chen, C. Y. Wang, and S. M. Fu, Production of tumor necrosis factor/cachetin by human B cell lines and tonsillar B cells, *J. Exp. Med.*, *168*:1539 (1988).

12. P. Rieckmann, F. D'Allesandro, R. P. Nordan, A. S. Fauci, and J. H. Kehrl, IL-6 and tumor necrosis-α. Autocrine and paracrine cytokines involved in B cell function, *J. Immunol.*, *146*:3462–3468 (1991).

13. F. T. Cordingley, A. Bianchi, A. V. Hoffbrand, J. E. Reittie, H. E. Heslop, A. Vyakarnam, M. Turner, A. Meager, and M. K. Brenner, Tumor necrosis factor as an autocrine tumor growth factor for chronic B cell malignancies, *Lancet, i*:969–971 (1988).

14. A. C. M. Bianchi, H. E. Heslop, H. G. Drexler, F. T. Cordingley, M. Turner, W. C. P. De Mel, A. V. Hoffbrand, and M. K. Brenner, Effects of TNF and αIFN on chronic B cell malignancies, *Nouv. Rev. Fr. Hematol.*, *30*:317–319 (1988).

15. W. Digel, M. Stefanic, W. Schoniger, C. Buck, A. Raghavachar, N. Frickhofen, H. Heimpel, and F. Porzsolt, Tumor necrosis factor induces proliferation of neoplastic B cells from chronic lymphocytic leukemia, *Blood, 73*:1242–1246 (1989).

16. C. Buck, W. Digel, W. Schoniger, M. Stefanic, A. Ragnavachar, H. Heimpel, and F. Porzsolt, Tumor necrosis factor-alpha, but not lymphotoxin, stimulates growth of tumor cells in hairy cell leukemia, *Leukemia, 4*(6):431–434 (1990).

17. W. Digel, W. Schoniger, M. Stefanic, H. Janssen, C. Buck, M. Schmid, A. Raghavachar, and F. Porzsolt, Receptors for tumor necrosis factor on neoplastic B cells from chronic lymphocytic leukemia are expressed in vitro but not in vivo, *Blood, 76*(8):1607–1613 (1990).

18. R. Foa, M. Massaia, S. Cardona, et al., Production of tumor necrosis factor-alpha by B-cell chronic lymphocytic leukemia cells: A possible regulatory role of TNF in the progression of the disease, *Blood, 76*:393–400 (1990).

19. N. Taniguchi, H. Kuratsune, A. Kanamaru, et al., Inhibition against CFU-C and CFU-E colony formation by soluble factor(s) derived from hairy cells, *Blood, 73*:907–913 (1989).

20. A. Lindemann, W. D. Ludwig, W. Oster, R. Mertelsmann, and F. Hermann, High-level secretion of tumor necrosis factor-alpha contributes to hematopoietic failure in hairy cell leukemia, *Blood, 73*(4):880–884 (1988).

21. R. Michalevicz, R. Porat, M. Vechoropoulos, S. Baron, M. Yanoov, Z. Cydowitz, and S. Shibolet, Restoration of in vitro hematopoiesis in B-chronic lymphocytic leukemia by antibodies to tumor necrosis factor, *Leuk. Res., 15*: 111–120 (1991).

22. T. Hahn, G. Kuminsky, L. Bassous, Y. Barak, and A. Berrebi, Tumor necrosis factor in B chronic lymphocytic leukemia (letter), *Br. J. Haematol., 71*:299 (1989).

23. C. Weiss, B. Stehle, A. D. Ho, and W. Hunstein, Serum levels of tumor necrosis factor-α in hairy cell leukemia, *Blood, 74*:321–322 (1989).

24. R. J. Ford, L. Yoshimura, J. Morgan, et al., Growth factor-mediated tumor cell proliferation in hairy cell leukemia, *J. Exp. Med., 162*:1093–1098 (1985).

25. A. Biondi, V. Rossi, R. Rassan, T. Barbui, S. Buttoni, M. Sironi, A. Mantovani, and A. Rambaldi, Constitutive expression of the interleukin-6 gene in chronic lymphocytic leukemia, *Blood, 73*:1279–1284 (1989).

26. C. Billard and J. Wietzerbin, On the mechanism of action of interferon-alpha in hairy cell leukemia, *Eur. J. Cancer, 26*:67–69 (1990).

27. H. E. Heslop, A. C. M. Bianchi, F. T. Cordingley, et al., Effects of α-interferon on autocrine growth factor loops in B lymphoproliferative disorders, *J. Exp. Med., 172*:1729–1734 (1990).

28. Y. Levy, J. P. Fermand, S. Navarro, et al., Interleukin-6 dependence of spontaneous in vitro differentiation of B cells from patients with IgM gammopathy, *Proc. Natl. Acad. Sci. USA, 87*:3309 (1990).

29. T. Hahn and A. Berrebi, Tumor necrosis factor accelerates autocrine growth of B chronic lymphocytic leukemia cells through interleukin-6, *Blood, 76(1)*: 96a (1990).

30. M. T. Kawano, T. Hirano, T. Matsuda, et al., Autocrine generation and essential requirement for BSF-2/IL-6 for human multiple myeloma, *Nature, 322*:83–86 (1988).

31. B. Klein, X.-G. Zhang, M. Jourdan, et al., Paracrine rather than autocrine regulation of myeloma-cell growth and differentiation by interleukin-6, *Blood, 73*:517 (1989).

32. H. Jernberg, M. Pattersson, T. Kishimoto, and K. Nilsson, Heterogeneity in response to interleukin-6 (IL-6) expression of IL-6 and IL-6 receptor mRNA

in a panel of established human multiple myeloma cell lines, *Leukemia, 5*: 255–265 (1991).

33. C. G. Freeman, A. S. Freedman, S. N. Rabinowe, J. M. Segil, J. Horowitz, K. Rosen, J. F. Whitman, and L. M. Nadler, Interleukin 6 gene expression in normal and neoplastic B cells, *J. Clin. Invest., 83*:1512–1518 (1989).
34. N. Tohoyama, H. Karasuyama, and T. Tada, *J. Exp. Med., 171*:389–400 (1990).
35. R. Bataille, M. Jourdan, X.-G. Zhang, and B. Klein, Serum levels of interleukin-6, a potent myeloma cell growth factor, as a reflect of disease severity in plasma cell dyscrasias, *J. Clin. Invest., 84*:2008–2011 (1989).
36. H. Ludwig, D. M. Nachbaur, E. Fritze, et al., Interleukin-6 as a prognostic factor in multiple myeloma, *Blood, 77*:2794–2795 (1991).
37. V. Pistoa, F. Cozzolino, A. Rubartelli, M. Torcia, S. Roncello, and M. Ferrarini, In vitro production of interleukin 1 by normal and malignant human B lymphocytes, *J. Immunol., 136*:1688–1692 (1986).
38. C. Uggla, M. Aguilar-Santelises, A. Rosen, H. Mellstedt, and M. Jondal, Spontaneous production of interleukin-1 activity by chronic lymphocytic leukemia cells, *Blood, 70*:1851 (1987).
39. F. Morabito, E. F. Prasthofer, N. E. Dunlap, C. E. Gross, and A. B. Tilden, Expression of myelomonocytic antigens on chronic lymphocytic leukemia B cells correlates with their ability to produce interleukin-1, *Blood, 70*:1750–1757 (1987).
40. M. Aguilar-Sentelises, J. F. Amador, H. Mellstedt, and M. Jondal, Low IL-1β production in leukemic cells from progressive B cell chronic lymphocytic leukemia (B-CLL), *Leuk. Res., 13*:937–942 (1989).
41. M. Aguilar-Santelises, R. Magnusson, S. B. Svenson, A. Loftenius, B. Anderson, H. Mellstedt, and M. Jondal, Expression of interleukin-1α, interleukin-1β and interleukin 6 in chronic lymphocytic leukaemia (B-CLL) cells from patients at different stages of disease progression, *Clin. Exp. Immunol., 84*:422–428 (1991).
42. A. A. Ghaderi, P. Richardson, C. Cardone, M. J. Milsum, N. Ling, S. Gillis, J. Ledbetter, and J. Gordon, Stimulation of B-chronic lymphocytic leukemia populations by recombinant interleukin-4 and other defined growth-promoting agents, *Leukemia, 2*:165–170 (1988).
43. G. Cimino, L. Annino, F. Giona, et al., Serum interleukin-1 beta levels correlate with neoplastic bulk in hairy cell leukemia, *Leukemia, 5*:602–605 (1991).
44. L. P. Ruco, A. Stoppacciaro, M. Valtieri, et al., Absence of natural killer activity and interleukin-1 release in IKTM1 + spleen hairy cells, *Clin. Immunol. Immunopathol., 26*:47–55 (1983).
45. S. D. Griffiths and J. C. Cawley, The effect of cytokines, including IL-1, IL-4 and IL-6 in hairy cell proliferation/differentiation, *Leukemia, 4*:337–340 (1990).
46. F. Cozzolino, M. Torcia, D. Aldinucci, et al., Production of interleukin-1 by bone marrow myeloma cells, *Blood, 74*:380–387 (1989).
47. F. M. Uckun, D. E. Mayers, A. S. Fauci, et al., Leukemia B cell precursors constitutively express functional receptors for human IL-1, *Blood, 74*:761–776 (1989).

48. J. R. Quesada, J. Reuben, J. T. Manning, E. M. Hersh, and J. U. Gutterman, Alpha interferon for induction of remission in hairy cell leukemia, *N. Engl. J. Med., 310*:15–18 (1984).

49. M. J. Ratain, H. M. Golomb, J. W. Vardiman, et al., Relapse after interferon alfa-2b therapy for hairy-cell leukemia; analysis of prognostic variables, *J. Clin. Oncol., 6*:1714–1721 (1988).

50. R. G. Steis, J. W. Smith, W. J. Urba, et al., Loss of interferon antibodies during prolonged continuous interferon-α2a therapy in hairy cell leukemia, *Blood, 77*:792–798 (1991).

51. M. J. O'Connell, J. P. Colgan, M. M. Oken, et al., Clinical trials of recombinant leucocyte A interferon as initial therapy for favorable histology non-Hodgkin's lymphomas and chronic lymphocytic leukemia. An Eastern Cooperative Oncology Group pilot study, *J. Clin. Oncol., 4*:128–136 (1980).

52. H. W. L. Ziegler-Heitbrock, R. Schlag, D. Fleiger, et al., Favorable response of early stage B CLL patients to treatment with IFN-α_2, *Blood, 73*:1426–1430 (1989).

53. C. Rozman, E. Montserrate, N. Vinolas, A. Urbano-Ispizua, J. M. Ribera, T. Gallart, and C. Compernolle, Recombinant alpha interferon in the treatment of B chronic lymphocytic leukemia in early stages, *Blood, 71*:1295–1298 (1988).

54. G. A. Pangalis and E. Griva, Recombinant alfa-2b-interferon therapy in untreated stages A and B chronic lymphocytic leukemia, *Cancer, 61*:869–872 (1988).

55. K. A. Foon, G. C. Bottino, P. G. Abrams, et al., Phase II trial of recombinant leucocyte A interferon in patients with advanced chronic lymphocytic leukemia, *Am. J. Med., 78*:216–220 (1985).

56. F. Mandelli, G. Avvisati, S. Amadori, et al., Maintenance treatment with recombinant interferon alfa-2b in patients with multiple myeloma responding to conventional induction chemotherapy, *N. Engl. J. Med., 322*:1430–1434 (1990).

57. H. Mellstedt, A. Osterborg, M. Bjorkholm, et al., Induction treatment with alpha-interferon in multiple myeloma; An interim report from MGCS, *Eur. J. Hematol., 51*:124–128 (1989).

58. M. M. Oken, R. A. Kyle, P. R. Greipp, et al., Chemotherapy plus interferon (rIFNα_2) in the treatment of multiple myeloma, *Proc. ASCO*, 116.

59. C. G. E. Price, A. Z. S. Rohatiner, W. Steward, et al., Interferon α_{2b} as initial therapy in combination with Chlorambucil and as maintenance therapy in follicular lymphoma, *Ann. Oncol.*, in press (1991).

60. S. D. Griffiths and J. C. Cawley, The beneficial effects of α-IFN in hairy cell leukemia are not attributable to NK cell mediated cytotoxicity, *Leukemia, 1*: 372–376 (1987).

61. F. T. Cordingley, A. V. Hoffbrand, and M. K. Brenner, Cytokine-induced enhancement of the susceptibility of hairy cell leukaemia lymphocytes to natural killer cell lysis, *Br. J. Haematol., 70*:37–41 (1988).

62. K. A. Paganelli, S. S. Evans, T. Han, and H. Ozer, B cell growth factor-induced proliferation of hairy cell lymphocytes and inhibition by type I interferon in vitro, *Blood, 67*:937–942 (1986).

63. E. Genot, C. Billard, F. Sigaux, C. Mathoit, L. Degos, E. Falcoff, and J. P. Kolb, Proliferative response of hairy cells to B cell growth factor (BCGF): In vivo inhibition by interferon-α and in vitro effects of interferon-α, -β and -γ, *Leukemia, 1*:590–596 (1987).

64. C. Billard, D. Ferbus, F. Sigaux, et al., Action of interferon-alpha on hairy cell leukemia: Expression of specific receptors and (2'-5') oligo (A) synthetase in tumor cells from sensitive and resistant patients, *Leuk. Res., 12*:11–18 (1988).

65. W. C. P. De Mel, A. V. Hoffbrand, F. J. Giles, et al., Alpha interferon therapy for haematological malignancies: Correlation between *in vivo* induction of the 2'-5' oligoadenylate system and clinical response, *Br. J. Haematol., 74*:452–456 (1990).

66. M. G. Rosenblum, B. L. Maxwell, M. Talpaz, et al., In vivo sensitivity and resistance of chronic myelogenous leukemia cells to α-interferon: Correlation with receptor binding and induction of 2'5'-oligoadenylate synthetase, *Cancer Res., 46*:4848–4852 (1986).

67. C. Dani, N. Mechti, M. Piechaczyk, et al., Increased rate of degradation of c-myc mRNA in interferon-treated Daudi cells, *Proc. Natl. Acad. Sci. USA, 82*:4896–4899 (1985).

68. D. Caput, B. Beutler, S. Hartog, A. Brown-Shimer, and A. Cerami, Identification of a common nucleotide sequence in the untranslated region of mRNA molecules specifying inflammatory mediators, *Proc. Natl. Acad. Sci. USA, 83*:1670 (1986).

69. S. W. Pelz and J. Ross, Autogenous regulation of histone mRNA decay by histone proteins in a cell-free system, *Mol. Cell. Biol., 7*:4345–4356 (1987).

70. G. Shaw and R. A. Kamen, A conserved AU sequence from the 3' untranslated region of GM-CSF mRNA mediates selective mRNA degradation, *Cell, 46*:659 (1986).

71. W. C. P. De Mel, A. V. Hoffbrand, D. Catovsky, A. B. Mehta, G. C. Ihra, and K. Ganeshaguru, Increase in 2'5'-oligoadenylate synthetase caused by deoxycoformycin, *Br. J. Haematol., 74* (suppl.):6 (1990).

72. F. Lauria, G. P. Bagnara, L. Catani, et al., The inhibitory effect of serum from hairy cell leukaemia patients on normal progenitor cells may disappear following prolonged treatment with alpha-interferon, *Br. J. Haematol., 72*: 497–501.

4

Chromosome Abnormalities in B-Cell Chronic Lymphocytic Leukemia

Gunnar Juliusson and Gösta Gahrton
Karolinska Institute at Huddinge Hospital, Huddinge, Sweden

INTRODUCTION

Chromosome analysis has been a prerequisite for the identification of gene abnormalities in hematologic malignancies. The Philadelphia chromosome described in 1960 (1) enabled the characterization of the bcr/abl hybrid gene (2), and the translocation between chromosomes 14 and 18 consistently found in follicular lymphomas (3) guided the identification of the bcl-2 gene (4) and gene product (5).

Furthermore, chromosome abnormalities have proved to be important prognostic markers in acute leukemia of both the lymphoblastic (6) and nonlymphoid (7) types.

Chromosome analysis requires metaphase cells. This is usually not a great problem in acute leukemias, blastic lymphomas, or chronic myelocytic leukemia. However, in chronic lymphocytic leukemia (CLL) it is a major obstacle, since the tumor cells have an extremely low mitotic index, and therefore mitogen activation in vitro (8) is a necessity.

The banding (9) is essential for the identification of chromosome abnor-

This paper was written for the International Working Party on Chromosomes in Chronic Lymphocytic Leukemia. Participants in the IWCCLL are listed at the end of this chapter.

malities. Without banding, the size of the chromosome and localization of the centromere enables the sorting of the chromosomes into different groups; however, the distinction between normal chromosomes of similar sizes, e.g., number 13 and 14, or number 21 and 22, requires banding. Even more, in the characterization of chromosome breaks, translocations and subtle changes, banded metaphase cells of optimal quality are required. Unfortunately, it seems that tumors often provide metaphase cells of poor quality, which may hamper the identification of marker chromosomes and structural abnormalities. In fact, the metaphase cells of the best quality in tumor material may often be residual normal cells contaminating the cell sample.

However, despite these difficulties, methodological improvements have made it possible to identify with high accuracy clonal chromosomal abnormalities in hematological tumors, including CLL.

MITOGEN ACTIVATION OF CLL CELLS AND CYTOGENETIC TECHNIQUES

Normal peripheral blood lymphocytes consist mainly of T cells, which are readily brought into mitosis by in-vitro cultivation with the T-cell mitogen phythemagglutinin (10). This technique was previously used also in CLL, although CLL in 95% of the cases is a B-cell disorder. Thus, the evaluated cells in the early studies were most likely residual normal T cells (11), and for a long period CLL was claimed to lack abnormal chromosomes (12). The breakthrough in the chromosome analysis of CLL cells came by the ability to induce mitosis in the leukemic cells in vitro (8), using the techniques developed by immunologists for the activation of normal B cells (13). B-cell mitogen activation soon became known as a prerequisite for chromosome analysis in B-CLL. The most frequently used mitogens have been lipopolysaccharide from *E. coli*, tetradecanoyl-phorbol-acetate, cyto-chalasin B, Epstein-Barr virus, and pokeweed mitogen. These mitogens might be used alone or in various combinations. The presence of occasional T cells is important for the mitogenic action. Phythemagglutinin may be used if one keeps in mind that the effect on B cells is mediated by T-cell-derived cytokines. Extensive T-cell depletion before culture in order to avoid chromosome analysis of contaminating cells mostly precludes the mitoses of the leukemia cells. B-cell growth factors, supernatants from mixed lymphocyte cultures or other types of "conditioned" media, or allo-geneic normal mononuclear cells (14) might also be used. Unstimulated bone marrow cell cultures are also reported to give rise to metaphases from the leukemic cells (15). However, the optimal culture procedure is not known, since there has been no large study comparing the success rates regarding both mitotic index and percentage abnormal metaphases with different culture techniques. It is recommended that one set up multiple cultures, since it seems that no single mitogen is best for every case. However, it is rarely seen that a specific clone is picked up in one culture, whereas a completely different clone is stimulated by another mitogen. The culture technique usually includes incubation of 2 million cells per milliliter of serum-containing medium with mitogens in humidified air with 5% CO_2, and harvested on day 3 to day 5. The cells are then treated with colchicine to arrest them in metaphase, and with hypotonic potassium chloride solution to spread the chromosomes. The cells are fixed in methanol/acetic acid and air-dried on slides. Banding is performed with quinacrine mustard [Q banding (9)] or Giemsa [G banding]. Several slides from different cell cultures are scanned for the presence of good-quality metaphases, and karyotyping is performed on cells from slides where the cell activation seems to have been successful. In some patients it takes a very large number of evaluated cells to identify a clonal chromosomal abnormality, whereas in others a specific aberration is found in all cells studied, regardless of the culture technique used. Repeated samplings might in a small part of the patients result in the identification of a previously undetected clone. However, cells that defy cell division in vitro once, often continue to do so (16).

A clonal chromosomal abnormality is defined as two metaphases with the identical structural abnormality or trisomy, or three metaphases with loss of the same chromosome (17). In this and many previous studies (18,19), the clone was considered cytogenetically normal if there were at least 10 metaphases evaluated without the finding of a clonal abnormality. This is an arbitrary distinction, since a much larger number of evaluated metaphases may be needed to pick up clonal changes. Some patients have one or sometimes several metaphases with abnormal chromosomes without fulfilling the criteria for a clonal change, and their karyotypes are thus designated normal. If fewer than 10 metaphases can be evaluated, the karyotype is regarded as not evaluable.

CHROMOSOME ABNORMALITIES IN B-CLL

The chromosome analysis of the first successfully activated B-CLL cells were in 1979 showing a t(11;14) translocation (20), an abnormality that later led to the cloning of the proposed oncogene bcl-1 (21). However, already in 1980 it was found that a trisomy of chromosome 12 was the most frequent abnormality in B-CLL (22,23). This finding is confirmed beyond doubt in several studies (see review in Ref. 24), as well as in the present cooperative study. However, it was not until 1987 that the second most common abnormality was identified, i.e., the deletions of parts of the long arm of chromosome 13 (25), including the retinoblastoma suppressor oncogene (26).

CLL is the most common leukemia in the Western world. Most patients have large amounts of tumor cells readily available through simple venipuncture. Treatment is often delayed because of an indolent initial course of the disease, and leukemia cells are often easy to sample also following treatment, since standard treatment rarely induces a complete remission from CLL. Furthermore, the patients are generally long-lived, although most of them are old. All these factors should facilitate the collection of chromosome data in CLL, in comparison with acute leukemia, where chemotherapy eradicates the leukemic cells from the circulation mostly within weeks from diagnosis, or nonleukemic lymphoma, in which surgical biopsies are needed for a satisfactory cell yield. However, the difficulties with mitogen stimulation and CLL cell cultures have in the past made most institutions reluctant to resort to the laborious CLL chromosome studies.

In order to gain more information in a shorter time about the incidence and clinical implications of chromosome abnormalities in CLL, and to overcome variations due to small numbers of studied patients the 4th International Workshop on CLL in Paris 1988 (27) invited all institutions worldwide with an active interest in CLL chromosomes to participate in a working party. Clinical, phenotypic, and chromosome data were collected through a report form. The results of the first compilation, comprising 433 patients from five European centers, were published in 1990 (19). The number of patients in the study has now increased to 662, with 11 participating institutions.

IWCCLL STUDY

Both clinical and cytogenetic data from at least one occasion were available from 649 patients, and these patients were analyzed for survival and incidence of specific chromosome abnormalities. In addition, 13 patients selected for the presence of structural abnormalities on chromosome 13 were reported from one institution (Minneapolis); these are included only in the analysis of specific chromosome 13 breakpoints (see Fig. 3). The interpretation of the karyotypes was performed by the referring institution. In most cases phenotypic data of the CLL cells were available, and the commitment to the B-cell lineage was always documented.

Clonal abnormalities were found in the cells of 311 patients, with the number of chromosomal aberrations shown in Fig. 1. Balanced transloca-

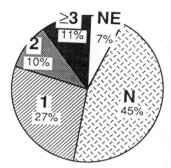

Figure 1 Patients according to number of chromosomal abnormalities. NE, not evaluable due to insufficient number of metaphases (n = 45); N, normal karyotype, i.e., at least 10 evaluable metaphases without a clonal abnormality (n = 293); 1, single chromosomal abnormality (n = 176); 2, two clonal chromosomal abnormalities (n = 64); ≥3, three or more clonal abnormalities (n = 71).

tions were regarded as single abnormalities, despite the two chromosome breakpoints involved. There were 293 cytogenetically normal patients, and 45 cases considered cytogenetically nonevaluable.

Numerical Abnormalities

The most common abnormality was trisomy 12, which was found in 112 patients (19% of evaluable patients and 36% of those with clonal abnormalities). Numerical abnormalities involving other chromosomes were less frequent. Trisomy 3 was found in 14 patients, +18 in 7, +8 in 5, +21 in 5, +19 in 3, and +22 in 3 patients. Monosomies most frequently involved chromosome 17, which was seen in 14 patients. Loss of one X chromosome was seen in 8 females and 1 male. Monosomy of chromosomes 13, 8, 9, and 18 was found in 9, 9, 8, and 8 patients, respectively. Monosomy 21 was seen in 7 cases, −14 in 6, −4 in 5, and −5 in 5 patients.

Structural Abnormalities

The number of patients with structural clonal abnormalities involving specific chromosomes is shown in Fig. 2. Most commonly affected were chromosomes 13, 14, 11, and 6. The involved specific chromosome bands are shown in detail in Figs. 3 through 7. The specific chromosome regions most commonly involved in structural abnormalities were 13q14, 14q32, 13q12, 11q13, and 13q22.

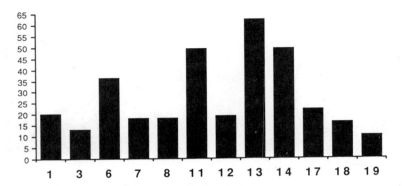

Figure 2 Number of patients with structural clonal chromosomal abnormalities involving specified chromosomes.

Chromosome 12

Trisomy 12 was by far the most common abnormality, whereas structural abnormalities on chromosome 12 are rare. Since the breakpoint sites might be clues to important genes localized on chromosome 12, these breakpoints are shown in Fig. 7. In four cases a breakpoint at 12q13 was seen. The suggested localization of important genes to chromosome 12 bands q13 to q22 was previously deduced from a single patient with a duplication of this

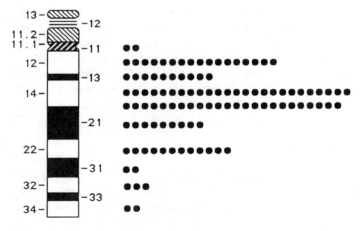

Figure 3 Map of chromosome 13. Each dot indicates one patient with an identified structural abnormality assigned to that specific band. There are two rows of dots for band 13q14.

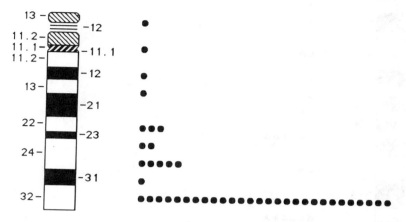

Figure 4 Map of chromosome 14. Each dot indicates one patient with an indentified structural abnormality assigned to that specific band.

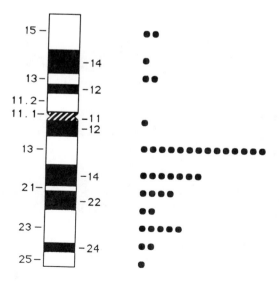

Figure 5 Map of chromosome 11. Each dot indicates one patient with an identified structural abnormality assigned to that specific band.

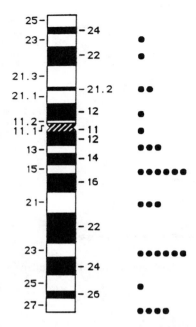

Figure 6 Map of chromosome 6. Each dot indicates one patient with an identified structural abnormality assigned to that specific band.

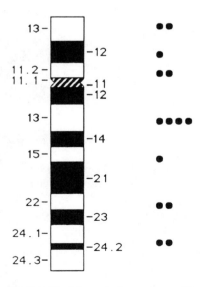

Figure 7 Map of chromosome 12. Each dot indicates one patient with an identified structural abnormality assigned to that specific band.

90

region (28). Three other patients have shown translocations between 12q13 and the centromeric region of chromosome 17 (24): in two cases 17p13, and in one case 17p11. One of these cases had the translocated marker chromosome in addition to two normal chromosomes 12, thus forming a trisomy of the chromosome 12 region distal to 12q13 (shown in Ref. 16). Another patient had a mosaicism with either +12 or +del(12)(q22). Recently, a case with the karyotype 47,XX,+i(12q) was reported (29), thus showing a quadruplication of genes localized to the long arm of chromosome 12. Thus, given the high frequency of trisomy 12 and the low incidence of structural abnormalities on chromosome 12, it is noticeable that a high proportion of the structural abnormalities on chromosome 12 results in partial trisomies, with the common region q13 to q22. Continuing studies of genes localized to these regions should therefore be of particular interest.

Chromosome 13

The most common structural abnormality in CLL (19,24,25) involves the site of the retinoblastoma gene, 13q14 (26). In the present study, cells from 19 patients had chromosome translocations with 13q14 as one of the breakpoints; however, the corresponding breakpoints were highly variable. Only four sites occurred in translocations with 13q14 twice, i.e., 14q13, 14q24, 14q32, and 19p13. Ten patients had translocations involving chromosome 13 with breakpoints at another band than q14, with no recurrent corresponding chromosome region. One patient had a translocation between both her chromosomes 13, with breakpoints at q31 and q34.

Interstitial deletions involving 13q were found in 35 patients, and, interestingly, in all but one the site of the retinoblastoma gene was deleted. The most common specific deletion was del(13) (q12q14), which was found in 13 cases.

Terminal 13q deletions were found in 5 cases; the breakpoints were 13q14, 13q21, and 13q22, respectively, and unidentified in 2 cases.

Chromosome 14

Structural abnormalities on chromosome 14 most commonly involved 14q32, the site of the genes for the immunoglobulin heavy chains. Rearrangements of this huge set of genes are compulsory for lymphoid stem cells differentiating into the B-cell lineage, and 14q32 is a very common translocation breakpoint in all kinds of B-cell tumors, without specificity for B-CLL. The donor chromosome for the 14q+ markers in this study was most commonly number 11, with the breakpoint at the proposed bcl-1 oncogene at 11q13 (21), which was found in 14 cases. The other breakpoint sites involved in 14q32 translocations were 1p22, 2p14, 2p16, 2p22, 7q22, 8q24, 12q15, 13q14, 18q13, 18q21, and 19q13. A breakpoint on chromosomes 11 and 19, respectively, with undefined exact localization was found in two cases, and the donor chromosome was unknown in 3 cases. Thus, translocations juxtaposing the immunoglobulin heavy chain gene to the myc, bcl-2, and bcl-3 genes, respectively, occur rarely in B-CLL.

Most of the other structural abnormalities involving chromosome 14 were terminal deletions with breakpoints at bands q22 to q24.

The site for the T-cell receptor alpha gene, 14q11, which is a common breakpoint in T-cell CLL and other T-cell tumors (30), was never in this study involved in structural abnormalities.

Chromosome 11

The site of the bcl-1 oncogene, 11q13 (21), is the most frequent breakpoint on chromosome 11, and the break is mostly a part of an 11;14-translocation. One patient had a terminal deletion with a break at 11q13. Another patient had breaks at 11q13 on both chromosomes; one was a part of translocation with 14q32 and the other with 17p13. In contrast, most of the breakpoints distal to 11q13 were involved in deletions. All six patients with breakpoints at 11q14 were deletions; four of them were terminal deletions, and two were interstitial deletions with the other breakpoint at 11q21 and 11q23, respectively. All but one of the 10 patients with breakpoints at 11q21 to q24 had 11q deletions: One was an interstitial q21q23, and the others were terminal. A t(11;13)(q23;q14) translocation was seen in one patient.

Chromosome 6

Deletions were the most common abnormalities involving chromosome 6. The interstitial deletion q15q23 was found in 3 patients, and q13q27, q15q27, and q21q27 were found in 1 patient each. Four patients had 6;13-translocations, but the breakpoint on chromosome 6 was different in every case. Two different 6;7-translocations were also found. Thus, structural abnormalities commonly involve chromosome 6, but the breakpoints are spread over the whole of the chromosome.

Chromosome 17

An isochromosome 17q was found in 5 patients. Band q13 was involved in translocations in 4 patients; two of them were translocated to 12q13, one to 11q13, and one to 1p36.

Chromosome 19

Four patients had translocations involving chromosome 19 band p13. Interestingly, the translocation partner was a well-known chromosome region in three of them, 13q14 in two cases (one of them as a part of a three-way translocation also including Yq11), and 11q13 in one.

The locus of the bcl-3 gene (31), i.e., 19q13 (32), was involved in t(14; 19)(q32;q13) translocations in 2 patients, and in another 4 patients the other breakpoint was at 2q22, 3q11, 8p11, and 12p11, respectively.

Single Chromosomal Abnormalities

In more than half of all patients with clonal abnormalities, a single chromosomal change was identified. In analogy with the findings in chronic myelocytic leukemia and follicular lymphoma, it seems reasonable to believe that clues to the pathogenetic mechanisms of CLL could be found in such cases.

Trisomy 12 and structural abnormalities involving chromosome 13 appear to be most important, since these aberrations frequently occur as single ones. A slightly lower fraction of patients with single changes were found among those with aberrations involving chromosomes 6 and 11. In contrast, 80% of the structural abnormalities of chromosome 14 were accompanied by additional aberrations (Fig. 8).

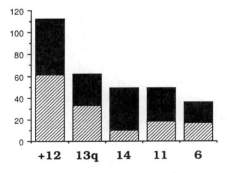

Figure 8   Number of patients with trisomy 12 and structural chromosome abnormalities involving chromosome 13q, 14, 11, and 6. Striped area indicates number of patients with single abnormalities. Solid area those with two or more abnormalities. Full height of bar indicates total number of patients with specified abnormality.

Normal Karyotypes

In about half of the patients, no clonal abnormality is seen. In a small proportion of them, no evaluable metaphases could be found despite repeated attempts to induce mitosis. In a somewhat larger proportion of the patients, there are occasional cells with chromosomal abnormalities. In these cases, an extended search might help to identify more cells, fulfilling the criteria for a clonal change. However, it is not likely that the true incidence of trisomy 12 is much higher than what is found using conventional chromosome analysis. This view is supported by studies using the restriction fragment length polymorphism (RFLP) technique on genes localized to chromosome 12, which permits the determination of the copy number of the studied genes in interphase cells. Trisomy 12, as indicated by RFLP, was shown to be present in almost 100% of the cells in some patients, although a minor fraction of the metaphases had trisomy 12 in the chromosome analysis. However, RFLP suggesting trisomy 12 was never found in patients with normal or not-evaluable karyotype (33), indicating that CLL cells with trisomy 12 are rarely undetected because of an inability to enter mitosis. However, other chromosomal abnormalities may well be present in patients with apparent normal or not-evalubale karyotype. The genetic changes may either be too small to be detectable with conventional cytogenetics, or the fraction of the abnormal cell population that enters mitosis may be unsufficient. Further studies with molecular genetic techniques will certainly elucidate this issue.

CHROMOSOMES DURING DISEASE PROGRESSION

Although clonal evolution with additional chromosome abnormalities and the development of new clones do occur in CLL, these changes are rare, even during disease progression. We have studied a mean of 3.7 samples from 41 patients during a mean interval of 4.2 years. Six patients (15%) showed changes of the karyotype, and 5 (12%) showed an abnormal clone only once (16). Similar results were achieved by Nowell and co-workers (34), and recently by Oscier and co-workers, who found karyotypic evolution in 18 of 112 patients (16%) during a mean sampling interval of 2.9 years (35).

Thus, the specific chromosomal abnormality appears to be achieved very early in the malignant transformation. Complex karyotypes in CLL are not generally the result of karyotypic evolution over a long period of time, and are not usually associated with end-stage disease. This is in contrast to the acquisition of additional chromosome abnormalities at transformation of chronic myelogeneous leukemia and follicular lymphoma. Chromosome data in CLL, achieved at diagnosis or at any time during the course of the disease, are therefore well suited for prognostic use.

PROGNOSTIC IMPLICATIONS OF CHROMOSOME ABNORMALITIES: PREVIOUS AND PRESENT STUDIES

It has become increasingly clear that chromosome studies have prognostic importance in CLL. Patients with Rai stage 0 disease have a higher frequency of normal karyotypes than those with Rai stages 1–4, without clear progression within the stages (24). Multivariate analyses have shown that clinical stage and cytogenetic studies are independent prognostic variables (19).

Trisomy 12 and Prognosis

As early as 1982, it was found by Robèrt and co-workers that patients with trisomy 12 developed a therapy-demanding disease earlier than patients without clonal abnormalities (36). This was corroborated by Sadamori's finding in 1984 of 4 patients with trisomy 12 requiring treatment within 1 year, in contrast to patients with normal karyotypes (37). Life-table (38) analyses (18), also comparing patients with single abnormalities only (39), confirmed the early need for treatment in patients with trisomy 12. However, the difference in overall survival of patients with and without trisomy 12 was not significant, but suggestive if patients with single abnormalities only were compared (24). If low-risk patients [Rai stage 0–2 (40)] were compared, patients with a single $+12$ abnormality had a poorer survival than those with normal karyotype ($p < 0.03$) (41).

In the first IWCCLL study (19), the number of patients with single chromosomal abnormalities was large enough to enable a significant separation of the survival curves for patients (all stages) with trisomy 12 (median, 5.4 years) and other aberrations (median, 8.6 years), as compared to those with normal karyotypes (median, 14 years). Very similar survival curves were found in the now updated and expanded patient material (Figs. 9 and 10).

Trisomy 12 thus seems to have an adverse impact on survival in otherwise low-risk patients. However, the survival of patients with poor-prognostic factors, such as multiple chromosome abnormalities and advanced clinical stage, is not further impaired by the presence of trisomy 12.

Normal Versus Abnormal Karyotype and Prognosis

Following the initial observation of a shorter therapy-free survival in CLL patients with trisomy 12 (36), and the finding that the karyotype had prog-

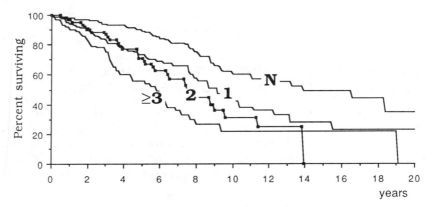

Figure 9 Overall survival according to number of clonal chromosomal abnormalities. N, normal karyotype (n = 293); 1, single chromosomal abnormalities (n = 176); 2, two abnormalities (n = 64); ≥3, three or more chromosomal abnormalities (n = 71).

nostic implications in acute leukemia (7), the search for prognostic associations to karyotype began. Tin Han and co-workers first showed that patients with any clonal abnormality had poorer survival than those with normal karyotypes (42), and we were able to show an increasingly poor

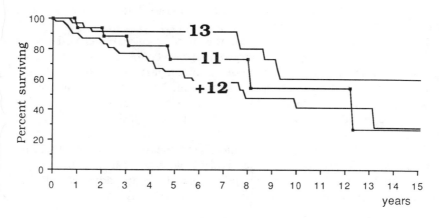

Figure 10 Overall survival according to karyotype, patients with single chromosomal abnormalities only. 11, structural abnormalities involving chromosome 11 (n = 18); +12, trisomy of chromosome 12 (n = 61); 13, structural abnormalities involving chromosome 13 (n = 33).

prognosis with an increasing complexity of the karyotype (18,43). These findings were also confirmed in the first (19) and also in the extended (Fig. 9) collaborative IWCCLL study.

Structural Abnormalities and Prognosis

In the first IWCCLL study it was found that patients with structural abnormalities involving the long arm of chromosome 13 had a similar survival as those with a normal karyotype, i.e., a better survival than patients with other chromosomal abnormalities (19). This was true also when studying patients with abnormalities involving only band 13q14, or those with 13q-changes as single abnormalities (Fig. 10). Structural 13q-abnormalities are commonly found as single abnormalities (Fig. 8), in contrast to the structural changes involving 14q. Abnormalities involving 14q are associated with a poor survival (19,44), but this is probably attributed to its presence in complex karyotypes. The 10 patients with single 14q abnormalities had a longer survival than those with single trisomy 12, and no worse prognosis than other patients with single abnormalities. Patients with structural abnormalities involving chromosome 6 seemed to have a similar survival (Fig. 11) as those with 13q-abnormalities. Patients with chromosome 11 changes seemed to have an intermediate survival among the group of patients with clonal abnormalities (Fig. 10). However, the prognostic information from single abnormalities involving chromosomes 6, 11, and 14 is uncertain because of limited number of patients.

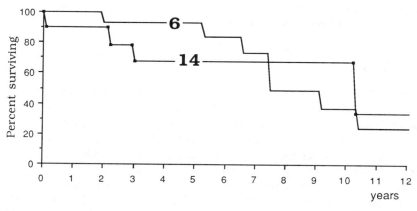

Figure 11   Overall survival according to karyotype, patients with single chromosomal abnormalities only. 6, structural abnormalities involving chromosome 6 (n = 17); 14, structural abnormalities involving chromosome 14 (n = 10).

Abnormal-to-Normal Metaphase Ratio and Prognosis

We noted in 1985 that patients with a high proportion of metaphases with clonal abnormalities had a poorer prognosis than patients with a high proportion of normal metaphases (45). This finding was confirmed from Roswell Park Memorial Institute (46), and by multivariate Cox regression (47) analyses (19,43). Of greatest interest is that patients with a small proportion of metaphases with trisomy 12 and a high percentage of normal metaphases were found to have the chromosomal abnormality in almost 100% of the interphase cells, when studied by RFLP and scanning densitometry (48). This result can only be interpreted as a preferential stimulation of a minor proportion of residual normal cells by the mitogens used. The results are fully compatible with those of Knuutila and co-workers (11,49), who used membrane markers on metaphase cells for a simultaneous phenotype and chromosome analysis. Thus, the prognostic association of the percentage abnormal metaphases would imply a better survival of patients who have normal cells that respond better to mitogen stimulation, compared to patients with no or unresponsive normal cells. Alternatively, this reflects our previous finding that proliferating CLL-cells, as indicated by a high thymidine uptake, are associated with poor prognosis (43,50,51). A combination of these alternatives seems to be a likely explanation for these prognostic findings.

Nonevaluable Cytogenetics and Prognosis

In only 45 cases (7%) were chromosome studies considered nonevaluable. Overall, this group appears to have an intermediate prognosis, which relates to the clinical heterogeneity of the cases.

GENE STUDIES

No relevant gene on chromosome 12, and no pathogenetic mechanism by which the occurrence of trisomy 12 may lead to the development of CLL, is as yet documented. We are still left with the hypothesis that the 50% increase from two to three copies of unidentified genes localized on chromosome 12 would alter the life span or the cell control mechanisms in the affected pre-B cell leading to the expanding CLL cell clone. None of the known oncogenes localized to chromosome 12 seems to be responsible. The low incidence of structural abnormalities on chromosome 12 also seems puzzling, and it is intriguing that a high proportion of these structural abnormalities results in partial duplications of chromosome 12, with the common region q13 to q22. It might be speculated that collaborating genes on chromosome 12 are needed for the leukemogenesis, and that randomly occurring structural changes on chromosome 12 rather disturb this collaboration of the involved genes than enhance the pathogenetic mechanism.

The bcl-2 gene, however, seems to be involved in some instances. This involvement is rarely documented by cytogenetic techniques in CLL, in contrast to follicular lymphomas, where 18q21 translocations are frequently seen (3). The breakpoint of the bcl-2 gene (52) in CLL seems to be in the first exon (53), and the translocation seems to prefer the immunoglobulin light-chain genes (54).

The retinoblastoma gene (26) is shown to be involved in CLL in the meaning that frequently one of the alleles is deleted (19,25). The pathogenesis of tumors related to antioncogenes are associated with the inactivation of both alleles, which so far is not shown by cytogenetic techniques in CLL, but was recently found with molecular techniques in 1 of 40 patients studied (55). Furthermore, decreased amounts of retinoblastoma protein and mRNA has also recently been found in the CLL cells of some patients (56). These data might indicate a role for the retinoblastoma protein in the pathogenesis of CLL. Another possibility is that a hitherto unknown (anti-onco-) gene of importance to CLL pathogenesis also is located at 13q14, and that the loss of the retinoblastoma gene is an irrelevant coincidence due to the close proximity to the relevant gene.

SUMMARY

Cytogenetic techniques in CLL cells have shown two major chromosome abnormalities with a probable pathogenetic role, i.e., trisomy 12, and deletions of 13q14. Terminal deletions of the long arm of chromosome 11 and 6 might also be significant, whereas 14q+ marker chromosomes are common additional abnormalities without significance by themselves. Of interest is that the finding of trisomy 12 indicates poor survival, whereas 13q deletions and normal karyotypes indicate good prognosis. Complex karyotypes are more commonly found at diagnosis than developing during the course of the disease, and are adverse prognostic signs.

PARTICIPANTS IN THE INTERNATIONAL WORKING PARTY ON CHROMOSOMES IN CLL

Gunnar Juliusson and Gösta Gahrton, Karolinska Institute at Huddinge Hospital, Huddinge, Sweden

David Oscier and Margaret Fitchett, Royal Victoria Hospital, Bournemouth, United Kingdom

Fiona Ross, Western General Hospital, Edinburgh, United Kingdom
Vasantha Brito-Babapulle and Daniel Catovsky, Royal Marsden Hospital,
London, United Kingdom
Sakari Knuutila and Erkki Elonen, University of Helsinki, Helsinki, Fin-
land
Monika Lechleitner, University of Innsbruck, Insbruck, Austria
Joseph Tanzer, Hôpital Jean-Bernard, Cédex, France
Michèle Schoenwald, Hôpital de la Source, Cédex, France
Gian Luigi Castoldi and Antonio Cuneo, Arcispedale S. Anna, Ferrara,
Italy
Peter Nowell, University of Pennsylvania, Philadelphia, Pennsylvania
LoAnn Peterson and Neil Kay, Hennepin County Medical Center, Minne-
apolis, Minnesota

REFERENCES

1. P. C. Nowell and D. A. Hungerford, A minute chromosome in human chronic
   granulocytic leukemia, *Science, 132*:1497 (1960).
2. R. Kurzrock, J. U. Gutterman, and M. Talpaz, The molecular genetics of
   Philadelphia chromosome-positive leukemias, *N. Engl. J. Med., 319*:990
   (1988).
3. J. J. Yunis, M. M. Oken, M. E. Kaplan, K. M. Ensrud, R. R. Howe, and A.
   Theologides, Distinctive chromosomal abnormalities in histologic subtypes of
   non-Hodgkin's lymphoma, *N. Engl. J. Med., 307*:1231 (1982).
4. Y. Tsujimoto, L. R. Finger, J. Yunis, P. C. Nowell, and C. M. Croce, Cloning
   of the chromosome breakpoint of neoplastic B cells with the t(14;18) chromosome translocation, *Science, 226*:1097 (1984).
5. Z. Chen-Levy, J. Nourse, and M. L. Cleary, The bcl-2 candidate proto-
   oncogene product is a 24-kilodalton integral-membrane protein highly expressed in lymphoid cell lines and lymphomas carrying the t(14;18) translocation, *Mol. Cell. Biol., 9*:701 (1989).
6. C. D. Bloomfield, A. I. Goldman, G. Alimena, et al., Chromosomal abnormalities identify high-risk and low-risk patients with acute lymphoblastic leukemia, *Blood, 67*:415 (1986).
7. J. J. Yunis, R. D. Brunning, R. B. Howe, and M. Lobell, High-resolution
   chromosomes as an independent prognostic indicator in adult acute non-
   lymphocytic leukemia, *N. Engl. J. Med., 311*:812 (1984).
8. K.-H. Robert, E. Möller, G. Gahrton, H. Eriksson, and B. Nilsson, B-cell
   activation of peripheral blood lymphocytes from patients with chronic lymphatic leukemia, *Clin. Exp. Immunol., 33*:302 (1978).
9. T. Caspersson, G. Lomakka, and L. Zech, The 24 fluorescence patterns of the
   human metaphase chromosomes — Distinguishing characters and variability,
   Hereditas, 67:89 (1971).
10. D. Rowlands, R. Daniele, P. Nowell, and H. Wurzel, Characterization of

lymphocyte subpopulations in chronic lymphocytic leukemia, *Cancer, 34*:1962 (1974).

11. K. Autio, E. Elonen, L. Teerenhovi, and S. Knuutila, Cytogenetic and immunologic characterization of mitotic cells in chronic lymphocytic leukaemia, *Eur. J. Haematol., 39*:289 (1987).

12. P. E. Crossen, Giemsa banding patterns in chronic lymphocytic leukaemia, *Humangenetik, 27*:151 (1975).

13. G. Möller (ed.), Lymphocyte activation by mitogens, *Transplant. Rev., 11* (1972).

14. P. Nowell, T. V. Shankey, J. Finan, D. Guerry, and E. Besa, Proliferation, differentiation, and cytogenetics of chronic leukemic B lymphocytes cultured with mitomycin-treated normal cells, *Blood, 57*:444 (1981).

15. Y. Ueshima, J. M. Haren, M. L. Bird, and J. D. Rowley, Culture conditions in chronic lymphocytic leukemia: Relationship to karyotype, *Leukemia, 3*:192 (1989).

16. G. Juliusson, K. Friberg, and G. Gahrton, Consistency of chromosomal aberrations in chronic B-lymphocytic leukemia. A longitudinal cytogenetic study of 41 patients, *Cancer, 62*:500 (1988).

17. ISCN, An international system for human cytogenetic nomenclature, *Cytogenet. Cell Genet., 21*:309 (1978).

18. G. Juliusson, K.-H. Robèrt, Å. Öst, K. Friberg, P. Biberfeld, B. Nilsson, L. Zech, and G. Gahrton, Prognostic information from cytogenetic analysis in chronic B-lymphocytic leukemia and leukemic immunocytoma, *Blood, 65*:134 (1985).

19. G. Juliusson, D. G. Oscier, M. Fitchett, F. M. Ross, G. Stockdill, M. J. Mackie, A. C. Parker, G. L. Castoldi, A. Cueno, S. Knuutila, E. Elonen, and G. Gahrton, Prognostic subgroups in B-cell chronic lymphocytic leukemia defined by specific chromosomal abnormalities, *N. Engl. J. Med., 323*:720 (1990).

20. G. Gahrton, L. Zech, K.-H. Robèrt, and A. G. Bird, Mitogenic stimulation of leukemic cells by Epstein-Barr virus, *N. Engl. J. Med., 301*:438 (1979).

21. Y. Tsujimoto, E. Jaffe, J. Cossman, J. Gorham, P. C. Nowell, and C. M. Croce, Clustering of breakpoints on chromosome 11 in human B-cell-neoplasms with the t(11;14) chromosome translocation, *Nature, 315*:340 (1986).

22. G. Gahrton, K.-H. Robèrt, K. Friberg, L. Zech, and A. G. Bird, Extra chromosome 12 in chronic lymphocytic leukemia, *Lancet, i*:146 (1980).

23. G. Gahrton, K.-H. Robèrt, K. Friberg, L. Zech, and A. G. Bird, Nonrandom chromosomal aberrations in chronic lymphocytic leukemia revealed by polyclonal B-cell-mitogen stimulation, *Blood, 56*:640 (1980).

24. G. Juliusson, and G. Gahrton, Chromosomal aberrations in B-cell chronic lymphocytic leukemia. Pathogenetic and clinical implication, *Cancer Genet. Cytogenet., 45*:143 (1990).

25. M. Fitchett, M. J. Griffiths, D. G. Oscier, S. Johnson, and M. Seabright, Chromosome abnormalities involving band 13q14 in hematologic malignancies, *Cancer Genet. Cytogenet., 24*:143 (1987).

26. J. J. Yunis and N. Ramsay, Retinoblastoma and subband deletion of chromosome 13, *Am. J. Dis. Child., 132*:161 (1978).
27. 4th International Workshop on Chronic Lymphocytic Leukaemia, *Nouv. Rev. Fr. Hématol., 30*:261 (1988).
28. G.Gahrton, K.-H. Robèrt, K. Friberg, G. Juliusson, P. Biberfeld, and L. Zech, Cytogenetic mapping of the duplicated segment of chromosome 12 in lymphoproliferative disorders, *Nature, 297*:513 (1982).
29. H. Xiao, A. W. Block, J. Romano, B. Dadley, and T. Han, i(12q) in B-cell chronic lymphocytic leukemia, *Cancer Genet. Cytogenet., 50*:171 (1990).
30. C. M. Croce, M. Isobe, A. Palumbo, J. Puck, J. Ming, D. Tweardy, J. Erikson, M. Davis, and G. Rovera, Gene for alpha-chain of human T-cell receptor: Location on chromosome 14 region involved in T-cell neoplasms, *Science, 227*:1044 (1985).
31. T. W. McKeithan, J. D. Rowley, T. B. Shows, and M. O. Diaz, Cloning of the chromosome translocation breakpoint junction of the t(14;19) in chronic lymphocytic leukemia, *Proc. Natl. Acad. Sci. USA, 84*:9257 (1987).
32. Y. Ueshima, M. L. Bird, J. W. Vardiman, and J. D. Rowley, A 14;19 translocation in B-cell chronic lymphocytic leukemia: A new recurring chromosome aberration, *Int. J. Cancer, 36*:287 (1985).
33. S. Einhorn, T. Meeker, G. Juliusson, K. Burvall, and G. Gahrton, No evidence of trisomy 12 or t(11;14) by molecular genetic techniques in chronic lymphocytic leukemia cells with a normal karyotype, *Cancer Genet. Cytogenet., 48*:183 (1990).
34. P. C. Nowell, L. Moreau, P. Growney, and E. C. Besa, Karyotypic stability in chronic B-cell leukemia, *Cancer Genet. Cytogenet., 33*:155 (1988).
35. D. Oscier, M. Fitchett, T. Herbert, and R. Lambert, Karyotypic evolution in B-cell chronic lymphocytic leukaemia, *Genes, Chromosomes & Cancer, 3*:16 (1991).
36. K.-H. Robèrt, G. Gahrton, K. Friberg, L. Zech, and B. Nilsson, Extra chromosome 12 and prognosis in chronic lymphocytic leukaemia, *Scand. J. Haematol., 28*:163 (1982).
37. N. Sadamori, T. Han, J. Minowada, and A. A. Sandberg, Clinical significance of cytogenetic findings in untreated patients with B-cell chronic lymphocytic leukemia, *Cancer Genet. Cytogenet., 11*:45 (1984).
38. R. Peto, M. C. Pike, P. Armitage, et al., Design and analysis of randomized trials requiring prolonged observation of each patient. II. Analysis and examples, *Br. J. Cancer, 35*:1 (1977).
39. G. Juliusson, K.-H. Robèrt, and G. Gahrton, Cytogenetic abnormalities in chronic lymphocytic leukemia, *N. Engl. J. Med., 311*:123 (1984).
40. K. R. Rai, A.Sawitsky, E. P. Cronkite, A. D. Chanana, R. N. Levy, and B. S. Pasternack, Clinical staging of chronic lymphocytic leukemia, *Blood, 46*:219 (1975).
41. G. Juliusson, and G. Gahrton, Prognostic implication of trisomy 12 and non-trisomy 12 karyotypes in B cell chronic lymphocytic leukemia. *Blood, 66*:470 (1985).
42. T. Han, H. Ozer, N. Sadamori, et al., Prognostic importance of cytogenetic

abnormalities in patients with chronic lymphocytic leukemia, *N. Engl. J. Med., 310*:288 (1984).

43. G. Juliusson, Immunological and cytogenetic studies improve prognosis prediction in chronic B-lymphocytic leukemia: A multivariate analysis of 24 variables, *Cancer, 58*:688 (1986).

44. S. Pittman, and D. Catovsky, Prognostic significance of chromosome abnormalities in chronic lymphocytic leukemia, *Br. J. Haematol., 58*:649 (1984).

45. G. Juliusson, and G. Gahrton, Abnormal/normal metaphase ratio and prognosis in chronic B-lymphocytic leukemia, *Cancer Genet. Cytogenet., 18*:307 (1985).

46. T. Han, H. Ozer, L. Emrich, N. Sadamori, K. Ohtaki, G. A. Gomez, E. S. Henderson, M. L. Bloom, and A. A. Sandberg, Prognostic importance of abnormal metaphases in chronic lymphocytic leukemia, *Proc. Am. Soc. Clin. Oncol., 4*:168 (abstr.) (1985).

47. D. R. Cox, Regression model and life tables, *J. Roy. Stat. Soc., B34*:187 (1972).

48. S. Einhorn, K. Burvall, G. Juliusson, G. Gahrton, and T. C. Meeker, Molecular analyses of trisomy 12 in chronic lymphocytic leukemia, *Leukemia, 3*:871 (1989).

49. S. Knuutila, E. Elonen, L. Teerenhovi, et al., Trisomy 12 in B-cells of patients with B-cell chronic lymphocytic leukemia, *N. Engl. J. Med., 314*:865 (1986).

50. G. Juliusson, K.-H. Robèrt, B. Nilsson, and G. Gahrton, Prognostic value of B-cell mitogen-induced and spontaneous thymidine uptake in vitro in chronic B-lymphocytic leukaemia cells, *Br. J. Haematol., 60*:429 (1985).

51. G. Juliusson and G. Gahrton, Clinical implications of CLL cell proliferation in vitro, *Nouv. Rev. Fr. Hématol., 30*:399 (1988).

52. Y. Tsujimoto and C. M. Croce, Analysis of the structure, transcripts, and protein products of bcl-2, the gene involved in human follicular lymphoma, *Proc. Natl. Acad. Sci. USA, 83*:5214 (1986).

53. M. Adachi, J. Cossman, D. Longo, C. M. Croce, and Y. Tsujimoto, Variant translocation of the bcl-2 gene to immunoglobulin lambda light chain gene in chronic lymphocytic leukemia, *Proc. Natl. Acad. Sci. USA, 86*:2771 (1989).

54. M. Adachi, A. Tefferi, P. R. Greipp, T. J. Kipps, and Y. Tsujimoto, Preferential linkage of bcl-2 to immunoglobulin light chain gene in chronic lymphocytic leukemia, *J. Exp. Med., 171*:559 (1990).

55. A. M. Ginsberg, M. Raffeld, and J. Cossman, Inactivation of the retinoblastoma gene in human lymphoid neoplasms, *Blood, 77*:833 (1991).

56. N.E. Kay, L. C. Peterson, and E. Ranheim, Molecular and protein analysis of the retinoblastoma (13q12-14) locus in a subset of B-CLL patients with a retinoblastoma locus abnormality, 5th International Workshop on CLL, Sitges (Barcelona), April 26–28, 1991 (T. Vallespi and E. Montserrat, eds.), Abstract book, p. 17.

5

Oncogenes in Chronic Lymphocytic Leukemia

Yoshihide Tsujimoto
The Wistar Institute of Anatomy and Biology, Philadelphia, Pennsylvania

Tumorigenesis involves several processes by which genes are altered. A partic-ular group of genes, oncogenes, are responsible for tumorigenesis, and their deregulation by genetic alteration can lead normal cells toward a fully malig-nant state. Because the genetic changes in oncogenes are conserved during tumorigenesis, we are able to identify the oncogenes from malignant cells, and to analyze them to understand the process of tumorigenesis.

METHODS OF IDENTIFYING ONCOGENES

Retroviral Strategy

We know that an acute transforming retrovirus contains a unique transform-ing gene (v-oncogene) within its genome and that other slow-transforming retroviruses can activate a cellular oncogene (c-oncogene) by retroviral inser-tion. By analyzing the genome of an acute transforming virus and the DNA near the retroviral integration sites, we are able to identify oncogenes. Thus, retroviral research has provided us with a tool to search for oncogenes (1).

DNA Transfection Methods (2)

The introduction of oncogene(s) by transfection can morphologically trans-form an appropriate recipient cell such as mouse NIH3T3, or primary

105

fibroblast cell of rat embryo. Other transfected oncogenes can confer tumorigenicity on cells in athymic nude mice without any morphological transformation. By serial cycles of DNA transfection, one can identify and clone a gene that is responsible for morphological transformation or tumorigenicity. The DNA transfection method has been widely and successfully used to identify many of the oncogenes we know at the present time.

Analysis of Chromosomal Abnormalities

Human neoplastic cells are often associated with nonrandom chromosomal aberrations. A well-accepted concept is that chromosomal aberrations deregulate cellular oncogenes and, as a result, contribute to neoplastic transformation of normal cells. The best-analyzed chromosome aberrations thus far are the c-myc activating chromosome translocations in Burkitt's lymphoma and the c-abl activating chromosome translocation in chronic myelogenous leukemia (see Ref. 3 for review).

A number of chromosome translocations and inversions in B and T cells directly involve the immunoglobulin (Ig) and T-cell receptor (TCR) loci, respectively, and the DNA probes from these loci are available. Therefore, the oncogenes activated by the chromosome translocations and inversions in B- and T-cell tumors can be obtained molecularly by cloning the breakpoints of chromosome abnormalities using the Ig and TCR probes and subsequently analyzing the DNA region linked to the Ig and TCR loci. The number of such second-generation oncogenes or candidates identified by this method (bcl-2, bcl-3's, tcl-3, lyl-1, pbx, scl/tal/tcl-5, etc.) is increasing dramatically. The advantage of analyzing chromosomal abnormalities is that the chromosome translocations allow us to identify genes involved in one of many steps of tumorigenesis in vivo and that may not be identified by the conventional, retroviral, DNA transformation, or tumorigenicity methods.

STRATEGY TO IDENTIFY ONCOGENES INVOLVED IN CLL

In the search for oncogenes crucial to chronic lymphocytic leukemia (CLL) genesis, great advances have been made through study of chromosome abnormalities, especially reciprocal chromosome translocations found in CLL.

Analysis of Known Oncogenes and DNA Transfection

One approach to the study of CLL cells is using oncogenes identified by the first two methods described in the previous section. Abnormal expression, rearrangements, or mutations of known oncogenes can be analyzed in CLL cells. This procedure has been used with the ras and bcl-2 genes in CLL. Several groups of investigators have examined the possible involvement of ras gene activation (oncogenic mutation) in B-CLL with a positive outcome (4–6). Rearrangement of the bcl-2 gene in B-CLL will be discussed below. A second approach is to transfect appropriate recipient cells (NIH3T3) with DNA obtained from CLL cells, and to look for morphologically transformed cells in tissue culture or tumorigenic cells in nude mice. Oncogene(s) can be isolated as described above. Transfection assay has been used to identify many oncogenes involved in human tumors, but it has been unproductive for CLL.

Search for CLL Oncogenes by Tracing Chromosomal Abnormalities

A considerable number of nonrandom chromosome abnormalities have been described in CLL of B- and T-cell origin. The most prominent example of chromosomal abnormality in B-cell CLL is trisomy 12 (7). Although trisomy 12 must provide a growth advantage to CLL cells, perhaps by somehow involving an oncogene, any feasible method to analyze the role of trisomy 12 is unfortunately not available. Since many chromosome translocations and inversions associated with B- and T-cell CLL directly involve Ig and TCR loci, respectively, involved oncogenes can be identified by cloning the breakpoints of chromosome abnormalities, using DNA probes from Ig and TCR loci, and subsequently analyzing the DNA region physically linked to the Ig and TCR regions.

The best-characterized recurrent chromosome abnormalities associated with CLL are chromosome translocations t(11;14)(q13;q32) and t(14; 19)(q32;q13.1). Both translocations directly involve the immunoglobulin heavy-chain gene at chromosome 14 band q32, as commonly seen in other B-cell neoplasms. In the following section (also see Table 1), we describe four chromosome translocations analyzed thus far in CLL, and the oncogenes involved.

EXAMPLES OF ONCOGENES INVOLVED IN CLL GENESIS

t(11;14)(q13;q32) Translocation/bcl-1 Gene

We took advantage of the availability of the immunoglobulin heavy-chain gene probe, and cloned the breakpoint of the t(11;14) translocation from CLL (8). The analogy to Burkitt's lymphoma, in which the c-myc gene is activated by specific chromosome translocations t(8;14), t(2;18) and t(8;22), was used to hypothesize that a new protooncogene, bcl-1 (*B*-cell *l*eukemia/ *l*ymphoma-1) resided on chromosome 11 band q13 near the breakpoint (8).

Table 1 Oncogenes Involved in CLL

Oncogene	Chromosomal location (abnormality involved)	Incidence	Gene product	References
bcl-1	11q13 t(11;14)(ql3;q32)	A few percent	Cyclin?	8, 21, 22
bcl-2	18q21 t(14;18)(q32;q21)	5–10%	Block apoptosis	37, 45, 46
bcl-3	19q13.1 t(14;19)(q32;q13.1)	A few percent	SW16/CD2 motif	69, 70, 71
tcl-1 (putative)	14q32 t(14;14)(q11;q32)	?	?	78, 79
Rb (anti-oncogene)	13q14 deletion	A few percent	Nuclear protein	81

However, extensive search for a transcription unit around the breakpoint failed. Failure to detect a gene might be due to the considerable heterogeneity of breakpoints of the t(11;14) translocation on chromosome 11 (8–11) and to the location of the bcl-1 gene at quite a distance from the original breakpoint clustering region.

Several oncogenes, including Int-2 (12), Hstf1 (13), and Sea (14), have been mapped cytogenetically in the same region as the t(11;14) breakpoint region (bcl-1 locus), and some of the oncogenes are coamplified with the bcl-1 locus in human mammary tumors (15) and head and neck squamous carcinoma (16). One of those genes has been a candidate for identification as the bcl-1 oncogene. However, since the expression of Hstf1 and Int-2 genes is not detectable in the CLL with t(11;14) translocation (Y. Tsujimoto, unpublished result), it is likely that they are not the bcl-1 gene. Since the Sea oncogene was mapped further away on the telomeric side of the Int-2 gene, it is very unlikely that the Sea gene is involved in CLL. Some mammary tumor cases showed bcl-1 amplification but not amplification of Int-2, Hstf1, or Sea oncogenes (15), indicating that these oncogenes are not involved in mammary tumors either. Although different oncogenes could be involved in CLL and mammary tumors, if the same gene is involved, it must be between the Int-2/Hstf-1 and bcl-1 loci, a distance estimated at less than 1000 kb (17).

Another candidate for the bcl-1 oncogene recently emerged from the study of parathyroid adenoma. Parathyroid adenomas are common benign neoplasms; rare cases have been described with the rearranged parathyroid hormone gene (PTH) at chromosome 11 band p15 (18). The PTH rearrangement has been shown to be the result of fusion of the PTH and chromosome 11 band q13 loci (18). The probe from chromosome 11q13 was developed and used to identify a transcription unit, named PRAD1 (*para*thyroid *ade*noma). This gene is overexpressed in a subset of parathyroid tumors and, more interestingly, in all cases thus far tested of centrocytic lymphoma (a subset of intermediate lymphoma) with a high incidence of t(11;14)(q13;q32) translocation (19,20) and B-CLL with the t(11;14)(q13; q32) translocation (21). The control cell lines, including CLL without the t(11;14) and follicular lymphoma and lymphoblastoid cell lines, revealed a very low level of PRAD1 gene expression (21). Thus, the PRAD1 gene is a likely candidate for the bcl-1 gene involved in the t(11;14) translocation. The PRAD1 gene has been mapped more than 100 kb away from the original major breakpoint clustering region of the t(11;14) translocation (Arnold and Tsujimoto, unpublished). The primary structure of the PRAD1 protein, deduced from the DNA sequence, revealed distant homology to cyclin (22). Although the function of this gene product remains to be experimentally elucidated, the PRAD1 protein might be involved in cell cycle control.

The involvement of the bcl-1 gene is not restricted to B-CLL, but is known to be associated with other B-cell tumors such as some cases of diffuse B-cell lymphoma (23) and multiple myeloma (24).

t(18;22)(q21;q11) and t(2;18)(p11;q21)/bcl-2 gene

The bcl-2 gene (25–28) is at chromosome 18q21 and was originally identified through the study of the t(14;18)(q21;q32) translocation, which is a hallmark of follicular lymphoma (29,30). Use of the Ig heavy-chain gene probe allowed us to clone the breakpoint of the t(14;18) translocation and develop DNA probes from chromosome 18q21. Using chromosome 18q21 probes, we and others identified a transcription unit (bcl-2). Subsequent studies have revealed that involvement of the bcl-2 gene rearrangement is not restricted to the follicular lymphoma but is seen in other B-cell tumors, namely, in approximately 30% of diffuse large cell lymphomas that carry the t(14;18) translocation (31), in pre-B-cell leukemia with t(14;18) (32), and in B-cell CLL (33–35,82). The rearrangements of the bcl-2 gene are clustered at three different regions around the gene. In the case of the t(14; 18) translocation, which results in the juxtaposition of the bcl-2 and Ig heavy-chain loci (25,27,28,36), the majority of the breaks (more than 60%) occur within the 3′ noncoding region of the bcl-2 gene (major breakpoint clustering region) and 20% in the 3′ flanking region (minor clustering region) (26,37,38). The consequence of the t(14;18) translocation is deregulation of the bcl-2 gene expression (39,40).

The involvement of the 5′ end of the bcl-2 gene is rather rare in follicular lymphoma (41,42) but is seen at a significant frequency (approximately 5–10%) in B-CLL (35,82). In B-CLL, the bcl-2 rearrangements have been shown molecularly to be the result of reciprocal chromosome translocation between the bcl-2 and Ig light-chain genes (33–35). Although no description of karyotypic abnormalities, t(2;18) and t(18;22), corresponding to the bcl-2 rearrangements in CLL was reported in spite of extensive studies, we have recently succeeded in demonstrating the presence of the t(18;22) and t(2;18) reciprocal chromosome translocations together with evidence of the bcl-2/Ig light-chain gene juxtapositions at the molecular level in B-CLL (43,44). Deregulated expression of the bcl-2 gene in CLL with t(2;18) and t(18;22) is expected but not yet experimentally demonstrated.

There seems a striking difference in the molecular mechanism of the chromosome translocations between with the 5′ region of the bcl-2 gene in CLL and within the 3′ region of the gene in follicular lymphoma. The t(14;18) translocation (3′ break) has been proposed, on the basis of several common features, to be mediated by the recombination machinery of the Ig gene rearrangement (36), while the t(2;18) and t(18;22) translocations (5′ break) seem to be facilitated by the presence of the potential Z-DNA (left-handed) elements (45). Possible involvement of Z-DNA elements in other chromosome translocations has also been reported (46).

The bcl-2 gene has a unique structure and consists of two major exons (5′ and 3′) (47) separated by an intron of about 370 kb (39). The 5′ exon itself produces several species of mRNA without the 3′-exon sequences (47; Tsujimoto, unpublished). The transcription starts at multiple initiation sites (39) and mRNA is processed at different poly-A sites (47). The occasional removal, by splicing, of a region 220 bp from the 5′ noncoding region of the bcl-2 gene (39) indicates that the 5′ exon could be divided into two exons. Thus, the bcl-2 gene is transcribed into heterogeneous species of mRNA. Since the major breakpoint clustering region of the t(14;18) translocation is within the 3′ untranslated region of the bcl-2 gene, the translocation results in production of chimeric mRNA consisting of the bcl-2 and Ig heavy-chain genes (39,48).

Since the splicing donor site is within the 5′ exon, two different gene products are made. One, bcl-2α (26 kD), is derived from the spliced 5′ and 3′ exons, and the other, bcl-2β (21 kD), from the 5′ exon (47). The bcl-2α and -β are identical except for their carboxyl terminal portions. The bcl-2 gene is well conserved among species, including mouse, hamster, and chicken (26,49; Tsujimoto, unpublished). The primary sequence of the bcl-2 protein does not reveal a significant homology with any known proteins.

The bcl-2α protein, a predominant product of the bcl-2 gene, is a membrane protein (50,51) and has recently been localized in a mitochondrial inner membrane (52). The hydrophobic amino acids at the carboxyl terminus of the bcl-2α protein are considered responsible for the membrane localization (50,51).

A variety of bcl-2 gene transfer experiments have shown that the bcl-2α protein has the unique characteristic of providing prolonged survival to human and mouse hematopoietic cells in the absence of a required growth factor(s) (53). Interestingly, this positive role of bcl-2 protein is restricted to certain types of cells. The bcl-2 protein provides prolonged survival, in the absence of the required growth factor, to IL-3-dependent mouse myeloid and pro-B-cell lines (53,54) and to IL-7-dependent mouse pre-B-cell lines (55) and Epstein-Barr virus immortalized human B-lymphoblast cell lines (56–58) but not to an IL-2-dependent mouse T-cell line or to an IL-6-dependent mouse myeloma cell line (54). In the cases of EBV-B cells and IL-7-dependent mouse pre-B-cell lines, we have shown that the better survival conferred by bcl-2 protein is not specific to the absence of the required growth factor but is more general to a variety of stress conditions including heat shock and certain drugs (55,59). Using the mouse IL-3-dependent pro-B-cell line and IL-7-dependent mouse pre-B-cell lines, it has been shown that the bcl-2 protein, directly or indirectly, blocks the programmed cell death (apoptosis) (52,55). Cell death in metazoans can be characterized as either "accidental" (necrosis) or "programmed" (apoptosis). The former refers to death in cells subjected to wide deviations from normal homeostasis, such as might be induced by toxins, anoxia, or depletion of energy-producing pathways. Apoptosis, on the other hand, refers to cell death that is the expected outcome of the normal functioning of a particular cell system. Apoptosis is characterized by early changes in the nuclear membrane and chromatin condensation, followed by DNA fragmentation in integral multiples of a nucleosome unit (180 base pairs). Apoptosis requires de-novo protein synthesis, and therefore inhibitors of RNA transcription and protein synthesis block apoptosis.

A lymphadenopathy similar to human follicular lymphoma is developed by bcl-2 transgenic mice (60,61). The abnormality detected in the hematopoietic compartments of transgenic mice is an expansion of a pool of small IgM/IgD B cells in the spleen and, more dramatically, in the bone marrow (61,62). All these cells are in the resting stage (G_0/G_1) and could respond to mitogenic stimulations. Some lines of bcl-2 transgenic mice also developed abnormalities in their T cells (63). The T lymphocytes from these mice revealed increased survival in tissue culture without growth factors (63). It has been reported that bcl-2 cooperates with the c-myc gene to produce immortalized pre-B-cell lines from bone marrow culture in vitro (53) and also to produce more aggressive tumors in the bcl-2 transgenic mice (64).

The cooperation of the bcl-2 and c-myc genes in aggressive human tumors is well documented, as is the presence of two characteristic chromosome translocations, t(14;18) and t(8;14) (32,65–68). The synergistic effect of c-myc and bcl-2 was also documented in myc/bcl-2 double-transgenic mice which were produced by a cross between the bcl-2 and myc transgenic mice (63). The myc/bcl-2 mice showed white cell counts 50- to 100-fold higher than the normal controls, and the white cells were all large and therefore presumably proliferating, unlike those in the bcl-2 transgenic mice. The myc/bcl-2 transgenic mice with hyperproliferation of pre-B and B cells developed tumors much faster then myc transgenic mice and, surprisingly, the tumors derived from a cell with the hallmark of a primitive hematopoietic cell, perhaps lymphoid committed stem cells (61). The synergy was not observed between N-ras and bcl-2 genes (63).

A widely accepted role of the bcl-2 gene in neoplastic transformation of B lymphocytes is that the bcl-2 gene product does not have any dominant role in cell proliferation but the activation of the bcl-2 gene prolongs survival of B cells and, as a result, the chance of any secondary change, which is more critical for tumorigenesis per se, is increased. This idea has been experimentally demonstrated in our pre-B-cell line system, in which the bcl-2 infected cell lines but not control cells produced IL-7-independent cell lines in the absence of IL-7 in the medium (55).

t(14;19)(q32;q13) Translocation/bcl-3 Gene

The bcl-3 gene is a putative oncogene located at chromosome 19 band q13. The bcl-3 gene was identified by the study of the t(14;19) reciprocal chromosome translocation infrequently associated with the B-cell CLL (69–71). The breakpoint of the t(14;19) translocation was molecularly cloned using the Ig heavy-chain gene DNA as probe and subsequently a transcription unit (bcl-3 gene) was identified near the breakpoint on chromosome 19. Five cases of CLL with the t(14;19) translocation have been analyzed, and the breakpoint in IgH locus is within one of two Sα regions. In three cases, the break on chromosome 19 is immediately upstream of the bcl-3 gene (McKeithan, personal communication).

The bcl-3 gene is about 11.5 kb in size, comprising 9 exons (McKeithan, personal communication). The bcl-3 mRNA is present in a wide variety of tissues. The gene is virtually silent in unstimulated but dividing cells, whereas it is rapidly turned on by phorbol ester (PMA) and PHA stimulation (McKeithan, personal communication). This suggests that the bcl-3 gene product is not required for proliferation but is involved in an early phase of lymphocytic activation.

The predicted bcl-3 protein contains 446 amino acid residues (47 kD). A unique feature of the bcl-3 protein is that it consists of seven tandem copies of a sequence of about 33 amino acids. This repeat shares some degree of homology with the SW16/CDC2 motif (71). The SW16/CDC2 motif is found in other proteins, including CDC10, SW41, and SW46 in yeast, all of which regulate events occurring at the initiation of new cell cycle (72,73). The bcl-3 gene is the first known oncogene to contain the SW16/CDC2 motif. This suggests that the bcl-3 protein is involved in the control of the cell cycle, which is consistent with the observation of gene activation in normal lymphocytes as described above. However, the SW16/CDC2 motif is also present in the cytoplasmic domain of transmembrane proteins including Notch protein in *Drosophila*, and lin-12 and glp-1 proteins in *C. elegans,* and all are involved in cell differentiation (71). Recently, two other proteins (Xotch and Ankyrin) with similar motifs have also been identified from *Xenopus* and human cDNA, respectively (74,75). Thus the SW16/CDC-2 motifs are found in two apparently different kinds of proteins. Although it is still premature to speculate about the function of the bcl-3 protein in normal and neoplastic B lymphocytes, it might be a transcription activation factor.

t(14;14)(q11;q32)/tcl-1 Gene

Although lymphocytic neoplasms of T-cell origin are considerably less common than their B-cell counterparts, nonrandom chromosome translocations and inversions are also present in many of these cases. These abnormalities often directly involve the TCR loci.

Ataxia telangiectasia is characterized by cerebellar ataxia, variable levels of T-cell immunodeficiency, and hypersensitivity to ionizing radiation. In ataxia telangiectasia, both nonrandom chromosome translocations and lymphoid malignancies are frequent events (76). Preleukemic clonal expansion of cells carrying specific chromosomal abnormalities, such as the inv14(q11;q32) inversion or t(14;14)(q11;q32) translocation, are often observed in these patients (77). The t(14;14) translocation carried by T-cell CLL developed by ataxia telangiectasia patients has been studied molecularly (78,79). The breakpoint at 14q11 was within the TCRα locus, and the breakpoint at 14q32 was centromeric to the Ig heavy-chain locus. The putative oncogene tcl-1 (*T* cell *l*eukemia/*l*ymphoma) has been postulated at the chromosome 14q32 region. The same gene might be involved in another chromosome translocation t(7;14)(q35;q32), which is associated with T-cell acute lymphoblastic leukemia because of the breakpoints at chromosome 14q32 of two different translocations apparently only 250 kb apart (78).

Although the tcl-1 gene remains to be identified, it might provide useful information concerning an early step of tumorigenesis because the t(14;14) translocation is seen in preleukemic monoclonal cells of ataxia telangiectasia patients.

MODE OF ACTIVATION OF ONCOGENES

Oncogenes and oncogene candidates identified through chromosome translocations are associated with Ig and TCR genes, and therefore the mode of oncogene activation could be either qualitative (mutations) or quantitative change. The only available information is provided by bcl-2. The primary result of the translocation is to deregulate transcription of the bcl-2 gene (39,40), but not to introduce mutations in the bcl-2 gene (80). Since the translocated bcl-2 gene is transcribed at a higher level than the normal counterpart in follicular lymphoma (39,40), the cis element(s), the most likely enhancer sequence(s) within the Ig locus, is thought to be responsible for deregulation of the bcl-2 gene. However, the direct involvement of the cis elements in gene activation has not been demonstrated experimentally in the bcl-2 translocation or even for the c-myc translocations, the major role of which is also deregulation of the c-myc gene expression by cis elements in the Ig loci. One of the best ways to confirm the involvement of cis elements in the oncogene activation might be "knock-out experiments," in which the cis element of interest is deleted in tumor cell lines and one measures the bcl-2 or c-myc gene expression level.

PERSPECTIVE

All Burkitt's lymphomas are known to carry one of three chromosome translocations, all of which directly involve the c-myc oncogene. Most follicular lymphomas and chronic myelogenous leukemia carry the bcl-2 and c-abl oncogene activation, respectively. Why is there not a consistent involvement of a single oncogene in B-CLL instead of the irregular involvement of bcl-1, bcl-2, or bcl-3? CLL that carries any of these oncogenes has no unique clinical feature as compared to other CLLs whose bcl-1, bcl-2, and bcl-3 are not deregulated, although more careful investigation has to be carried out. B-CLL may emerge as a heterogeneous disease. Alternatively, there might be significant differences of susceptibility of the involved oncogenes to the translocations among different B-cell tumors; for example, during follicular lymphomagenesis there might be a stage in which the bcl-2 becomes highly susceptible to the translocation. Maybe the processes of CLL genesis, affected by the bcl-1, -2, and -3 oncogenes, can be bypassed by other events. Since the bcl-1 and bcl-2 genes are involved in B-cell tumors other than CLL, the tumorigenesis process contributed by the activation of these genes might not be unique to the CLL as described in the bcl-2 gene section. Since no consistent chromosome abnormality is implicated in CLL, the discovery approach based on chromosome abnormalities might not be particularly fruitful with respect to identifying an oncogene consistently involved in CLL.

Recessive oncogenes have become of great interest in the last several years, and most efforts in this field have been made with solid tumors. However, it is conceivable that recessive oncogenes are also important in hematopoietic tumor development. As far as this author is aware, there are few studies along this line. Recently, CLL cells were found with abnormalities of the retinoblastoma (Rb) locus (81). One case of CLL deleted the 5′ part of the Rb gene and the other case revealed an abnormal size of Rb mRNA. Although the incidence of Rb locus abnormality in CLL is extremely low (about 2 out of 40 cases tested), it might be sufficient to encourage us to study more extensively the involvement of recessive oncogene in the pathogenesis of CLL.

Another approach to CLL genesis could be to isolate genes expressed specifically in CLL using differential screening or subtraction library techniques. The problem with this approach is the lack of a quick assay to isolated genes by their functions in tumorigenesis and the difficulty in finding the right normal counterpart of CLL.

Although no consistent chromosome abnormalities have been found, the study of chromosome aberrations could be the most promising way to dissect the pathogenesis of CLL. The extensive study of chromosome abnormalities associated with CLL will probably result in discovery of a number of new oncogenes. Study of these oncogenes, together with those described here and recessive oncogenes, may unveil aspects of CLL genesis that will finally lead us to a full understanding of the molecular basis of CLL genesis.

REFERENCES

1. H. E. Varmus, Form and function of retroviral proviruses, *Science, 216*:812 (1982).
2. G. M. Cooper, Cellular transforming genes, *Science, 218*:801 (1982).
3. F. G. Haluska, Y. Tsujimoto, and C. M. Croce, Oncogene activation by chromosome translocation in human malignancy, *Ann. Rev. Genet., 21*:321 (1987).
4. A. Neri, D. M. Knowles, A. Greco, F. McCormick, and R. Dalla-Favera, Analysis of RAS oncogene mutation in human lymphoid malignancies, *Proc. Natl. Acad. Sci. USA, 85*:9268 (1988).

5. P. J. Browett, K. Ganeshaguru, A. V. Hoffbrand, and J. D. Norton, Absence of Kirsten-ras oncogene activation in B-cell chronic lymphocytic leukemia, *Leukemia Res., 12*:25 (1988).

6. P. J. Browett and J. D. Norton, Analysis of ras gene mutation and methylation state in human leukemias, *Oncogene, 4*:1029 (1989).

7. G. Gahrton, G. Juliusson, K-H. Robert, and K. Friberg, Chromosomal aberrations in chronic lymphocytic leukemia, in *Chronic Lymphocytic Leukemia* (A. Polliack and D. Catovsky, eds.), Harwood Academic Publishers, pp. 289–304 (1988).

8. Y. Tsujimoto, J. J. Yunis, L. Onorato-Showe, J. Erickson, P. C. Nowell, and C. M. Croce, Molecular cloning of the chromosomal breakpoint of B-cell lymphomas and leukemias with the t(11;14) chromosome translocation, *Science, 224*:1403 (1984).

9. Y. Tsujimoto, E. Jaffe, J. Cossman, J. Gorham, P. C. Nowell, and C. M. Croce, Clustering of breakpoints on chromosome 11 in human B-cell neoplasms with the t(11;14) chromosome translocation, *Nature, 315*:340 (1985).

10. P. H. Rabbitts, J. Douglas, P. Fischer, E. Nacheva, A. Karpas, D. Catovsky, J. V. Melo, R. Baer, M. A. Stinson, and T. H. Rabbitts, Chromosome abnormalities at 11q13 in B cell tumors, *Oncogene, 3*:99 (1988).

11. T. C. Meeker, J. C. Grimaldi, R. O'Rourke, E. Louie, G. Juliusson, and S. Einhorn, An additional breakpoint region in the bcl-1 locus associated with the t(11;14)(q13;q32) translocation of B-lymphocytic malignancy, *Blood, 74*: 1801 (1989).

12. G. Casey, R. Smith, D. McGillivary, G. Peters, and C. Dickson, Characterization and chromosome assignment of the human homolog of int-2, a potential proto-oncogene, *Mol. Cell. Biol., 6*:502 (1986).

13. M. Yoshida, W. Wada, H. Satoh, T. Yoshida, H. Sakamoto, K. Miyagawa, J. Yokota, T. Koda, M. Kakinuma, T. Sugimura, and M. Terada, Human Hst1 (Hstf1) gene maps to chromosome band 11q13 and coamplifies with the Int2 gene in human cancer, *Proc. Natl. Acad. Sci. USA, 85*:4861 (1988).

14. B. P. Williams, J. P. Shipley, N. K. Spurr, D. R. Smith, M. J. Hayman, and P. N. Goodfellow, A human sequence homologous to v-sea maps to chromosome 11, band q13, *Oncogene, 3*:345 (1988).

15. C. Theillet, J. Adnane, P. Szepetowski, M-P. Simon, P. Jeanteur, D. Birnbaum, and P. Gaudray, Bcl-1 participates in the 11q13 amplification found in breast cancer, *Oncogene, 5*:147 (1990).

16. J. R. Berenson, J. Yang, and R. A. Mickel, Frequent amplification of the bcl-1 locus in head and neck squamous cell carcinoma, *Oncogene, 4*:1111 (1989).

17. C. Nguyen, D. Roux, M. G. Mattei, O. de Lapeyriere, M. Goldfarb, D. Birnbaum, and B. R. Jordan, The FGF-related oncogenes hst and int-2, and the bcl-1 locus are contained within one megabase in band q13 of chromosome 11, while the fgf-5 oncogene maps to 4q21, *Oncogene, 3*:703 (1988).

18. A. Arnold, H. G. Kim, R. D. Gaz, R. L. Eddy, Y. Fukushima, M. G. Byers, T. B. Shows, and H. M. Kronenberg, Molecular cloning and chromosomal mapping of DNA rearranged with the parathyloid hormone gene in a parathyloid adenoma, *J. Clin. Invest., 83*:2034 (1987).

19. M. E. Williams, C. D. Westermann, and S. H. Swerdlow, Genotypic characterization of centrocytic lymphoma: frequent rearrangement of the chromosome 11 bcl-1 locus, *Blood, 76*:1387 (1990).
20. D. D. Weisenburger, W. G. Sanger, J. O. Armitage, and D. T. Purtilo, Intermediate lymphocytic lymphoma: Immunophenotypic and cytogenetic findings, *Blood, 69*:1617 (1987).
21. C. L. Rosenberg, E. Wong, A. E. Bale, Y. Tsujimoto, N. L. Harris, and A. Arnold, Overexpression of PRAD1 (D11S287E), a candidate bcl-1 breakpoint-region oncogene in centrocytic lymphomas, Submitted.
22. T. Motokura, T. Bloom, H. G. Kim, H. Juooner, J. V. Ruderman, H. M. Kronenberg, and A. Arnold, A novel cyclin encoded by a bcl1-linked candidate oncogene, *Nature, 350*:512 (1991).
23. J. J. Yunis, The chromosomal basis of human neoplasia, *Science, 221*:227 (1983).
24. H. van den Berghe, K. Vermaelen, A. Louwagie, A. Criel, C. Mecucci, and J.-P. Vaerman, High incidence of chromosome abnormalities in IgG3 myeloma, *Cancer Genet. Cytogenet., 11*:381 (1984).
25. Y. Tsujimoto, L. R. Finger, J. Yunis, P. C. Nowell, and C. M. Croce, Cloning of the chromosome breakpoint of neoplastic B cells with the t(14;18) chromosome translocation, *Science, 266*:1097 (1984).
26. Y. Tsujimoto, J. Cossman, E. Jaffe, and C. M. Croce, Involvement of the bcl-2 gene in follicular lymphoma, *Science, 228*:1440 (1985).
27. M. L. Cleary and J. Sklar, Nucleotide sequence of a t(14;18) chromosomal breakpoint in follicular lymphoma and demonstration of a breakpoint cluster region near a transcriptionally active locus on chromosome 18, *Proc. Natl. Acad. Sci. USA, 82*:7439 (1985).
28. A. Bakhshi, J. P. Jensen, P. Goldman, J. J. Wright, O. W. McBridge, A. L. Epstein, and S. J. Korsmeyer, Cloning the chromosomal breakpoint of t(14; 18) human lymphoma: Clustering around J_H on chromosome 14 and near a transcriptional unit on 18, *Cell, 41*:899 (1985).
29. S. Fukuhara, J. D. Rowley, D. Variakojis, and H. M. Golomb, Chromosome abnormalities in poorly differentiated lymphocytic lymphoma, *Cancer Res., 39*:3119 (1979).
30. J. J. Yunis, M. M. Oken, A. Theologides, B. B. Howe, and M. E. Kaplan, Recurrent chromosomal defects are found in most patients with non-Hodgkin's lymphoma, *Cancer Genet. Cytogenet., 13*:17 (1984).
31. M-S. Lee, M. B. Blick, S. Pathak, J. M. Trujillo, J. J. Butler, R. L. Katz, P. McLaughlin, F. B. Hagemeister, W. S. Velasquez, A. Goodacre, A. Cork, J. U. Gutterman, and F. Cabanillas, The gene located at chromosome 18 band q21 is rearranged in uncultured diffuse lymphomas as well as follicular lymphomas, *Blood, 70*:90 (1987).
32. L. Pegoraro, A. Palumbo, J. Erickson, M. Fauda, B. Giovanazzo, B. S. Emanuel, G. Rovera, P. C. Nowell, and C. M. Croce, A 14;18 and 8;14 chromosome translocation in a cell line derived from an acute B-cell leukemia, *Proc. Natl. Acad. Sci. USA, 81*:7166 (1984).
33. M. Adachi, J. Cossman, C. M. Croce, and Y. Tsujimoto, Variant translocation of the bcl-2 gene to Igλ in a chronic lymphocytic leukemia, *Proc. Natl. Acad. Sci. USA, 86*:2771 (1989).

34. M. Adachi and Y. Tsujimoto, Juxtaposition of human bcl-2 and immunoglobulin lambda light chain gene in chronic lymphocytic leukemia is the result of a reciprocal chromosome translocation between chromosome 18 and 22. *Oncogene, 4*:1073 (1989).

35. M. Adachi, A. Tefferi, P. R. Greipp, T. Kipps, and Y. Tsujimoto, Preferential linkage of bcl-2 to immunoglobulin light chain gene in chronic lymphocytic leukemia, *J. Ext. Med., 171*:559 (1990).

36. Y. Tsujimoto, J. Gorham, J. Cossman, E. Jaffe, and C. M. Croce, The t(14;18) chromosome translocation involved in B-cell neoplasms result from mistakes in VDJ joining, *Science, 229*:1390 (1985).

37. M. L. Cleary, N. Galili, and J. Sklar, Detection of a second t(14;18) breakpoint cluster region in human follicular lymphomas, *J. Exp. Med., 164*:315 (1986).

38. L. M. Weiss, R. A. Warnke, J. Sklar, and M. L. Cleary, Molecular analysis of the t(14;18) chromosomal translocation in malignant lymphomas, *N. Engl. J. Med., 317*:1185 (1987).

39. M. Seto, U. Jaeger, R. D. Hockett, W. Graninger, S. Bennett, P. Goldman, and S. J. Korsmeyer, Alternative promoters and exons, somatic mutation and deregulation of the Bcl-2-Ig fusion gene in lymphoma, *EMBO J., 7*:123 (1988).

40. J. C. Reed, Y. Tsujimoto, S. F. Epstein, M. Cuddy, T. Slabiak, P. C. Nowell, and C. M. Croce, Regulation of bcl-2 gene expression in lymphoid cell lines containing normal #18 or t(14;18) chromosome, *Oncogene Res., 4*:271 (1989).

41. Y. Tsujimoto, M. M. Bashir, I. Givol, J. Cossman, E. Jaffe, and C. M. Croce, DNA rearrangements in human follicular lymphoma can involve the 5′ or the 3′ region of the bcl-2 gene, *Proc. Natl. Acad. Sci. USA, 84*:1329 (1987).

42. H. Osada, M. Seto, R. Ueda, N. Emi, N. Takagi, Y. Obata, T. Suchi, and T. Takahashi, bcl-2 gene rearrangement analysis in Japanese B cell lymphoma; novel bcl-2 recombination with immunoglobulin κ chain gene, *Jpn. J. Cancer Res., 80*:711 (1989).

43. S. Tashiro, M. Takechi, M. Kikuchi, Y. Tsujimoto, and N. Kamada, t(18;22) translocation with juxtaposition of bcl-2 and immunoglobulin λ light chain genes in chronic lymphocytic leukemia, Submitted.

44. S. Tashiro, M. Takechi, H. Aso, K. Takauchi, T. Kyo, H. Dohy, N. Kamada, and Y. Tsujimoto, 2;18 translocation in chronic lymphocytic leukemia with juxtaposition of bcl-2 and immunoglobulin κ light chain genes, Submitted.

45. M. Adachi and Y. Tsujimoto, Potential Z-DNA elements surround the breakpoints of chromosome translocation within the 5′ flanking region of bcl-2 gene, *Oncogene, 5*:1653 (1990).

46. T. Boehm, L. Mengle-Gaw, U. R. Kees, N. Spurr, I. Lavenir, A. Forster, and T. H. Rabbitts, Alternating purine-pyrimidine tracts may promote chromosomal translocations seen in a variety of human lymphoid tumors, *EMBO J., 8*:2621 (1989).

47. Y. Tsujimoto and C. M. Croce, Analysis of the structure, transcripts, and protein products of bcl-2, the gene involved in human follicular lymphoma, *Proc. Natl. Acad. Sci. USA, 83*:5214 (1986).

48. M. L. Cleary, S. D. Smith, and J. Sklar, Cloning and structural analysis of cDNA for bcl-2 and a hybrid bcl-2/immunoglobulin transcript resulting from the t(14;18) translocation, *Cell, 47*:19 (1986).

49. M. Negrini, E. Silini, C. Kozak, Y. Tsujimoto, and C. M. Croce, Molecular analysis of mbcl-2: Structure and expression of the murine gene homologous to the human gene involved in follicular lymphoma, *Cell, 49*:455 (1987).

50. Y. Tsujimoto, N. Ikegaki, and C. M. Croce, Characterization of the protein product of bcl-2, the gene involved in human follicular lymphoma, *Oncogene, 2*:3 (1987).

51. Z. Chen-Levy and M. L. Cleary, Membrane topology of the bcl-2 proto-oncogenic protein demonstrated in vitro, *J. Biol. Chem., 265*:4929 (1990).

52. D. Hockenbery, G. Nunez, C. Milliman, R. D. Schrelber, and S. J. Korsmeyer, Bcl-2 is an inner mitochondrial membrane protein that blocks programmed cell death, *Nature, 348*:334 (1990).

53. D. L. Vaux, S. Cory, and J. M. Adams, Bcl-2 gene promotes heamatopoietic cell survival and co-operates to immortalize pre-B cells, *Nature, 335*:440 (1988).

54. G. Nunez, L. London, D. Hockenbery, M. Alexander, J. P. McKearn, and S. J. Korsmeyer, Deregulated bcl-2 gene expression selectively prolongs survival of growth factor-deprived hematopoietic cell lines, *J. Immunol., 144*: 3602 (1990).

55. Y. Tsujimoto, K. Endo, and G. Borzillo, In preparation.

56. Y. Tsujimoto, Overexpression of the human bcl-2 gene product results in growth enhancement of Epstein-Barr virus-immortalized B cells, *Proc. Natl. Acad. Sci. USA, 86*:1958 (1989).

57. G. Nunez, M. Seto, S. Seremetis, D. Ferrero, G. Grignani, S. J. Korsmeyer, and R. Dalla-Favera, Growth- and tumor-promoting effects of deregulated bcl-2 in human B-lymphoblastoid cells, *Proc. Natl. Acad. Sci. USA, 86*:4589 (1989).

58. J. C. Reed, S. Haldar, M. P. Cuddy, C. M. Croce, and D. Makover, Deregulated bcl-2 expression enhances growth of a human B cell line, *Oncogene, 4*: 1123 (1989).

59. Y. Tsujimoto, Stress-resistance conferred by high level of bcl-2α protein in human B lymphoblastoid cell, *Oncogene, 4*:1331 (1989).

60. T. J. McDonnell, N. Deane, F. M. Platt, G. Nunez, U. Jaeger, J. P. McKearn, and S. J. Korsmeyer, Bcl-2-immunoglobulin transgenic mice demonstrate B cell survival and follicular lymphoproliferation, *Cell, 57*:79 (1989).

61. A. Strasser, A. W. Harris, M. L. Bath, and S. Cory, Novel primitive lymphoid tumors induced in transgenic mice by cooperation between myc and bcl-2, *Nature, 348*:331 (1990).

62. T. J. McDonnell, F. M. Platt, D. Hockenberry, L. London, J. P. McKearn, and S. J. Korsmeyer, Deregulated bcl-2-immunoglobulin transgene expands a resting but responsive immunoglobulin M and D-expressing B-cell population, *Mol. Cell. Biol., 10*:1901 (1990).

63. A. Strasser, A. W. Harris, D. L. Vaux, E. Webb, M. L. Bath, A. G. Elefanty, J. M. Adams, and S. Cory, Abnormalities of the immune system induced

by dysregulated bcl-2 expression in transgenic mice, *Curr. Topics Microbiol. Immunol.*, in press.

64. T. J. McDonnell and S. J. Korsmeyer, Progression from lymphoid hyperplasia to high-grade malignant lymphoma in mice transgenic for the t(14;18), *Nature, 349*:254 (1991).

65. G. L. Mufti, T. J. Hamblin, D. G. Oscier, and S. Johnson, Common ALL with pre-B cell features showing (8;14) and (14;18) chromosome translocations, *Blood, 62*:1142 (1983).

66. C. E. Gauwerky, F. G. Haluska, Y. Tsujimoto, P. C. Nowell, and C. M. Croce, Evolution of B-cell malignancy: Pre-B-cell leukemia resulting from myc activation in a B-cell neoplasm with a rearranged bcl-2 gene, *Proc. Natl. Acad. Sci. USA, 85*:8548 (1988).

67. D. deLong, B. M. H. Voetdijk, G. C. Beverstock, G. J. B. van Ommen, R. Willemze, and P. M. Kluin, Activation of the c-myc oncogene in a precursor-B-cell blast crisis of follicular lymphoma, presenting as composite lymphoma, *N. Engl. J. Med., 318*:1373 (1988).

68. M. Thangavelu, O. Olopade, E. Beckman, J. W. Vardiman, R. A. Larson, T. W. McKeithan, M. M. Le Beau, and J. D. Rowley, Clinical, morphologic, and cytogenetic characteristics of patients with lymphoid malignancies characterized by both t(14;18)(q32;q21) and t(8;14)(q21;q32) or t(8;22)(q24;q11), *Genes Chromosomes Cancer, 2*:147 (1990).

69. T. W. McKeithan, J. D. Rowley, T. B. Shows, and M. O. Diaz, Cloning of the chromosome translocation breakpoint junction of the t(14;19) in chronic lymphocytic leukemia, *Proc. Natl. Acad. Sci. USA, 84*:9257 (1987).

70. T. W. McKeithan, H. Ohno, and M. O. Diaz, Identification of a transcriptional unit adjacent to the breakpoint in the 14;19 translocation of chronic lymphocytic leukemia, *Genes Chromosomes Cancer, 1*:247 (1990).

71. H. Ohno, G. Takimoto, and T. W. McKeithan, The candidate proto-oncogene bcl-3 is related to genes implicated in cell lineage determination and cell control, *Cell, 60*:991 (1990).

72. L. Breeden and K. Nasmyth, Similarity between cell-cycle genes of budding yeast and fission yeast and the Notch gene of *Drosophila, Nature, 329*:651 (1987).

73. L. Breeden and K. Nasmyth, Cell cycle control of the yeast HO gene: Cis- and trans-acting regulators, *Cell, 48*:389 (1987).

74. C. Coffman, W. Harris, and C. Kintner, Xotch, the *Xenopus* homolog of *Drosophila* Notch, *Science, 249*:1438 (1990).

75. S. E. Lux, K. M. John, and V. Bennett, Analysis of cDNA for human erythrocyte ankyrin indicates a repeated structure with homology to tissue-differentiation and cell-cycle control proteins, *Nature, 344*:36 (1990).

76. A. M. R. Taylor, in *Ataxia Telangiectagia: A Cellular and Molecular Link Between Cancer, Neuropathology and Immune Deficiency* (B. A. Bridges and D. F. Harnder, eds.), John Wiley, New York, pp. 53–81 (1982).

77. R. S. Sparkes, R. Como, and D. W. Golde, Cytogenetic abnormalities in ataxia telangiectasia with T-cell chronic lymphocytic leukemia, *Cancer Gent. Cytogenet., 1*:329 (1980).

78. G. Russo, M. Isobe, R. Gatti, J. Finan, O. Batuman, K. Huebner, P. C. Nowell, and C. M. Croce, Molecular analysis of a t(14;14) translocation in leukemic T-cells of an ataxia telangiectasia patient, *Proc. Natl. Acad. Sci. USA, 86*:602 (1989).

79. M. P. Davey, V. Bertness, K. Nakahara, J. P. Johnson, O. W. McBride, T. A. Waldmann, and I. R. Kirsch, Juxtaposition of the T-cell receptor α-chain locus (14q11) and a region (14q32) of potential importance in leukemogenesis by a 14;14 translocation in a patient with T-cell chronic lymphocytic leukemia and ataxia telangiectasia, *Proc. Natl. Acad. Sci. USA, 85*:9287 (1988).

80. C. Hua, M. Raffeld, H-S. Ko, P. Fast, A. Bakhshi, and J. Cossman, Mechanism of bcl-2 activation in human follicular lymphoma, *Oncogene, 5*:233 (1990).

81. A. M. Ginsberg, M. Raffeld, and J. Cossman, Inactivation of the retinoblastoma gene in human lymphoid neoplasms, *Blood, 4*:833 (1991).

82. S. Raghoebier, J. H. J. M. van Krieken, J. C. Kluin- Nelemans, A. Gills, G. J. B. van Ommen, A. M. Ginsberg, M. Raffeld, and Ph. M. Kluin, Oncogene rearrangements in chronic B-cell leukemia, *Blood, 177*:1560 (1991).

6

Immunologic and Therapeutic Implications of Anti-Idiotype Antibodies

Thomas J. Kipps
University of California, San Diego, La Jolla, California

Anti-idiotypic antibodies are useful tools in the analysis and possible immunotherapy of B-cell chronic lymphocytic leukemia (CLL). Anti-idiotypic antibodies have facilitated our analyses of Ig gene expression in CLL, providing us with insight into the cytogenesis of this disease. Also, these reagents may detect variable region determinants of the surface Ig expressed by all cells within a leukemia B-cell population. As such, these determinants may be excellent targets for immunotherapy (1–5). Further development in our knowledge of idiotype expression in CLL may allow us to devise new immunotherapeutic strategies for this common adult leukemia.

GENETICS OF IMMUNOGLOBULIN DIVERSITY

Immunoglobulin Gene Rearrangement

The antibody variable region is formed through the juxtaposition of two polypeptide immunoglobulin chains that are encoded by gene complexes on different chromosomes. (6–8). During B-cell ontogeny, discontinuous genetic elements within these gene complexes undergo a series of rearrangements to generate the exons that ultimately may encode the heavy and light chains of the Ig molecule (9–12). The first Ig gene rearrangements generally occur within the heavy-chain gene complex. At least 24 minigenes, termed diversity segments (D) (13–16), are located between the heavy-chain variable region genes (V_H genes) and six functional J_H minigenes (17,18). One or more D segments may rearrange and become juxtaposed with a single J_H element (19,20). The generated DJ_H complex then may rearrange with one of hundreds of different V_H genes (14,21–23) to form a V_HDJ_H exon that may encode the variable portion of the antibody heavy chain (19,20). Subsequent to successful V_HDJ_H rearrangements, one of approximately 70 kappa V genes (V_κ genes) (24–30) may undergo rearrangement to one of five J_κ minigenes (18), this producing an exon that may encode that kappa light-chain variable region (18,31,32). Should these gene rearrangements fail to generate a functional $V_\kappa J_\kappa$ exon, one of approximately 70 lambda light-chain V genes (V_λ genes) (33,34) may rearrange with one of apparently four functional J_λ-C_λ complexes (35–40) to generate the genes necessary for lambda light-chain expression. The final products of such genetic gymnastics are the genes required for efficient synthesis of the heavy and light chains of the Ig molecule.

Somatic Hypermutation

Following successful Ig gene rearrangement, a highly specialized process may introduce mutations in the expressed Ig V genes (41–43). This process is designated somatic hypermutation. Somatic hypermutation is not active in all B cells and apparently may not be triggered by mitogen-induced B-cell activation (44). However, during discrete stages of B-cell differentiation, hypothetical "mutases" may be expressed that can permute the rearranged Ig V genes (43,45,46). Expressed Ig V genes may incur new mutations at rates as high as 10^{-3} base substitutions per base pair per generation over several cell divisions, particularly during the secondary humoral immune response to antigen (41,42,46). Such mutations apparently are clustered in the region spanning from 300 bp 5′ of the rearranged variable region exon to approximately 1 kb 3′ of the rearranged minigene J segment (47). Subsequent selection of the Ig encoded by such mutated Ig V genes may enhance the frequency of nonconservative base substitutions in the DNA sequences encoding the combining site(s) for antigen (45,48–52). This process enhances tremendously the diversity of the humoral immune repertoire.

IMMUNOGLOBULIN VARIABLE REGION STRUCTURE

Immunoglobulin Variable Region Subgroups

Despite the large number of different Ig variable regions that can be generated through the above mechanisms, each Ig polypeptide may be assigned to one of a relatively small number of variable region subgroups (53). Comparisons of the amino acid sequences of a large number of different monoclonal Ig proteins reveal four segments of limited amino acid sequence diversity between different Ig heavy- or light-chain variable regions (53). These segments are designated the Ig variable region frameworks (FR) (Fig. 1). Each Ig polypeptide may be assigned to one of a relatively small number of variable region subgroups based on the primary structure of its first three FRs. Moreover, each subgroup has characteristic FR sequences that serve to distinguish it from other variable region subgroups. Initially, human heavy chains were divided into three subgroups, while kappa or lambda light chains were divided into four or six subgroups, respectively (53).

A recent review of over 60 human Ig lambda light-chain variable region sequences resulted in revision of the lambda light-chain subgroup classification (54). All lambda light-chain sequences previously used to define the six lambda light-chain subgroups (53) were argued to fall actually into four main subgroups. Sequences previously assigned to subgroups IV and V were reclassified as belonging to subgroups III and II, respectively (54). In addition, three previously nonassigned lambda light-chain sequences that did not satisfy structural criteria for any of these four subgroups (33,55–57) were each assigned to represent a new subgroup, designated as IV, V, or VII (54). This new schemata brings the total number of lambda light-chain subgroups to seven.

Satisfying expectations that immunoglobulin subgroups defined families of highly related antibody variable region genes (V genes), variable region amino acid subgroup homologies are found to extend to the nucleic acid sequence level (21,22,30,58–64). Cloned Ig V genes whose deduced amino acid sequences belong to a given subgroup generally share greater than

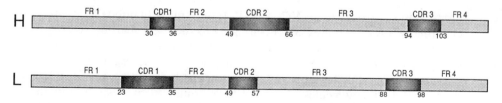

Figure 1 Schematic diagrams depicting the framework regions (FRs) and complementarity determining regions (CDRs) of the immunoglobulin heavy chain (H) or light chain (L). The first, second and third CDRs are labeled CDR1, CDR2, CDR3, respectively. Similarly, the first through fourth framework regions are labeled FR1, FR2, FR3, and FR4. The amino acid residues that define the borders between these regions are numbered at the bottom of each diagram, according to Kabat et al. [1].

80% nucleic acid sequence homology. One exception to this generalization resulted in the designation of a new heavy-chain variable gene subgroup (23,65). The deduced amino acid sequences for several newly defined heavy-chain V genes (V_H genes) were noted to have features typical of heavy-chain variable regions of the V_H2 subgroup. However, these newly identified V_H genes were noted to have less than 70% homology with previously defined "V_H2 genes." As such, these V_H genes were assigned to a new V_H gene subgroup, designated V_H4. Isolation of additional V_H genes has divulged two additional V_H gene subgroups that were not identified at the amino acid level, designated V_H5 and V_H6 (22,66,67). The V_H genes of V_H5 subgroup are most similar to members of the V_H1 subgroup, and the single-copy V_H6 gene is most related to V_H genes of the V_H4 subgroup. However, unlike the noted protein sequence homologies between variable regions encoded V_H2 or V_H4 genes, the deduced amino acid FR sequences of V_H5 or V_H6 genes are subgroup specific.

Features of the primary structure that serve to distinguish immunoglobulin subgroups may be detected serologically (68–72). Crystallographic data of Ig variable regions indicate that amino acids within the first and third FR regions of either the light or heavy chain form beta bends on the external surface of the molecule (73–77). These regions form relatively compact structures on the external solvent-accessible face of the antibody molecule that are not adjacent to the classic antibody-combining site for antigen. Thus, amino acid differences noted between the different variable region subgroups should be amenable to recognition by anti-subgroup antibodies.

Using isolated monoclonal kappa or lambda light chains as immunogens, Solomon and colleagues generated rabbit antisera that were each rendered specific for an Ig light-chain subgroup through extensive absorption with human Ig of irrelevant variable region subgroups (72,78–80). These investigators developed antisera specific for each of the four kappa light-chain variable region subgroups ($V_\kappa1$, $V_\kappa2$, $V_\kappa3$, or $V_\kappa4$), or each of five lambda light-chain subgroups ($V_\lambda1$, $V_\lambda2$, $V_\lambda3$, $V_\lambda4$, or $V_\lambda6$). All lambda light chains classified via Kabat et al. (53) as belonging to the $V_\lambda5$ subgroup react with antisera specific for the $V_\lambda2$ subgroup, providing serologic data supporting the need to reorganize the lambda light-chain variable region subgroups (see above) (54). Furthermore, a few murine mAb generated against intact immunoglobulin molecules also have been found to have specificity for human Ig variable region subgroups (81,82). In addition, antisera, each specific for one of the kappa variable region subgroups (83) or heavy-chain variable region subgroups (84,85), have been generated using synthetic peptides corresponding to subgroup-specific primary amino acid sequences in the first FR region of the V_κ region or V_H region, respectively. Thus, the epitope(s) within the FRs may serve to distinguish Ig molecules with respect to their variable region subgroup.

Immunoglobulin Idiotypes

Anti-subgroup antibodies, however, need to be distinguished from anti-idiotypic antibodies. Positioned between the FR regions are three segments of extreme hypervariability in both light- and heavy-chain sequences (53). The third hypervariable region is generated through the recombinatorial process joining the antibody light-chain V gene with the J segment, in the case of the light chain, or the V_H gene with the somatically generated DJ_H segment of the antibody heavy chain (9,13,14,31,86). The diversity in the first and second hypervariable region reflects in part germline DNA-encoded differences between disparate antibody V genes, a diversity often noted even between V genes of the same subgroup (21,22,30,58–64).

Affinity labeling and crystallographic studies have substantiated earlier contentions that the hypervariable regions on both chains fold together to form the antigen combining site (73–77). Hence, these regions of hypervariability are designated the complementarity-determining regions, or CDRs (Fig. 1). During an immune response, somatic hypermutation subsequent to V gene rearrangement also may play an important role in increasing the amino acid sequence diversity noted within these regions (discussed above). During secondary immune responses, extensive amino acid substitutions may occur in the CDRs. In contrast, amino acid replacement mutations are noted to be much less frequent in the framework regions than would be anticipated if the nucleic acid substitutions were occurring randomly. As a consequence, the subgroup determinants that characterize an entire variable region subgroup may be relatively resilient to the process of somatic hypermutation. On the other hand, the CDRs may form determinants of unique specificity that contribute to the epitopes recognized by anti-idiotypic antibodies.

Cross-Reactive Idiotypes

Despite the tremendous potential for diversity in Ig V gene expression and genetic polymorphisms, antibodies produced by B-cell malignancies of unrelated persons may share common idiotypic determinants. Initially identified using highly absorbed heterologous antisera (87), and then more recently using murine mAbs (82,88–90), these common idiotopes, designated cross-reactive idiotopes or CRIs, were defined initially on IgM autoantibodies, such as rheumatoid factors (RFs). That such CRIs are not internal images reflecting a common antigen-binding activity, however, initially was suggested by protein-sequence data demonstrating that the light- or heavy-chain variable regions of CRI-bearing immunoglobulins may have highly homologous primary structure (91–96).

Patients with CLL and related small lymphocytic CD5 B-cell lymphomas frequently have neoplastic cells that express autoantibody-associated CRIs.

In an early study of over 30 CLL patients, 5 of 20 (25%) with kappa light-chain-expressing CLL had malignant cells that expressed the 17.109 CRI (97,98). Furthermore, approximately 20% of both kappa and lambda light-chain-expressing CLL were found to react with G6 (99,100), a mAb specific for an Ig heavy-chain-associated CRI present on several RF paraproteins (89). Yet an additional mAb specific for a distinct rheumatoid factor (RF) heavy-chain-associated CRI, named Lc1 (100–102), labeled neoplastic Ig-expressing B cells from 7 of 56 (13%) patients with CLL and related B-cell lymphomas (100). Another 2 cases (4%) in this study were found to have malignant cells reactive with B6, a third mAb specific for an autoantibody-heavy-chain-associated CRI that is distinct from either the G6-CRI or Lc1-CRI (100,103). Recently, other investigators have found additional CRIs that also are expressed frequently in CLL and related B-cell neoplasms (104,105).

IMMUNOLOGIC IMPLICATIONS OF CRI EXPRESSION IN CLL

Nonrandom V_H Gene Expression in CLL

The frequent expression of such autoantibody-associated CRIs in CLL implies that Ig V gene expression in this disease is highly restricted. Nucleic acid sequence analyses reveal that G6-reactive leukemic cells from unrelated CLL patients express nearly identical V_H1 genes (106). These V_H genes are homologous to a V_H1 gene frequently used by human fetal splenocytes, designated 51p1 (67). Despite expressing homologous V_H genes, however, G6-reactive leukemic cells may express markedly different D segments and utilize J_H3, J_H4, J_H5, or J_H6 gene segments. Comparisons of the deduced amino acid sequences of G6-reactive CLL and those of G6-negative antibody heavy chains encoded by V_H1 genes suggests that the G6-CRI in CLL is relatively resilient to substitutions within CDR3, but affected by permutations within CDR1 and CDR2. Thus the frequent expression of the G6-CRI implies that the V_H1 gene, 51p1, may be used by the leukemia cells from a sizable proportion of patients with CLL.

In order to evaluate the frequency at which V_H1 genes undergo Ig gene recombination in CLL independent of CRI expression, we used consensus oligonucleotides corresponding to all V_H1 leader sequences and J_H minigenes to amplify the V_H1 genes juxtaposed with DJ_H through Ig gene rearrangement in the leukemia cell DNA from 44 randomly selected and newly screened patients with common CLL. Using the polymerase chain reaction, we amplified rearranged V_H1 genes in 39% of these samples (17/44) (Duffy, Johnson, Kobayashi, and Kipps, unpublished observations). Fifteen (88%) of these rearranged V_H1 genes were functional. The overall frequency of functional V_H1 genes (34%) is lower than the frequency of

V_H1 gene expression noted in CLL by some investigators [i.e., 5/11 (45%) (107)], but higher than that noted by others [e.g., 6/34 (18%) (108) and 6/40 (15%) (109)]. However, evaluation of the differences noted in these surveys using the Student's t test indicates that they apparently do not reach significance ($p > 0.01$), suggesting that they may represent chance variations in sampling.

In any case, analyses of the nucleotide sequence of these rearranged V_H1 gene reveals a biased use of the 51p1 gene that encodes the G6-CRI. Although 51p1 is but one of an estimated 35–80 genes that belong to the V_H1 gene family, two-thirds (10/15) of the functionally rearranged V_H1 genes were homologous to 51p1. Two of the 15 (13%) functionally rearranged V_H1 were homologous to another germline V_H1 gene, designated V35. V35 is peculiar in that it is the closest V_H1 gene to the D and J_H gene complexes (110). As 51p1 apparently is rearranged and expressed more often than V35, proximity to the D and J_H loci evidently does not solely determine the frequency of V_H gene rearrangements.

Other studies also have noted restriction in the V_H genes used in CLL. For example, the V_H genes belonging to the largest and generally most frequently used V_H gene family, V_H3, apparently account for a relatively small proportion of the V_H genes used in CLL (111,112). However, the relatively small V_H subgroups, V_H4 and V_H5, and the single-copy V_H6 gene appear proportionately overrepresented in the Ig V_H gene rearrangements detected in CLL (107,109,111,113). Conceivably, development of anti-idiotypic antibodies to the proteins encoded by these V_H genes may detect additional CRIs that are frequently expressed in this disease.

In fact, a few anti-CRI mAbs have been developed that recognize the protein product of conserved Ig V_H4 genes. The mAb Lc1 detects a "supra-typic CRI" associated with the expression of a sub-subset of V_H4 genes (103), namely, $V_H4.11$ (114)/V71-4 (21), $V_H4.18$ (114)/V72-1 (23), and V_H71-2 (23). As noted above, in one survey, over 10% of the CLL patients tested had leukemia cells reactive with this mAb (100). In addition, another mAb, designated 9G4, reacts with the protein product of $V_H4.21$ (115), a V_H gene that frequently encodes IgM cold agglutinins. In contrast to Lc1, however, the expression frequency of this CRI in CLL may be less than a few percent (T. J. Hamblin, personal communication). This contrasts also with the relatively frequent expression of this CRI noted during early B-cell ontogeny (116), suggesting that the repertoire of expressed Ig V genes in CLL may be distinct from that expressed in early B-cell development.

Kappa Light-Chain V Gene Rearrangement

Similarly, Ig V_κ gene rearrangement in CLL apparently is not random. 17.109-reactive leukemia cells from unrelated CLL patients express very

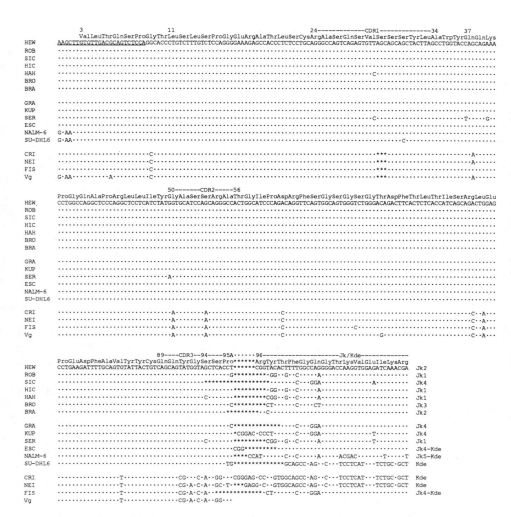

Figure 2 Nucleic acid sequences of kappa light chain variable regions. The name of each sequence is listed to the left. All sequences are compared with HEW. Dots (·) indicate homology with the HEW sequence. Asterisks (*) designate gaps that were introduced to maximize sequence homology. Sequences HEW, ROB, SIC, HIC, HAH, SRO, BRA are the kappa light chain variable region sequences of 17.109-reactive leukemia cells from unrelated patients with CLL. These sequences have ≥ 99% homology with *Humkv325*. Sequences GRA, KUP, SER, ESC, CRI, NEI, and FIS are the abortively rearranged and/or non-expressed kappa light chain variable regions of lambda light chain expressing chronic lymphocytic leukemia cells. Sequence SER has a C→T substitution, resulting in a stop codon (TAG) at amino acid position 37. Sequences NALM-6 and SU-DHL6 are the abortively rearranged kappa light chain variable regions of a pre-B cell cell line (NALM-6) and B cell line (SU-DHL6), respectively [2]. Also depicted is Vg, a germline V_x3

homologous Ig V_κ genes (117) (Fig. 2). These Ig V_κ genes are identical to a highly conserved germline $V_\kappa 3$ gene, designated Humkv325 (118). In the human haploid genome, Humkv325 is only one of approximately 70 V_κ genes that may undergo Ig gene rearrangement (30). Therefore, the frequent expression in CLL of the 17.109-CRI, and hence Humkv325, indicates that CLL B cells do not express V_κ genes at random.

At least two mechanisms may account for the frequent expression of certain Ig V genes in CLL. For example, some Ig V genes may encode Ig variable regions that are conducive to B-cell leukemogenesis. Alternatively, although not exclusively, certain Ig V genes simply may undergo Ig gene rearrangement more frequently than other Ig V genes, this contributing to their more common expression.

In order to study the frequency of Humkv325 gene rearrangement independent of its expression into protein, we isolated a DNA fragment upstream of Humkv325 to probe for nonfunctional Humkv325 Ig rearrangements in lambda light-chain-expressing CLL (λ-CLL) (119). We assembled 33 cases of common λ-CLL for analysis. Although most λ-CLL had kappa light-chain gene rearrangements on both alleles, 9 of the 33 samples (27%) had one kappa light-chain allele in the germline configuration. In 8 of the 33 (24%) λ-CLL, we identified Humkv325 Ig gene rearrangements. Using oligonucleotide primers specific for $V_\kappa 3$ genes and all J_κ minigenes or Kde, we performed PCR on all λ-CLL (119). PCR on each DNA sample with $V_\kappa 3$ gene rearrangements generated gene fragments of the expected size, which hybridized specifically with oligonucleotide probes corresponding to framework or complementarity-determining regions of the Humkv325 gene. Nucleic acid sequence analyses of representative samples confirmed that these DNA contained abortive Humkv325 gene rearrangements (Fig. 2). PCR of other λ-CLL did not generate any PCR product except in three cases. These three λ-CLL had abortive V_κ gene rearrangements involving another conserved $V_\kappa 3$ gene, designated Vg (Fig. 2). Similar to Humkv325, this conserved $V_\kappa 3$ gene frequently is found to encode the kappa light-chain variable region of IgM_κ autoantibodies (64,120,121). Despite the high de-

---

gene [3]. Sequences GRA, KUP, SER, ESC, NALM-6 and SU-DHL6, share greatest homology (>98%) with *Humkv325*, whereas sequences CRI, NEI, and FIS share greatest homology (≥99%) with Vg. Each kappa variable region except for Vg is rearranged with J_K, J_K-Kde or Kde, as listed at the end of each sequence (bottom right). Listed above the sequence, HEW, is the deduced amino acid sequence of HEW. Above this amino acid sequence are the amino acid numbers according to Kabat [1], and descriptors delineating CDR1, CDR2, CDR3 and the J_K and/or Kde sequences.

gree of sequence similarity between Vg and Humkv325 (Fig. 2), functionally rearranged VgJ$_\kappa$ exons do not encode kappa light-chain variable regions
that are recognized by 17.109 mAb.

These studies reveal a bias in V$_\kappa$ gene rearrangement that is independent
of protein expression. Theoretically, any one of 70 V$_\kappa$ genes may undergo
Ig rearrangement (30). Thus, if V$_\kappa$ gene rearrangement were random, the
chance of finding either Humkv325 or Vg gene rearrangements in λ-CLL
should be 1 in 70, or 1.4%. Moreover, the expected chance of Ig gene
rearrangements involving V$_\kappa$ genes other than Humkv325 (or Vg) should be
69/70, or 98.6%. Thus, the expected number of Humkv325 or Vg gene
rearrangements in the 57 Ig rearrangements detected in the 33 λ-CLL
should be less than 1 (0.8). On the other hand, the expected number of V$_\kappa$
gene rearrangements in these samples that involve genes other than
Humkv325 (or Vg) should be approximately 56 (56.2). However, in the
samples examined, we found 8 Humkv325 gene rearrangements, 49 non-
Humkv325 rearrangements, 3 Vg gene rearrangements, and 54 non-Vg gene
rearrangements. Chi-square analyses demonstrate that these observed values are greater than those that would be expected if V$_\kappa$ gene rearrangements
were truly random ($p = 0.0001$ for Humkv325, and $p = 0.0147$ for Vg).
Thus, independent of expression, Ig V$_\kappa$ gene rearrangement in CLL is not
random.

Lambda Light-Chain V Gene Subgroups

Recent studies suggest that the Ig lambda light-chain V gene (V$_\lambda$ gene) use
in CLL also may be restricted. One recent study described a panel of mAbs
generated against the variable region of a single IgG$_\lambda$ paraprotein (104).
Several of these mAbs apparently were specific for determinants located on
the lambda light chain of this paraprotein. Although it was not known if
such mAbs were anti-subgroup mAb or truly anti-CRI reagents, four of
the mAbs reacted with lambda-expressing leukemia cells from 5–29% of
patients with CLL. Efforts to characterize the molecular basis of the determinants recognized by these mAbs may reveal an Ig V$_\lambda$ gene(s) or Ig V$_\lambda$
gene subgroup that is frequently used in CLL. Using anti-subgroup antisera, Solomon and colleagues recently evaluated the neoplastic cell sIgs
from patients with CLL and related B-cell lymphomas (80). Of 12 neoplastic cell populations with sIg with λ light chains, seven (58%) were classified
as having light chains of Ig V$_\lambda$III subgroup, three (25%) were found to
have light chains of the Ig V$_\lambda$IV, and none were found to have light chains
of the Ig V$_\lambda$VI subgroup. This distribution contrasted with the distribution
noted among lambda light-chain Bence Jones proteins from patients with
multiple myeloma, in which less than 25% were of the Ig V$_\lambda$III subgroup,

fewer than 3% were of the Ig $V_\lambda IV$ subgroup, and over 10% were of the Ig $V_\lambda VI$ subgroup. Conceivably, such differences may reflect a distinction between CLL versus multiple myeloma in their use of Ig V_λ genes, similar to that noted for Ig V_κ genes and/or Ig V_κ gene subgroups (80,112). Such a distinction may be secondary to a restriction in the use of Ig V_λ genes in CLL, favoring expression of certain Ig V_λ genes that are not used substantially by other B-cell neoplasms and/or normal B-cell subsets.

Absence of Somatic Hypermutation in CLL

Given the enormous potential for Ig diversity through somatic mutation, however, nonrandom Ig V gene rearrangement simply may not account for the frequent expression in CLL of such autoantibody-associated CRIs as 17.109 or G6. As noted above, these mAbs react with determinants unique to Ig variable regions encoded by conserved Ig V genes that have not mutated substantially from the germline DNA. As such, these determinants serve to mark the expression of germline-encoded Ig V genes with little or no somatic mutation. Accordingly, the frequent expression of CRIs detected by such mAbs in CLL also suggests that the process of somatic hypermutation has not been activated in this adult B-cell leukemia. Consistent with this, we and others have not noted significant intraclonal diversity in the Ig V genes expressed in CLL (106,117,122,123).

In contrast, non-Hodgkin's lymphomas of follicular center cell origin demonstrate substantial intraclonal diversity in their expressed Ig V genes (reviewed in Ref. 124). Conceivably somatic mutation of the V genes expressed by these lymphomas may disrupt and destroy variable region determinants that are recognized by certain anti-CRI mAbs. Consistent with this, we find that autoantibody-associated CRIs, such as 17.109 or G6, are rarely expressed by these types of lymphomas (99). Unlike CLL, these lymphomas generally occur in younger individuals, do not express the CD5 surface antigen, and may be derived from a B-cell lineage(s) or stage(s) of differentiation distinct from that of conventional CLL (125,126).

Cytogenesis of CLL

Antibodies specific for a major CRI stain a subpopulation of lymphocytes that have a distinctive histologic distribution. Immunohistochemical studies on human tonsil reveal that antibodies specific for a major autoantibody-associated CRI stain a subpopulation of B cells that reside within the mantle zones surrounding the germinal centers of normal human tonsil. This distinctive distribution of CRI-reactive cells is noted in sections of every tonsil specimen examined to date (n > 24). In contrast, mAbs directed against variable region subgroup determinants stain a subpopulation of cells in both the mantle zones and germinal centers. Taking advantage of this anatomic distribution, we screened newly generated mAbs for their ability to bind exclusively a subset of mantle zone lymphocytes and identified reagents that react with novel CRIs that also may be expressed frequently in CLL (112). The overall success of these methods indicates that variable regions of the Igs produced by mantle-zone B cells may share idiotypic determinants with Igs expressed in B-cell CLL.

Differences in the expression frequencies of CRIs in B-cell malignancies may reflect apparent differences in the CRI expression frequencies of various subpopulations of normal B cells. As noted, each of these anti-CRI mAbs stains a subpopulation of mantle-zone lymphocytes but rarely any germinal-center B cells. Conceivably, germinal-center B cells may express V genes that differ from those expressed by mantle-zone B cells. Alternatively, though not exclusive of the former hypothesis, germinal-center B cells may express V genes that have undergone somatic hypermutation. In this regard, the paucity of CRI-positive cells in the germinal centers may mimic the low frequencies at which such CRIs are detected on Ig expressed by non-Hodgkin's lymphomas of presumed follicular center cell origin (99). The Ig V genes expressed by such lymphomas demonstrate intraclonal diversity in their expressed Ig V genes indicative of ongoing somatic mutation (127). Recent data suggest that this process is active in B cells located within the germinal centers of secondary B-cell follicles (128,129). Conceivably, somatic mutation of the V genes expressed by these lymphomas, and the germinal center cells from which they are derived, may disrupt and destroy variable region determinants that are recognized by certain anti-CRI mAbs. Consistent with this notion, mAbs specific for subgroup determinants, which are more resilient to the structural alterations induced by somatic hypermutation, stain cells in both the germinal centers and the surrounding mantle zones. Conceivably, lymphomas derived from such germinal-center B cells may retain this phenotype, accounting for the relatively high degree of intraclonal diversity observed in their expressed Ig V genes.

Similarly, the low level of noted Ig V gene mutations detected in CLL also may reflect the cytogenesis of this leukemia. CLL generally may be considered a malignancy of CD5 B cells (reviewed in Ref. 130). The latter constitute a small subpopulation of human B lymphocytes in the lymphoid organs and peripheral blood of normal adults (131–135). Four-color immunofluorescence analyses indicate that such CD5 B cells share the surface antigen phenotype of mantle-zone lymphocytes (136). In addition, these lymphocytes account for the great majority of B cells in the primary follicles of human fetal spleen (137,138), where high proportions of cells express these CRIs (139). Finally, independent clones of murine CD5 B cells are found to express identical Ig V genes without evidence for somatic mutation

(140,141). The antibodies encoded by such Ig V genes frequently are reactive with a variety of self-antigens, i.e., proteolytically processed erythrocyte membranes, denatured DNA, and/or the Fc portion of self-IgG (142–146). Stable expression of such Ig V genes with little or no somatic mutation may account for the finding that human CD5 B cells are enriched for cells that spontaneously may produce such IgM autoantibodies (147,148). In this light, the finding that most CLL patients have leukemia cells that express such IgM autoantibodies may be a reflection of the cytogenesis of this disease (98,149–151).

IMPLICATIONS OF ANTI-IDIOTYPES FOR IMMUNOTHERAPY

Immunotherapy of CLL

There are only a few published studies describing the use of anti-idiotypic antibodies to treat patients with CLL (104,152,153). In contrast to infusions with anti-CD5 mAbs, which produce rapid modulation of the CD5 surface antigen on the treated leukemia cells (154,155), immunotherapy with anti-idiotypic mAbs apparently may not result in rapid modulation of sIg or tumor cell activation (156). Significant reductions in the levels of circulating leukemia cells resulted from each infusion of anti-idiotypic mAb (156), or until resistance developed (152). However, in contrast to treatment of lymphomas of follicular center cell origin with anti-idiotypic antibodies (157), idiotype variants did not emerge after treatment with anti-idiotypic mAb, even after repeated mAb infusions over the course of 1 year's time (152,156). Rather, the development of resistance to therapy coincided with a decreased clearance rate of circulating id-anti-id immune complexes, reflecting perhaps a developing deficiency in host natural effector mechanism(s) (152). Such findings are consistent with the noted stability in Ig V gene expression of CLL B cells. In this regard, CLL actually may be more amenable to treatment with anti-idiotypic mAbs than B-cell lymphomas of follicular center cell origin.

Anti-CRI Antibodies for Immunotherapy

Anti-CRI may afford a partial answer to the problems associated with immunotherapy with monoclonal anti-idiotypic antibodies. The need to generate idiotypic-specific mAbs against each patient's malignant clone makes this form of therapy extremely costly, time consuming, and labor intensive (158). The requirement to tailor a unique reagent for each patient confounds clinical studies seeking to compare the role of immunoglobulin isotype, mode of mAb delivery, utility of antibody-toxin conjugates, and the relative advantages of single versus multiple mAb therapy. However, because CLL and related lymphomas apparently express a restricted Ig repertoire, batteries of anti-CRI mAbs may be developed suitable for the early diagnosis and possible future immunotherapy of a large number of patients with CD5 B-cell malignancies.

ACKNOWLEDGMENTS

The author is a Scholar of the Leukemia Society of America, funded in part by the Scott Helping Hand Fund. This work was supported in part by National Institutes of Health grant CA49870.

REFERENCES

1. R. G. Lynch, R. J. Graff, S. Sirisinha, E. S. Simms, and H. N. Eisen, Myeloma proteins as tumor-specific transplantation antigens, *Proc. Natl. Acad. Sci. USA, 69*:1540 (1972).
2. K. R. Schroer, D. E. Briles, J. A. Van Boxel, and J. M. Davie, Idiotypic uniformity of cell surface immunoglobulin in chronic lymphocytic leukemia. Evidence for monoclonal proliferation, *J. Exp. Med., 140*:1416 (1974).
3. G. T. Stevenson and F. K. Stevenson, Antibody to a molecularly-defined antigen confined to a tumour cell surface, *Nature, 254*:714 (1975).
4. G. T. Stevenson, E. V. Elliott, and F. K. Stevenson, Idiotypic determinants on the surface immunoglobulin of neoplastic lymphocytes: A therapeutic target, *Fed. Proc., 36*:2268 (1977).
5. G. Haughton, L. L. Lanier, G. F. Babcock, and M. A. Lynes, Antigen-induced murine B cell lymphomas. II. Exploitation of the surface idiotype as tumor specific antigen, *J. Immunol., 121*:2358 (1978).
6. S. Malcolm, P. Barton, C. Murphy, M. A. Ferguson-Smith, D. L. Bentley, and T. H. Rabbitts, Localization of human immunoglobulin kappa light chain variable region genes to the short arm of chromosome 2 by in situ hybridization, *Proc. Natl. Acad. Sci. USA, 79*:4957 (1982).
7. O. W. McBride, P. A. Hieter, G. F. Hollis, D. Swan, M. C. Otey, and P. Leder, Chromosomal location of human kappa and lambda immunoglobulin light chain constant region genes, *J. Exp. Med., 155*:1480 (1982).
8. I. R. Kirsch, C. C. Morton, K. Nakahara, and P. Leder, Human immunoglobulin heavy chain genes map to a region of translocations in malignant B lymphocytes, *Science, 216*:301 (1982).
9. S. Tonegawa, Somatic generation of antibody diversity, *Nature, 302*:575 (1983).
10. T. Honjo and S. Habu, Origin of immune diversity: genetic variation and selection, *Ann. Rev. Biochem., 54*:803 (1985).
11. J. G. Seidman and P. Leder, The arrangement and rearrangement of antibody genes, *Nature, 276*:790 (1978).

12. J. G. Seidman, A. Leder, M. Nau, B. Norman, and P. Leder, Antibody diversity, *Science, 202*:11 (1978).

13. H. Sakano, Y. Kurosawa, M. Weigert, and S. Tonegawa, Identification and nucleotide sequence of a diversity DNA segment (D) of immunoglobulin heavy-chain genes, *Nature, 290*:562 (1981).

14. U. Siebenlist, J. V. Ravetch, S. Korsmeyer, T. Waldmann, and P. Leder, Human immunoglobulin D segments encoded in tandem multigenic families, *Nature, 294*:631 (1981).

15. Y. Ichihara, H. Matsuoka, and Y. Kurosawa, Organization of human immunoglobulin heavy chain diversity gene loci, *EMBO J., 7*:4141 (1988).

16. L. Buluwela, D. G. Albertson, P. Sherrington, P. H. Rabbitts, N. Spurr, and T. H. Rabbitts, The use of chromosomal translocations to study human immunoglobulin gene organization: Mapping DH segments within 35 kb of the C mu gene and identification of a new DH locus, *EMBO J., 7*:2003 (1988).

17. J. V. Ravetch, U. Siebenlist, S. Korsmeyer, T. Waldmann, and P. Leder, Structure of the human immunoglobulin mu locus: Characterization of embryonic and rearranged J and D genes, *Cell, 27*:583 (1981).

18. P. A. Hieter, E. E. Max, J. G. Seidman, J. V. Maizel, Jr., and P. Leder, Cloned human and mouse kappa immunoglobulin constant and J region genes conserve homology in functional segments, *Cell, 22*:197 (1980).

19. G. D. Yancopoulos and F. W. Alt, Regulation of the assembly and expression of variable-region genes, *Ann. Rev. Immunol., 4*:339 (1986).

20. M. G. Reth, S. Jackson, and F. W. Alt, VHDJH formation and DJH replacement during pre-B non-random usage of gene segments, *EMBO J., 5*:2131 (1986).

21. M. Kodaira, T. Kinashi, I. Umemura, F. Matsuda, T. Noma, Y. Ono, and T. Honjo, Organization and evolution of variable region genes of the human immunoglobulin heavy chain, *J. Mol. Biol., 190*:529 (1986).

22. J. E. Berman, S. J. Mellis, R. Pollock, C. L. Smith, H. Suh, B. Heinke, C. Kowal, U. Surti, L. Chess, C. R. Cantor, and F. W. Alt, Content and organization of the human Ig VH locus: Definition of three new VH families and linkage to the Ig CH locus, *EMBO J., 7*:727 (1988).

23. K. H. Lee, F. Matsuda, T. Kinashi, M. Kodaira, and T. Honjo, A novel family of variable region genes of the human immunoglobulin heavy chain, *J. Mol. Biol., 195*:761 (1987).

24. D. L. Bentley and T. H. Rabbitts, Evolution of immunoglobulin V genes: Evidence indicating that recently duplicated human V kappa sequences have diverged by gene conversion, *Cell, 32*:181 (1983).

25. M. Pech, H. Smola, H. D. Pohlenz, B. Straubinger, R. Gerl, and H. G. Zachau, A large section of the gene locus encoding human immunoglobulin variable regions of the kappa type is duplicated, *J. Mol. Biol., 183*:291 (1985).

26. W. Lorenz, B. Straubinger, and H. G. Zachau, Physical map of the human immunoglobulin K locus and its implications for the mechanisms of VK-JK rearrangement, *Nucleic Acids Res., 15*:9667 (1987).

27. H. D. Pohlenz, B. Straubinger, R. Thiebe, M. Pech, F. J. Zimmer, and H. G. Zachau, The human V kappa locus. Characterization of extended immunoglobulin gene regions by cosmid cloning, *J. Mol. Biol., 193*:241 (1987).

28. B. Straubinger, E. Huber, W. Lorenz, E. Osterholzer, W. Pargent, M. Pech, H. D. Pohlenz, F. J. Zimmer, and H. G. Zachau, The human VK locus. Characterization of a duplicated region encoding 28 different immunoglobulin genes, *J. Mol. Biol., 199*:23 (1988).

29. A. Meindl, H. G. Klobeck, R. Ohnheiser, and H. G. Zachau, The V kappa gene repertoire in the human germ line, *Eur. J. Immunol., 20*:1855 (1990).

30. H. G. Zachau, The human immunoglobulin kappa locus and some of its acrobatics, *Biol. Chem. Hoppe-Seyler, 371*:1 (1990).

31. C. Brack, M. Hirama, R. Lenhard-Schuller, and S. Tonegawa, A complete immunoglobulin gene is created by somatic recombination, *Cell, 15*:1 (1978).

32. J. G. Seidman, M. M. Nau, B. Norman, S. P. Kwan, M. Scharff, and P. Leder, Immunoglobulin V/J recombination is accompanied by deletion of joining site and variable region segments, *Proc. Natl. Acad. Sci. USA, 77*: 6022 (1980).

33. M. L. Anderson, M. F. Szajnert, J. C. Kaplan, L. McColl, and B. D. Young, The isolation of a human Ig V lambda gene from a recombinant library of chromosome 22 and estimation of its copy number, *Nucleic Acids Res., 12*: 6647 (1984).

34. N. Yamasaki, S. Komori, and T. Watanabe, Complementary DNA for a human subgroup IV immunoglobulin lambda-chain, *Mol. Immunol., 24*:981 (1987).

35. P. Dariavach, G. Lefranc, and M. P. Lefranc, Human immunoglobulin C lambda 6 gene encodes the Kern + Oz − lambda chain and C lambda 4 and C lambda 5 are pseudogenes, *Proc. Natl. Acad. Sci. USA, 84*:9074 (1987).

36. J. A. Udey and B. B. Blomberg, Intergenic exchange maintains identity between two human lambda light chain immunoglobulin gene intron sequences, *Nucleic Acids Res., 16*:2959 (1988).

37. J. A. Udey and B. Blomberg, Human lambda light chain locus: Organization and DNA sequences of three genomic J regions, *Immunogenetics, 25*:63 (1987).

38. P. A. Hieter, G. F. Hollis, S. J. Korsmeyer, T. A. Waldmann, and P. Leder, Clustered arrangement of immunoglobulin lambda constant region genes in man, *Nature, 294*:536 (1981).

39. T. J. Vasicek and P. Leder, Structure and expression of the human immunoglobulin lambda genes, *J. Exp. Med., 172*:609 (1990).

40. T. R. Bauer, Jr., and B. Blomberg, The human lambda L chain Ig locus. Recharacterization of JC lambda 6 and identification of a functional JC lambda 7, *J. Immunol., 146*:2813 (1991).

41. D. McKean, K. Huppi, M. Bell, L. Staudt, W. Gerhard, and M. Weigert, Generation of antibody diversity in the immune response of BALB/c mice to influenza virus hemagglutinin, *Proc. Natl. Acad. Sci. USA, 81*:3180 (1984).

42. S. H. Clarke, K. Huppi, D. Ruezinsky, L. Staudt, W. Gerhard, and M. Weigert, Inter- and intraclonal diversity in the antibody response to influenza hemagglutinin, *J. Exp. Med., 161*:687 (1985).

43. T. Manser, L. J. Wysocki, M. N. Margolies, and M. L. Gefter, Evolution of antibody variable region structure during the immune response, *Immunol. Rev., 96*:141 (1987).

44. T. Manser, Mitogen-driven B cell proliferation and differentiation are not accompanied by hypermutation of immunoglobulin variable region genes, *J. Immunol., 139*:234 (1987).

45. G. M. Griffiths, C. Berek, M. Kaartinen, and C. Milstein, Somatic mutation and the maturation of immune response to 2-phenyl oxazolone, *Nature, 312*: 271 (1984).

46. N. S. Levy, U. V. Malipiero, S. G. Lebecque, and P. J. Gearhart, Early onset of somatic mutation in immunoglobulin VH genes during primary immune response, *J. Exp. Med., 169*:2007 (1989).

47. S. G. Lebecque and P. J. Gearhart, Boundaries of somatic mutation in rearranged immunoglobulin genes: Boundary is near the promoter, and 3′ boundary is approximately 1 kb V(D)J gene, *J. Exp. Med., 172*:1717 (1990).

48. T. Manser, S. Y. Huang, and M. L. Gefter, Influence of clonal selection on the expression of variable region genes, *Science, 226*:1283 (1984).

49. J. L. Claflin, J. Berry, D. Flaherty, and W. Dunnick, Somatic evolution of diversity among anti-phosphocholine antibodies induced with Proteus morganii, *J. Immunol., 138*:3060 (1987).

50. L. Wysocki, T. Manser, and M. L. Gefter, Somatic evolution of variable region structures during an immune response, *Proc. Natl. Acad. Sci. USA, 83*:1847 (1986).

51. C. Kocks and K. Rajewsky, Stepwise intraclonal maturation of antibody affinity through somatic hypermutation, *Proc. Natl. Acad. Sci. USA, 85*: 8206 (1988).

52. M. J. Shlomchik, A. Marshak-Rothstein, C. B. Wolfowicz, T. L. Rothstein, and M. G. Weigert, The role of clonal selection and somatic mutation in autoimmunity, *Nature, 328*:805 (1987).

53. E. Kabat, T. T. Wu, M. Reid-Miller, H. M. Perry, and K. S. Gottesmann, *Sequences of Proteins of Immunological Interest*, U.S. Government Printing Office, Bethesda, MD (1987).

54. P. Chuchana, A. Blancher, F. Brockly, D. Alexandre, G. Lefranc, and M. P. Lefranc, Definition of the human immunoglobulin variable lambda (IGLV) gene subgroups, *Eur. J. Immunol., 20*:1317 (1990).

55. S. Levy, E. Mendel, S. Kon, Z. Avnur, and R. Levy, Mutational hot spots in Ig V region genes of human follicular lymphomas, *J. Exp. Med., 168*:475 (1988).

56. N. Berinstein, S. Levy, and R. Levy, Activation of an excluded immunoglobulin allele in a human B lymphoma cell line, *Science, 244*:337 (1989).

57. D. Alexandre, P. Chuchana, F. Brockly, A. Blancher, G. Lefranc, and M. P. Lefranc, First genomic sequence of a human Ig variable lambda gene belonging to subgroup I. Functional genes, pseudogenes and vestigial se-

quences are interspersed in the IGLV locus, *Nucleic Acids Res., 17*:3975 (1989).

58. G. Matthyssens and T. H. Rabbitts, Structure and multiplicity of genes for the human immunoglobulin heavy chain variable region, *Proc. Natl. Acad. Sci. USA, 77*:6561 (1980).

59. G. Rechavi, D. Ram, L. Glazer, R. Zakut, and D. Givol, Evolutionary aspects of immunoglobulin heavy chain variable region (VH) gene subgroups, *Proc. Natl. Acad. Sci. USA, 80*:855 (1983).

60. N. Takahashi, T. Noma, and T. Honjo, Rearranged immunoglobulin heavy chain variable region (VH) pseudogene that deletes the second complementarity-determining region, *Proc. Natl. Acad. Sci. USA, 81*:5194 (1984).

61. D. L. Bentley, Most kappa immunoglobulin mRNA in human lymphocytes is homologous to a small family of germ-line V genes, *Nature, 307*:77 (1984).

62. H. G. Klobeck, A. Solomon, and H. G. Zachau, Contribution of human V kappa II germ-line genes to light-chain diversity, *Nature, 309*:73 (1984).

63. H. R. Jaenichen, M. Pech, W. Lindenmaier, N. Wildgruber, and H. G. Zachau, Composite human VK genes and a model of their evolution, *Nucleic Acids Res., 12*:5249 (1984).

64. M. Pech and H. G. Zachau, Immunoglobulin genes of different subgroups are interdigitated within the VK locus, *Nucleic Acids Res., 12*:9229 (1984).

65. B. A. Malynn, J. E. Berman, G. D. Yancopoulos, C. A. Bona, and F. W. Alt, Expression of the immunoglobulin heavy-chain variable gene repertoire, *Curr. Top. Microbiol. Immunol., 135*:75 (1987).

66. A. Shen, C. Humphries, P. Tucker, and F. Blattner, Human heavy-chain variable region gene family nonrandomly rearranged in familial chronic lymphocytic leukemia, *Proc. Natl. Acad. Sci. USA, 84*:8563 (1987).

67. H. W. Schroeder, Jr., J. L. Hillson, and R. M. Perlmutter, Early restriction of the human antibody repertoire, *Science, 238*:791 (1987).

68. C. Milstein, Linked groups of residues in immunoglobulin k chains, *Nature, 216*:330 (1967).

69. A. C. Wang, H. H. Fudenberg, and J. V. Wells, A new subgroup of the Kappa chain variable region associated with anti-Pr cold agglutinins, *Nature New Biol., 243*:126 (1973).

70. L. Hood and D. Ein, Immunologlobulin lambda chain structure: Two genes, one polypeptide chain, *Nature, 220*:764 (1968).

71. F. W. Tischendorf, M. M. Tischendorf, and E. F. Osserman, Subgroup-specific antigenic marker on immunoglobulin lambda chains: Identification of three subtypes of the variable region, *J. Immunol., 105*:1033 (1970).

72. A. Solomon, Light chains of immunoglobulins: Structural-genetic correlates, *Blood, 68*:603 (1986).

73. R. J. Poljak, Three-dimensional structure, function and genetic control of immunoglobulins, *Nature, 256*:373 (1975).

74. E. A. Padlan and D. R. Davies, Variability of three-dimensional structure in immunoglobulins, *Proc. Natl. Acad. Sci. USA, 72*:819 (1975).

75. D. M. Segal, E. A. Padlan, G. H. Cohen, S. Rudikoff, M. Potter, and D. R. Davies, The three-dimensional structure of a phosphorylcholine-binding

mouse immunoglobulin Fab and the nature of the antigen binding site, *Proc. Natl. Acad. Sci. USA, 71*:4298 (1974).

76. R. J. Poljak, X-ray diffraction studies of immunoglobulins, *Adv. Immunol., 21*:1 (1975).

77. P. M. Alzari, M. B. Lascombe, and R. J. Poljak, Three-dimensional structure of antibodies, *Ann. Rev. Immunol., 6*:555 (1988).

78. A. Solomon, Light chains of human immunoglobulins, *Methods Enzymol., 116*:101 (1985).

79. A. Solomon and D. T. Weiss, Serologically defined V region subgroups of human lambda light chains, *J. Immunol., 139*:824 (1987).

80. A. Solomon, D. T. Weiss, S. D. Macy, and R. A. Antonucci, Immunocytochemical detection of kappa and lambda light chain V region subgroups in human B-cell malignancies, *Am. J. Pathol., 137*:855 (1990).

81. J. L. Greenstein, A. Solomon, and G. N. Abraham, Monoclonal antibodies reactive with idiotypic and variable-region specific determinants on human immunoglobulins, *Immunology, 51*:17 (1984).

82. D. N. Posnett, R. Wisniewolski, B. Pernis, and H. G. Kunkel, Dissection of the human antigammaglobulin idiotype system with monoclonal antibodies, *Scand. J. Immunol., 23*:169 (1986).

83. G. J. Silverman, D. A. Carson, A. Solomon, and S. Fong, Human kappa light chain subgroup analysis with synthetic peptide-induced antisera, *J. Immunol. Methods, 95*:249 (1986).

84. G. J. Silverman, R. D. Goldfien, P. Chen, R. A. Mageed, R. Jefferis, F. Goni, B. Frangione, S. Fong, and D. A. Carson, Idiotypic and subgroup analysis of human monoclonal rheumatoid factors. Implications for structural and genetic basis of autoantibodies in humans, *J. Clin. Invest., 82*:469 (1988).

85. G. J. Silverman and D. A. Carson, Structural characterization of human monoclonal cold agglutinins: Evidence for a distinct primary sequence-defined VH4 idiotype, *Eur. J. Immunol., 20*:351 (1990).

86. P. Early, H. Huang, M. Davis, K. Calame, and L. Hood, An immunoglobulin heavy chain variable region gene is generated from three segments of DNA: VH, D and JH, *Cell, 19*:981 (1980).

87. H. G. Kunkel, V. Agnello, R. J. Winchester, J. D. Capra, and J. M. Kehoe, Cross-idiotypic specificity among monoclonal IgM proteins with anti-globulin activity, *Proc. Natl. Acad. Sci. USA, 71*:4032 (1974).

88. D. A. Carson and S. Fong, A common idiotope on human rheumatoid factors identified by a hybridoma antibody, *Mol. Immunol., 20*:1081 (1983).

89. R. A. Mageed, M. Dearlove, D. M. Goodall, and R. Jefferis, Immunogenic and antigenic epitopes of immunoglobulins XVII—Monoclonal antibodies reactive with common and restricted idiotopes to the heavy chain of human rheumatoid factors, *Rheumatol. Int., 6*:179 (1986).

90. J. L. Pasquali, A. M. Knapp, A. Farradji, and A. Weryha, Mapping of four light chain-associated idiotopes of a human monoclonal rheumatoid factor, *J. Immunol., 139*:818 (1987).

91. H. G. Kunkel, R. J. Winchester, F. G. Joslin, and J. D. Capra, Similarities

in the light chains of anti-gamma-globulins showing cross-idiotypic specificities, *J. Exp. Med., 139*:128 (1974).

92. D. W. Andrews and J. D. Capra, Complete amino acid sequence of variable domains from two monoclonal human anti-gamma globulins of the Wa cross-idiotypic group: Suggestion that the J segments are involved in the structural correlate of the idiotype, *Proc. Natl. Acad. Sci. USA, 78*:3799 (1981).

93. D. K. Ledford, F. Goni, M. Pizzolato, E. C. Franklin, A. Solomon, and B. Frangione, Preferential association of kappa IIIb light chains with monoclonal human IgM kappa autoantibodies, *J. Immunol., 131*:1322 (1983).

94. J. D. Capra and J. M. Kehoe, Structure of antibodies with shared idiotypy: The complete sequence of the heavy chain variable regions of two immunoglobulin M anti-gamma globulins, *Proc. Natl. Acad. Sci. USA, 71*:4032 (1974).

95. B. Pons-Estel, F. Goni, A. Solomon, and B. Frangione, Sequence similarities among kappa IIIb chains of monoclonal human IgM kappa autoantibodies, *J. Exp. Med., 160*:893 (1984).

96. J. D. Capra, J. M. Kehoe, R. C. Williams, Jr., T. Feizi, and H. G. Kunkel, Light chain sequences of human IgM cold agglutinins, *Proc. Natl. Acad. Sci. USA, 69*:40 (1972).

97. T. J. Kipps, S. Fong, E. Tomhave, P. P. Chen, R. D. Goldfien, and D. A. Carson, High-frequency expression of a conserved kappa light-chain variable-region gene in chronic lymphocytic leukemia, *Proc. Natl. Acad. Sci. USA, 84*:2916 (1987).

98. T. J. Kipps, S. Fong, E. Tomhave, P. P. Chen, R. D. Goldfien, and D. A. Carson, Immunoglobulin V gene utilization in CLL, in *Chronic Lymphocytic Leukemia: Recent Progress and Future Direction* (R. P. Gale and K. R. Rai, eds.), Alan R. Liss, New York, p. 115 (1987).

99. T. J. Kipps, B. A. Robbins, P. Kuster, and D. A. Carson, Autoantibody-associated cross-reactive idiotypes expressed at high frequency in chronic lymphocytic leukemia relative to B-cell lymphomas of follicular center cell origin, *Blood, 72*:422 (1988).

100. T. J. Kipps, B. A. Robbins, A. Tefferi, G. Meisenholder, P. M. Banks, and D. A. Carson, CD5-positive B-cell malignancies frequently express cross-reactive idiotypes associated with IgM autoantibodies, *Am. J. Pathol., 136*: 809 (1990).

101. M. Ono, C. G. Winearls, N. Amos, D. Grennan, A. Gharavi, D. K. Peters, and J. G. P. Sissons, Monoclonal antibodies to restricted and cross-reactive idiotopes on monoclonal rheumatoid factors and their recognition of idiotope-positive cells, *Eur. J. Immunol., 17*:373 (1987).

102. C. G. Winearls and J. G. P. Sissons, Use of idiotype markers for cellular detection of monoclonal rheumatoid factor, *Springer Semin. Immunopathol., 10*:67 (1988).

103. L. F. Pratt, R. Szubin, D. A. Carson, and T. J. Kipps, Molecular characterization of a supratypic cross reactive idiotype associated with IgM autoantibodies, *J. Immunol., 147*:2041 (1991).

104. P. G. Cachia, A. E. Dewar, A. S. Krajewski, G. Stockdill, L. C. Walker, and J. A. Habeshaw, Distribution of a set of idiotopes detected by a monoclonal antibody panel in 42 cases of chronic lymphocytic leukaemia: Definition of potential targets for immunotherapy, *Br. J. Haematol., 72*:150 (1989).

105. E. M. Swisher, D. L. Shawler, H. A. Collins, A. Bustria, S. Hart, C. Bloomfield, R. A. Miller, and I. Royston, The expression of shared idiotypes in chronic lymphocytic leukemia and small lymphocytic lymphoma, *Blood, 77*: 1977 (1991).

106. T. J. Kipps, E. Tomhave, L. F. Pratt, S. Duffy, P. P. Chen, and D. A. Carson, Developmentally restricted VH gene expressed at high frequency in chronic lymphocytic leukemia, *Proc. Natl. Acad. Sci. USA, 86*:5913 (1989).

107. L. Borche, A. Lim, J. L. Binet, and G. Dighiero, Evidence that chronic lymphocytic leukemia B lymphocytes are frequently committed to production of natural autoantibodies, *Blood, 76*:562 (1990).

108. M. Deane and J. D. Norton, Immunoglobulin heavy chain variable region family usage is independent of tumor cell phenotype in human B lineage leukemias, *Eur. J. Immunol., 20*:2209 (1990).

109. R. Mayer, T. Logtenberg, J. Strauchen, A. Dimitriu-Bona, L. Mayer, S. Mechanic, N. Chiorazzi, L. Borche, G. Dighiero, A. Mannheimer-Lory, B. Diamond, F. Alt, and C. Bona, CD5 and immunoglobulin V gene expression in B-cell lymphomas and chronic lymphocytic leukemia, *Blood, 75*:1518 (1990).

110. F. Matsuda, K. H. Lee, S. Nakai, T. Sato, M. Kodaira, S. Q. Zong, H. Ohno, S. Fukuhara, and T. Honjo, Dispersed localization of D segments in the human immunoglobulin heavy-chain locus, *EMBO J., 7*:1047 (1988).

111. M. Deane and J. D. Norton, Immunoglobulin heavy chain gene rearrangement involving V-V region recombination, *Nucleic Acids Res., 18*:1652 (1990).

112. O. Axelrod, G. J. Silverman, V. Dev, R. Kyle, D. A. Carson, and T. J. Kipps, Idiotypic cross reactivity of immunoglobulins expressed in Waldenstroms' macroglobulinemia, chronic lymphocytic leukemia, and mantle zone lymphocytes of secondary B cell follicles, *Blood, 77*:1484 (1991).

113. C. G. Humphries, A. Shen, W. A. Kuziel, J. D. Capra, F. R. Blattner, and P. W. Tucker, A new human immunoglobulin VH family preferentially rearranged in immature B-cell tumours, *Nature, 331*:446 (1988).

114. I. Sanz, P. Kelly, C. Williams, S. Scholl, P. Tucker, and J. D. Capra, The smaller human VH gene families display remarkably little polymorphism, *EMBO J., 8*:3741 (1989).

115. V. Pascual, K. Victor, D. Lelsz, M. B. Spellerberg, T. J. Hamblin, K. M. Thompson, I. Randen, J. Natvig, J. D. Capra, and F. K. Stevenson, Nucleotide sequence analysis of the V regions of two IgM cold agglutinins. Evidence that the VH4-21 gene segment is responsible for the major cross-reactive idiotype, *J. Immunol., 146*:4385 (1991).

116. F. K. Stevenson, G. J. Smith, J. North, T. J. Hamblin, and M. J. Glennie, Identification of normal B-cell counterparts of neoplastic cells which secrete cold agglutinins of anti-I and anti-i specificity, *Br. J. Haematol., 72*:9 (1989).

117. T. J. Kipps, E. Tomhave, P. P. Chen, and D. A. Carson, Autoantibody-associated kappa light chain variable region gene expressed in chronic lymphocytic leukemia with little or no somatic mutation. Implications for etiology and immunotherapy, *J. Exp. Med., 167*:840 (1988).

118. V. Radoux, P. P. Chen, J. A. Sorge, and D. A. Carson, A conserved human germline V kappa gene directly encodes rheumatoid factor light chains, *J. Exp. Med., 164*:2119 (1986).

119. L. Z. Rassenti, L. F. Pratt, P. P. Chen, D. A. Carson, and T. J. Kipps, Autoantibody-encoding kappa light chain genes frequently rearranged in lambda light chain expressing chronic lymphocytic leukemia, *J. Immunol., 147*:1060 (1991).

120. L. E. Silberstein, S. Litwin, and C. E. Carmack, Relationship of variable region genes expressed by a human B cell lymphoma secreting pathologic anti-Pr2 erythrocyte autoantibodies, *J. Exp. Med., 169*:1631 (1989).

121. M. M. Newkirk and J. D. Capra, Restricted usage of immunoglobulin variable-region genes in human autoantibodies, in *Immunoglobulin Genes* (T. Honjo, F. W. Alt, and T. Rabbitts, eds.), Academic Press, New York, p. 215 (1989).

122. L. F. Pratt, L. Rassenti, J. Larrick, B. Robbins, P. Banks, and T. J. Kipps, Immunoglobulin gene expression in small lymphocytic lymphoma with little or no somatic hypermutation, *J. Immunol., 143*:699 (1989).

123. T. C. Meeker, J. C. Grimaldi, R. O'Rourke, J. Loeb, G. Juliusson, and S. Einhorn, Lack of detectable somatic hypermutation in the V region of the Ig H chain gene of a human chronic B lymphocytic leukemia, *J. Immunol., 141*:3994 (1988).

124. R. Levy, S. Levy, M. L. Cleary, W. Carroll, S. Kon, J. Bird, and J. Sklar, Somatic mutation in human B-cell tumors, *Immunol. Rev., 96*:43 (1987).

125. M. Menon, H. G. Drexler, and J. Minowada, Heterogeneity of marker expression in B-cell leukemias and its diagnostic significance, *Leuk. Res., 10*: 25 (1986).

126. C. Liendo, L. Danieu, A. Al-Katib, and B. Koziner, Phenotypic analysis by flow cytometry of surface light chains and B and T cell antigens in lymph nodes involved with non-Hodgkin's lymphoma, *Am. J. Med., 79*:445 (1985).

127. R. Levy, S. Levy, S. L. Brown, S. Kon, and W. Carroll, Anti-idiotype antibodies reveal the existence of somatic mutation in human B cell lymphoma, *Monogr. Allergy, 22*:194 (1987).

128. M. Apel and C. Berek, Somatic mutations in antibodies expressed by germinal centre B cells early after primary immunization, *Int. Immunol., 2*:813 (1990).

129. J. Jacob, R. Kassir, and G. Kelsoe, In situ studies of the primary immune response to (4-hydroxy-3-nitrophenyl)acetyl. I. The architecture and dynamics of responding cell populations, *J. Exp. Med., 173*:1165 (1991).

130. T. J. Kipps, the CD5 B Cell, *Adv. Immunol., 47*:117 (1989).

131. F. Caligaris-Cappio, M. Gobbi, M. Bofill, and G. Janossy, Infrequent normal B lymphocytes express features of B-chronic lymphocytic leukemia, *J. Exp. Med., 155*:623 (1982).

132. M. Gobbi, F. Caligaris-Cappio, and G. Janossy, Normal equivalent cells of B cell malignancies: Analysis with monoclonal antibodies, *Br. J. Haematol., 54*:393 (1983).
133. N. Gadol and K. A. Ault, Phenotypic and functional characterization of human Leu1 (CD5) cells, *Immunol. Rev., 93*:23 (1986).
134. R. R. Hardy and K. Hayakawa, Development and physiology of Ly-1 B and its human homolog, Leu-1 B, *Immunol. Rev., 93*:53 (1986).
135. T. J. Kipps and J. H. Vaughan, Genetic influence on the levels of circulating CD5 B lymphocytes, *J. Immunol., 139*:1060 (1987).
136. T. J. Kipps and S. F. Duffy, Relationship of the CD5 B cell to human tonsillar lymphocytes that express autoantibody-associated cross reactive idiotypes, *J. Clin. Invest., 87*:2087 (1991).
137. M. Bofill, G. Janossy, M. Janossa, G. D. Burford, G. J. Seymour, P. Wernet, and E. Kelemen, Human B cell development. II. Subpopulations in the human fetus, *J. Immunol., 134*:1531 (1985).
138. J. H. Antin, S. G. Emerson, P. Martin, N. Gadol, and K. A. Ault, Leu-1 + (CD5 +) B cells. A major lymphoid subpopulation in fetal spleen: Phenotypic and functional studies, *J. Immunol., 136*:505 (1986).
139. T. J. Kipps, B. A. Robbins, and D. A. Carson, Uniform high frequency expression of autoantibody-associated cross reactive idiotypes in the primary B cell follicles of human fetal spleen, *J. Exp. Med., 171*:189 (1990).
140. I. Forster, H. Gu, and K. Rajewsky, Germline antibody V regions as determinants of clonal persistence and malignant growth in the B cell compartment, *EMBO J., 7*:3693 (1988).
141. D. Tarlinton, A. M. Stall, and L. A. Herzenberg, Repetitive usage of immunoglobulin VH and D gene segments in CD5 + Ly-1 B clones of (NZB NZW) F1 mice, *EMBO J., 7*:3705 (1988).
142. L. Reininger, P. Ollier, P. Poncet, A. Kaushik, and J. C. Jaton, Novel V genes encode virtually identical variable regions of six murine monoclonal anti-bromelain-treated red blood cell autoantibodies, *J. Immunol., 138*:316 (1987).
143. I. Sanz, P. Casali, J. W. Thomas, A. L. Notkins, and J. D. Capra, Nucleotide sequences of eight human natural autoantibody VH regions reveals apparent restricted use of VH families, *J. Immunol., 142*:4054 (1989).
144. M. Nakamura, S. E. Burastero, Y. Ueki, J. W. Larrick, A. L. Notkins, and P. Casali, Probing the normal and autoimmune B cell repertoire with Epstein-Barr virus. Frequency of B cells producing monoreactive high affinity autoantibodies in patients with Hashimoto's disease and systemic lupus erythematosus, *J. Immunol., 141*:4165 (1988).
145. I. Sanz, H. Dang, M. Takei, N. Talal, and J. D. Capra, VH sequence of a human anti-Sm autoantibody. Evidence that autoantibodies can be unmutated copies of germline genes, *J. Immunol., 142*:883 (1989).
146. R. Baccala, T. V. Quang, M. Gilbert, T. Ternynck, and S. Avrameas, Two murine natural polyreactive autoantibodies are encoded by nonmutated germ-line genes, *Proc. Natl. Acad. Sci. USA, 86*:4624 (1989).
147. P. Casali, S. E. Burastero, M. Nakamura, G. Inghirami, and A. L. Notkins,

Human lymphocytes making rheumatoid factor and antibody to belong to Leu-1 + and B-cell subset, *Science, 236*:77 (1987).

148. R. R. Hardy, K. Hayakawa, M. Shimizu, K. Yamasaki, and T. Kishimoto, Rheumatoid factor secretion from human Leu-1 + B cells, *Science, 236*:81 (1987).

149. J. L. Preud'homme and M. Seligmann, Anti-human immunoglobulin G activity of membrane-bound immunoglobulin M in lymphoproliferative disorders, *Proc. Natl. Acad. Sci. USA, 69*:2132 (1972).

150. P. Youinou, L. Mackenzie, B. M. Broker, D. I. Isenberg, A. Drogou-Lelong, A. Gentric, and P. M. Lydyard, The importance of CD5-positive B cells in nonorgan-specific autoimmune diseases, *Scand. J. Rheumatol. Suppl., 76*: 243 (1988).

151. B. M. Broker, A. Klajman, P. Youinou, J. Jouquan, C. P. Worman, J. Murphy, L. Mackenzie, R. Quartey-Papafio, M. Blaschek, P. Collins, S. Lal, and P. M. Lydyard, Chronic lymphocytic leukemic (CLL) cells secrete multispecific autoantibodies, *J. Autoimmun., 1*:469 (1988).

152. W. A. Allebes, F. W. Preijers, C. Haanen, and P. J. Capel, The development of non-responsiveness to immunotherapy with monoclonal anti-idiotypic antibodies in a patient with B-CLL, *Br. J. Haematol., 70*:295 (1988).

153. M. A. de Rie, D. J. van Heemstra, P. C. Huijgens, W. P. Zeijlemaker, T. A. Out, C. J. Melief, and A. E. von dem Borne, Production of mouse monoclonal antibodies for the analysis of idiotypes in serum of patients with chronic lymphatic leukaemia, *Br. J. Haematol., 68*:11 (1988).

154. R. O. Dillman, J. Beauregard, D. L. Shawler, S. E. Halpern, M. Markman, K. P. Ryan, S. M. Baird, and M. Clutter, Continuous infusion of T101 monoclonal antibody in chronic lymphocytic leukemia and cutaneous T-cell lymphoma, *J. Biol. Response Mod., 5*:394 (1986).

155. D. L. Shawler, J. Beauregard, S. E. Halpern, S. M. Baird, and R. O. Dillman, Tissue distribution and serum kinetics of T101 monoclonal antibody during passive anti-cancer therapy, *Clin. Immunol. Immunopathol., 41*:43 (1986).

156. W. Allebes, R. Knops, M. Herold, C. Huber, C. Haanen, and P. Capel, Immunotherapy with monoclonal anti-idiotypic antibodies: Tumour reduction and lymphokine production, *Leuk. Res., 15*:215 (1991).

157. T. Meeker, J. Lowder, M. L. Cleary, S. Stewart, R. Warnke, J. Sklar, and R. Levy, Emergence of idiotype variants during treatment of B-cell lymphoma with anti-idiotype antibodies, *N. Engl. J. Med., 312*:1658 (1985).

158. S. L. Giardina, R. W. Schroff, T. J. Kipps, C. S. Woodhouse, P. G. Abrams, H. C. Rager, A. C. Morgan, Jr., and K. A. Foon, The generation of monoclonal anti-idiotype antibodies to human B cell-derived leukemias and lymphomas, *J. Immunol., 135*:653 (1985).

7

Pathogenesis of the Immunodeficiency in B-Cell Chronic Lymphocytic Leukemia

Robert Foa
University of Torino, Torino, Italy

INTRODUCTION

In most patients suffering from B-cell chronic lymphocytic leukemia (B-CLL), the clinical course of the disease is associated with a variety of often severe complications, which include infections and secondary neoplasias. Infections are generally due to bacteria and are influenced by the degree of hypogammaglobulinemia. In the more advanced stages of the disease they may also be contributed by the neutropenia due to bone marrow failure and/or to cytotoxic therapy, and often result in terminal pneumonia. Overwhelming pneumococcal infection may occur after splenectomy; this worrying complication may be prevented by long-term prophylaxis with penicillin. Viral infections, resulting from a deficient cell-mediated immunity, may prove difficult to document because specific antibodies are not a reliable indicator of infection in B-CLL. Herpes zoster is common and can occasionally result in disseminated varicella zoster. A hemophagocytic syndrome resembling histiocytic medullary reticulosis has been reported and is probably due to intercurrent infections caused by DNA viruses.

Within the spectrum of B-cell chronic lymphoproliferative disorders, it has been clearly established that B-CLL patients are those who more frequently show at some stage during the course of their disease more or less severe signs of immunodeficiency. Studies carried out over the years have in fact progressively and convincingly established that multiple abnormalities may be encountered within the residual nonneoplastic B lymphocytes, as well as within the T- and cytotoxic cell compartments. Since these defects most often occur in the more advanced stages and since in B-CLL the clinical course of the disease is frequently complicated by infectious episodes, and since a higher-than-normal incidence of associated neoplasias has been reported, it has been suggested that the immunodeficiency associated with B-CLL may play a contributory role in the occurrence of some of these often fatal complications.

In this chapter we shall review the main findings that have led us to recognize the immunodeficient status of patients suffering from B-CLL and compare it with other closely related disorders. Attention will be focused on the possible involvement of these abnormalities in the course of the disease, as well as on their primary or secondary origin. Furthermore, in view of the progressive recognition of the close mechanisms that govern the process of cell-to-cell interaction, and of the important regulatory role played by different cytokines, the possibility that the latter may also be directly or indirectly involved in the pathogenesis of the immunodeficiency will be discussed. Finally, the role of treatment, as well as the potential of overcoming this often life-threatening situation, will be presented.

B-CELL ABNORMALITIES

For many years it has been well recognized that patients with B-CLL show a variable degree of hypogammaglobulinemia, with a progressive decrease of the levels of immunoglobulins (Ig), which may involve one, two, or all three main classes of Ig (1–4). The IgA are usually the first to be decreased, followed subsequently by a reduction in IgM and IgG (3,4). When the level of hypogammaglobulinemia has been correlated with the stage of the disease, it has been shown that the reduction in the levels of circulating Ig tends to worsen with the progression of the disease (3), thus rendering patients with advanced disease more susceptible to infective complications. A similar profound humoral immunodeficiency also occurs in B-cell chronic prolymphocytic leukemia (B-PLL) (5). Interestingly, in hairy cell leukemia (HCL), another closely related chronic B-cell disorder, the levels of serum Ig are most often within the normal range (6). As will be discussed below, the functional status of the T-cell compartment in HCL seems to differ considerably from that of B-CLL and B-PLL patients.

Also more frequently than in other B-cell disorders, in approximately 5–10% of B-CLL cases small monoclonal bands may be found in the serum.

These are most often IgM. Using more sensitive methods, it has been shown that small monoclonal bands of heavy or light Ig chains may be demonstrated in the serum and/or urine of a relatively high proportion of cases (7,8). Using such an approach, monoclonal proteins may be detected simultaneously in blood and urine in up to 25% of B-CLL cases. The Ig light chain of the monoclonal band corresponds to that expressed on the surface of the neoplastic B-cell clone.

Although the progressively depressed level of circulating Ig is contributed largely by the progressive decrease in normal B-cell function, following the overwhelming neoplastic B-cell expansion, over the last decade it has been clearly shown that other lymphocyte populations, namely the T-cell compartment, are most likely to play an important contributory role through multiple phenotypic and functional defects. This aspect will be dealt with in detail below, together with the possible involvement of specific cytokine networks.

T-CELL ABNORMALITIES

Phenotypic and functional abnormalities within the residual T-cell compartment of B-CLL patients have stimulated a considerable deal of interest over the years. This issue has gained relevance in the context of the rapidly developing evidence of the heterogeneity of normal T lymphocytes, and has become affordable as a consequence of the availability of the necessary tools to isolate the relatively small residual T-cell population in B-CLL. Thus, investigators are now able to carry out the appropriate tests to evaluate the phenotypic and functional features of the different T-cell subsets. The importance of this area of study has gained further credit in the same years owing to the progressive recognition of the close interactions between T- and B-cell populations and of the regulatory role played by T-cell subsets on the process of B-cell proliferation, differentiation, and maturation into antibody-producing plasma cells.

The first suggestion of an involvement of the T-cell compartment in B-CLL stemmed from the early recognition that while the percentage of T lymphocytes was always reduced in patients with B-CLL, the absolute number of T cells was instead increased (9). When these values were correlated with the clinical stage of the disease according to Rai's classification (10), it was found that the percentage of T lymphocytes progressively decreased as the stage increased, while the absolute number of circulating T cells tends to be significantly enhanced from the early stages of the disease (3). As mentioned above, the great methodological improvements in the 1980s allowed extensive studies aimed at investigating the features of this quantitative increase in T lymphocytes occurring in B-CLL. These have been addressed at unraveling both the phenotypic distribution of the different T-cell subsets, as well as the functional properties of such cells. Conclusions on the "functional" ability of the cells based solely on phenotypic analyses would not have been appropriate, and misleading interpretations could have been drawn.

T-Cell Subset Distribution

The first conclusive demonstration that a defect could in fact be identified within the T-cell population of B-CLL was reported by Kay et al. (11), who showed that the distribution of the circulating T-lymphocyte subsets based on the expression of the receptors for $T\mu$ (helper/inducer phenotype) and $T\gamma$ (suppressor/cytotoxic phenotype) was abnormal in the majority of B-CLL patients. In more detail, a significant increase in $T\gamma$ cells and a reduction in $T\mu$ cells has been described in the study reported above and was soon after confirmed in another report (12). Following the advent of monoclonal antibodies, these findings have been further confirmed and a correlation between T-cell subset distribution and clinical stage of the disease has been reported (13–15). While the percentage of circulating CD4-positive cells is usually reduced and that of CD8-positive cells is increased, with an overall decrease of the CD4 : CD8 ratio, the absolute number of both T-cell subsets is most often increased in patients throughout all stages of the disease. The possibility has also been suggested that this marked distributional abnormality of peripheral blood lymphocytes may be partially contributed by the preferential homing of CD4-positive cell subset in the bone marrow (16). While a similar phenotypic impairment appears to occur in B-PLL, the findings are less consistent in HCL, though an imbalanced CD4 : CD8 ratio has been described, particularly in patients with active disease (17).

More recent studies have shown that B-CLL patients have increased absolute numbers of phenotypically activated (DR +) CD4- and CD8-positive cells (18). The possibility, suggested by the same authors (18), that patients in early-stage disease may have elevated levels of circulating T-suppressor/inducer cells (CD45RA + , CD4 +), compatible with a clinical situation of chronic antigenic stimulation and accumulation of memory helper/inducer cells, has not been confirmed in a more recent report (19).

T-Cell Functional Studies

Necessarily, the phenotypic alterations observed within the T-cell population of B-CLL patients needed to be verified in a functional setting, in an attempt to clarify the true impact of these findings. The data accumulated over the years are consistent with the suggestion that, in B-CLL, several functional abnormalities take place within the residual T-cell population. These encompass a depressed or delayed response to mitogens and antigens (20,21), a diminished mixed lymphocyte reaction (22), and a reduced T-lymphocyte colony-forming capacity (23,24). Purification experiments have ruled out the possibility that these functional defects could be due simply to the dilution within the largely predominant neoplastic B-cell clone. Similarly to the T-cell subset distribution, the functional activity of the T lymphocytes also seems to decrease with disease progression, with a partial sparing in early-stage patients (25). When the issue of more specific functional properties was approached, evidence was provided (from a pokeweed-mitogen driven system) that a decreased helper capacity was present together with a normal or increased suppressor function (26–29).

Although these functional defects may well be operational in vivo, in view of the knowledge that the above-described functions are, in normal blood, largely a property of the CD4-positive subset and that the latter is proportionally decreased in the majority of B-CLL, work had to be performed to clarify whether the abnormalities observed could not be due simply to the reversed CD4 : CD8 ratio. The necessary purification experiments point, however, to a true defect within the helper T-cell subset, in terms of both in-vitro colony growth and helper capacity (24,29,30).

Though limited studies have been carried out in B-PLL, functional T-cell abnormalities similar to those observed in B-CLL have been reported (25). On the other hand, the scenery appears quite different in HCL, where the response to phytohemagglutinin (PHA), as well as the T-colony-forming capacity and helper activity, are usually preserved (31,32). As discussed below, it is tempting to suggest that these differences in T-cell functional repertoire between B-CLL/B-PLL and HCL may play a role in the different levels of circulating serum Ig observed in these conditions. The major phenotypic and functional properties of the T-cell compartment in the different chronic B-cell leukemias are summarized in Table 1.

A heterogeneous pattern of T-cell function has been observed in T-cell chronic lymphoproliferative disorders. Inevitably, the studies carried out are unable, in the great majority of cases, to discriminate between pathologic and residual normal T cells, since the latter usually cannot be isolated on the basis of the membrane phenotype. Thus, in general, the functional analyses performed in chronic T-cell disorders reflect the properties of the leukemic population. Table 2 illustrates the main phenotypic and functional characteristics in the different diseases. In the clonal expansions of granular lymphocytes (revealed by the monoclonal rearrangement of the T-cell receptor genes), which most often display a CD3+, CD4−, CD8+ membrane phenotype, the cells generally show a depressed response to PHA

Table 1 T- and Cytotoxic-Cell Compartment in B-Cell Chronic
Lymphoproliferative Disorders

Disease	CD4 : CD8 ratio	PHA TI[a]	Helper function	T-colony growth	NK[b]/K[c]	LAK[d]
B-CLL	Reversed	Low	Low	Low[e]	Low	Low
B-PLL	Reversed	Low	Low	Low	Low	Low
HCL	Reversed in active disease	Normal	Normal	Normal	Often low	Often low

[a]TI = transformation index.
[b]NK = natural killer.
[c]K = antibody-mediated killer.
[d]LAK = lymphokine activated killer.
[e]Partial sparing in stage 0 patients.

and T-colony growth, an absent or reduced helper function, and a heterogeneous suppressor function (33–35). T-cell prolymphocytic leukemia (T-PLL), adult T-cell leukemia/lymphoma (ATLL), and Sézary syndrome almost always express the CD4 antigen. Nonetheless, marked functional differences have been recorded with particular reference to the helper activity. In fact, while T-PLL may lack any functional capacity or display helper function (36), this is a characteristic feature of practically all Sézary syndromes (37,38). Rare cases with suppressor function have also been reported (39). ATLL cells, despite the expression of a CD4-positive phenotype, always reveal a suppressor function (40,41).

CYTOTOXIC COMPARTMENT

Several abnormalities have been reported within the cytotoxic compartment of B-CLL patients. These include a depressed natural killer (NK) and

Table 2 Phenotypic and Functional Features of T-Cell Chronic
Lymphoproliferative Disorders

Disease	CD4	CD8	PHA TI[a]	Help	Suppress	NK	K	LAK
LGL expansion[b]	−	+	−	−	−/+	−/+	+	−
T-PLL	+	−/+	−	+/−	−	−	−	−
ATLL	+	−	−	−	+	−	−	−
Sézary	+	−	−/+	+(−)	−(+)	−/+	−	−

[a]TI = transformation index.
[b]LGL = large granular lymphocytes.

antibody-mediated (K) killer activity (42,43), as well as a reduced capacity of the cytotoxic effector cells to bind the target (43). These defects of the cytotoxic compartment have been confirmed in B-CLL with the use of monoclonal antibodies. With the exception of the CD57 antigen, which shows a significantly higher expression in B-CLL compared to normal lymphocytes (15,42), other, more specific reagents have shown a markedly reduced reactivity in B-CLL (44). This reduced reactivity has been shown to correlate well with the NK function (44). On morphological grounds, the suggestion that NK cells in B-CLL may have defective azurophilic granules (45) helps to explain the depressed natural cytotoxic activity. Interestingly, it has been shown that a large proportion of CD4-positive cells in B-CLL are characterized by granular lymphocytes (46). This expanded population, barely found in normal subjects, may provide a further explanation for the numerous functional T-cell defects reported in B-CLL.

More recently, the lymphokine-activated killer (LAK) cell compartment has also been investigated in B-CLL. The results obtained indicate that B-CLL patients exhibit an overall significantly depressed LAK function against the NK-resistant Raji cell line compared to that of normal peripheral blood lymphocytes (47). More relevant in terms of control of tumor cell growth and of the potential clinical use of in-vivo IL-2-based immunotherapeutic protocols, leukemic B-CLL cells appear to be largely insensitive to the lytic action of autologous LAK effectors (47). Competition experiments carried in the same study suggest that the defect is not related to the recognition of the target, but rather to a postbinding lytic abnormality.

The analysis of the cytotoxic compartment in the other B- and T-cell chronic lymphoproliferative disorders has substantially shown similar results (Tables 1 and 2). Interestingly, while most untreated HCL patients display a significantly depressed NK function (48), this may be notably improved and frequently restored following prolonged treatment with interferon-α (49). This observation has not been so far reported in B-CLL. In practically all chronic lymphoid malignancies, the LAK compartment is markedly defective, in terms of both activity against allogeneic targets and autologous killing (47). In our experience, only in a proportion of HCL cases could we find some degree of lysis against the autologous pathologic cell population (47).

CYTOKINE NETWORK

The evidence that cytokines and/or growth factors may play a primary role in the process of growth, activation, and differentiation of normal and neoplastic hemopoietic cells has become a growing reality over the last few years. Support for this possibility has stemmed largely from the recognition of the close interactions between apparently distinct cell subsets based primarily on a cytokine network. The availability of cloned material, specific antibodies, bioassays and kits for serological or cell culture supernatants, probes for mRNA expression analyses, receptor determination tools, etc., allow one to verify the role played by cytokines and growth factors in the establishment and/or clinical course of acute and chronic leukemias.

In the context of chronic lymphoproliferative disorders, the possible involvement of different cytokines has been suggested. In B-CLL (50) it has been shown that IL-1 and IL-6 may be released by the leukemic clone and that the latter may also constitutively express the mRNA for IL-6 (51,52). Since neither IL-1 nor IL-6 seem to induce a proliferative signal on B-CLL cells, their role in this disease still needs to be fully understood. IL-4 has been suggested as an important regulatory factor, since it is capable of inhibiting the IL-2-dependent proliferation of B-CLL lymphocytes to a further extent than is observed with normal B cells (53). A relevant role for tumor necrosis factor (TNF) alpha as an autocrine growth factor in B-cell chronic lymphoproliferative disorders has been postulated. Based on detectable serum levels, constitutive release by the pathologic cells, mRNA expression, and proliferation experiments, it has been suggested that TNF-α may exert a regulatory effect on the leukemic clone in B-CLL (54,55).

With regard to the different cytokines and growth factors, it is likely that the IL-2 network may well play a relevant role in B-CLL, both in terms of a direct action on the neoplastic population and in the context of the topic of this chapter, in the pathogenesis or progression of the associated immunodeficiency. It has in fact been documented that the IL-2 produced by the T-cell population may be insufficient to exert its physiologic role on several functional properties of the T- and NK-cell compartment. This deficiency may be caused by a reduced availability of IL-2 due to its absorption by the overwhelming neoplastic B-cell clone (56) (and, as discussed below, by the increased levels of soluble IL-2 receptor), and may also be contributed to by a reduced production by the residual T-cell population (57). These findings are strengthened by the demonstration that exogenous recombinant IL-2 may markedly increase the in-vitro T-colony-forming capacity (58) and the cytotoxic function in B-CLL (59). The evidence that (a) IL-2 may induce a (co)stimulatory signal on B-CLL cells, particularly following a primary signal (60,61), (b) that IL-2 is capable of upregulating the expression of the p55 antigen of the IL-2 receptor on B-CLL cells (58), (c) that B-CLL cells may absorb IL-2 (56), and (d) that B-CLL cells may also release, upon activation, IL-2 (61), has raised the possibility that in B-CLL we may be facing an autocrine and/or paracrine loop involving IL-2. This possibility is further strengthened by the recent evidence that B-CLL cells may express, in addition to the p55 antigen (α subunit) of the IL-2 receptor (56,60), also the intermediate affinity p75 antigen (β subunit) (62,63, and personal data). Though the complete cytokine network still needs to be fully appreciated, the objective situation in untreated patients is such that each T lymphocyte is surrounded by approximately 10 neoplastic B cells, which, through a "sponge"-effect mechanism (outlined in Fig. 1), are capable of absorbing and consuming the T-cell-derived IL-2, thus contributing to the severe functional defects of the T and cytotoxic cells reported above. The overall possible role of IL-2 (as of the soluble IL-2 receptor described below) on both the neoplastic clone and on the accessory cells in B-CLL is represented schematically in Fig. 2.

SOLUBLE IL-2 RECEPTOR

The p55 subunit of the IL-2 receptor, which plays a crucial role in the process of lymphocyte proliferation, is not detectable on normal resting cells, but is expressed on the surface of activated T and B cells (64). In-vitro activated normal lymphoid cells may also release the IL-2 receptor from the surface in a soluble form (65). In chronic lymphoproliferative disorders, the p55 chain of the IL-2 receptor is constitutively expressed in ATLL (66), in HCL (67), and in a proportion of B-CLL cases (56,60). Since evidence has been provided that the soluble IL-2 receptor may bind to IL-2 (68), it is suggestive to postulate that in HCL this molecule may block IL-2, thus making it unavailable to exert its physiologic stimulation on the NK cells (69). The very high circulating levels of soluble IL-2 receptor reported in HCL (70) probably greatly favor this mechanism, and, in turn, the overall defective cell-mediated immunity taking place in this disorder (71). In fact, the values of soluble IL-2 receptor appear to be inversely correlated with the NK function of untreated patients with HCL (72). Furthermore, the levels of soluble IL-2 receptor greatly decrease or normalize after treatment with interferon-α (72), at a time when the NK function markedly improves (49).

Increased levels of soluble IL-2 receptor have also been reported in the serum of patients with B-CLL who are untreated or off therapy (73). In the same study, when the levels were correlated with the clinical stage, there was a trend toward lower values in patients with less invasive disease. Furthermore, functional studies revealed a better response to mitogens and helper capacity in those cases with the lowest serum levels of soluble IL-2 receptor (73). In view of the multiple T- and NK-cell defects recorded in B-CLL, it is likely that the higher-than-normal levels of soluble IL-2 receptor may interfere with the IL-2-mediated cell functions, thus downmodulat-

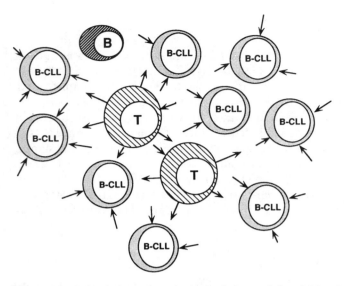

Figure 1 Schematic representation of the peripheral blood lymphocyte subset distribution in untreated B-CLL patients.

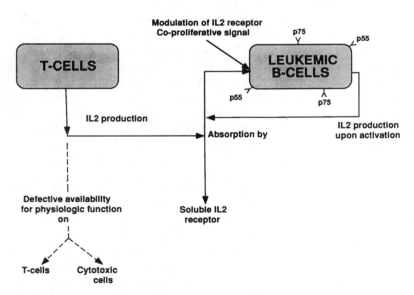

Figure 2 IL2 in B-CLL: through the overwhelming neoplastic B-cell population which may absorb IL2 and the elevated levels of soluble IL2 receptor, the T-cell produced IL2 may defectively exert its physiologic action on the residual T and cytotoxic cells. Furthermore, IL2 may also play a role on the neoplastic clone.

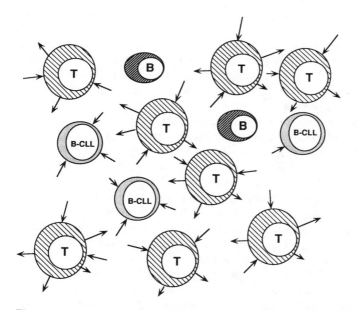

Figure 3 Schematic representation of the likely peripheral blood subset distribution in B-CLL patients following prolonged treatment.

ing the immune response, leading to defective immuneregulation, and, in turn, contributing to the profound immunodeficiency occurring in this disease.

CELL-TO-CELL INTERACTION

There is an endlessly growing body of supporting evidence that the different hemopoietic cell subsets are not isolated compartments, but rather closely interacting systems largely regulated by autocrine and paracrine cytokine and growth factor loops. This recognition is not restricted to normal blood and marrow cells but can be also extended to acute and chronic myeloid and lymphoid leukemias. In this respect the key question that needs to be answered is if and to what extent the numerous abnormalities encountered within the T, NK, and cytokine compartment in B-CLL can tie together, and what role they may play in the determinism or in the progression of the immunodeficiency correlated with B-CLL and, thus, in some of the clinical complications that are characteristically associated with this disease. In view of the clear role that T cells exert on the process of normal B-cell maturation and differentiation into terminal antibody-producing cells, and of the clear defect in helper activity documented within the T-cell population of B-CLL patients, it is most likely that this impairment in helper function will contribute to the progressive decrease in serum Ig observed in this disease. In turn, this defect will result in a higher risk of infectious complications. Again, it is worth recalling that both the serum Ig immunoparesis and the T-cell phenotypic and functional defects become more evident in the more advanced stages of the disease.

It is also likely that the multiple profound cytotoxic defects recorded in B-CLL patients, involving the NK, K, and LAK functions, may play a relevant role in the course of the disease. In terms of the neoplastic clone itself, the likelihood is that the severely depressed cytotoxic function, which is not adequately controlled by the immune system of the host, may contribute to the progression of the disease. With regard to the complications associated with B-CLL, the deficient killing machinery may contribute to the higher incidence of second neoplasias reported during the course of the disease (74,75), and of infective episodes. Furthermore, it has recently been reported that large granular lymphocytes from B-CLL patients are capable of downregulating the pokeweed mitogen-induced Ig secretion by normal B lymphocytes (76). In view of the suggestion that normal large granular lymphocytes appear to display a potent immunoregulatory activity on normal B cells, these findings further point to a defect of the NK compartment in B-CLL and provide evidence that this may play a negative regulatory role on the residual normal B-cell population.

ARE THE ABNORMALITIES OF THE T- AND CYTOTOXIC CELL COMPARTMENTS A PRIMARY OR A SECONDARY EVENT?

This question has been and still remains extremely important toward achieving a complete understanding of the pathogenesis of the multiple abnormalities recorded within the T- and cytotoxic cell compartments of patients will B-CLL. The evidence that the different phenotypic and functional defects often become apparent or worsen in the more advanced stages of the disease (13–15,25), and, in fact, that in the earlier stages there may be an at least partial sparing (25), would tend to favor the hypothesis that the heterogeneous immunoparesis most likely represents a secondary event occurring during the clinical course of the disease, rather than a primary event that may have led to a disregulation of the B-cell compartment. Furthermore, the possibility that the multiple T-cell abnormalities may be a consequence of their involvement as part of the neoplastic proliferation seems highly unlikely. This cell population lacks chromosome abnormalities and exhibits a heterozygous pattern of glucose 6-phosphate dehydrogenase. More recently, analyses at the DNA level aimed at evaluating the configuration of the T-cell receptor genes have shown that the possible presence of monoclonally rearranged cells, when present, occurs only in a small minority of cases (77 and personal data). Taken together, the findings so far accumulated favor the hypothesis of secondary T- and cytotoxic cell defects occurring as a consequence of the neoplastic event, which are thus unlikely to play an etiopathogenetic role in the establishment of B-CLL, but rather to play a potentially relevant part in the progressive hypogammaglobulinemia and in the complications associated with the disease. A similar situation of a secondary marked immunoparesis is a well-known feature taking place in patients with non-Hodgkin's lymphoma. Also in HCL the evidence that some of the abnormalities occur only in patients with active disease points to a secondary defect occurring in patients with B-cell chronic lymphoproliferative disorders.

CAN THE IMMUNODEFICIENCY BE MODIFIED BY TREATMENT?

A relevant aspect with obvious clinical implications is whether the multiple abnormalities within the T- and cytotoxic cell compartments can be influenced by treatment. This issue is conceptually important because, if an improvement could be convincingly documented, treatment might be considered for patients with documented immunologic abnormalities who otherwise may not be deemed eligible for treatment at all institutions. Some of the data reported suggest that, in a proportion of cases, treatment may affect some of the T-cell defects. This observation has been in the form of an improvement of the T-cell subset distribution following splenic irradiation (78,79) and splenectomy (80), and by an increase in the T-colony-forming capacity following chemotherapy (25). Phenotypic and functional changes have also been reported after treatment with a thymic product (81). Taken together, the overall data so far accumulated appear, however, rather anedoctal, and no study of an adequate number of cases has demonstrated conclusively that treatment consistently improves the immunodeficient status of B-CLL patients. Furthermore, no convincing evidence has been provided that treatment improves the levels of circulating Ig.

Biologically, prolonged treatment will significantly modify the ratio of B- and T-cell subsets in the patients, leading to a potentially normal or near-normal lymphocyte distribution (outlined in Fig. 3, following p. 155). Based on the above-reported data, it is conceivable that this effect may also lead to an improvement of the immunodeficiency. This entire issue will probably have to be readdressed on the basis of the encouraging clinical responses obtained in B-cell chronic lymphoproliferative disorders, including B-CLL, with new drugs, i.e., fludarabine and 2'-chlorodeoxyadenosine (82,83), or with a different therapeutic strategy aimed at a greater eradication of the disease using a protocol which contemplates prolonged therapy aimed at stopping treatment at the time of complete hematological remission (84). Finally, the recently reported in-vivo and in-vitro evidence of a potential synergistic action between chlorambucil and interferon-α in a proportion of B-CLL patients (85,86) makes this subgroup of patients a relevant category in which to reassess the immune status after treatment. This observation gains particular relevance in view of the well-known evidence that the marked clinicohematological improvements in patients with HCL following treatment with interferon-α are associated with an enhancement of the immune system, and in particular with an improvement or normalization of the NK function (49). In addition, there is the possibility that improving the circulating levels of serum Ig with treatment could influence the overall course of the disease (87).

CONCLUSIONS AND PERSPECTIVES

Little doubt exists that patients with B-CLL will suffer at some stage of their disease from a more or less severe situation of immunodeficiency. This is clearly shown by the decreased levels of serum Ig and by the multiple phenotypic and functional abnormalities within the T- and cytotoxic cell

Table 3 Immune Status in B-CLL Patients

1. Reduced serum Ig
2. Reduced percent of CD4+ cells, increased percent of CD8+ cells; reversed CD4/CD8 ratio → increases with disease progression
3. Increased absolute number of CD4+ and CD8+ cells throughout all stages
4. Reduced response to antigens and mitogens
5. Reduced NK, ADCC, and LAK activity
6. Reduced autologous LAK killing
7. Increased levels of soluble IL-2 receptor
8. Reduced IL-2 availability

compartments. The recognition of these defects has been made possible through the improved technological approaches capable of investigating the properties of specific lymphocyte subsets. Furthermore, these methodological advances have also allowed us to unravel the potential role played by the cytokine network in regulating numerous interacting mechanisms. The suggestion that the IL-2 produced by the T-cell population may be absorbed by the overwhelming neoplastic clone and/or blocked by the circulating soluble IL-2 receptor suggests for this cytokine a possible complexe role in B-CLL in terms of both a direct triggering effect on the leukemic B-cells and an indirect effect on the T- and cytotoxic cell compartments in terms of a defective availability of the molecule to exert its physiologic action on these lymphocyte subsets. These suggestions are further substantiated by in-vitro data showing that exogeous IL-2 may induce a proliferative signal on B-CLL cells and that it may considerably enhance the defective T- and NK-cell functions. The possible IL-2 involvement in B-CLL—as well as, for instance, the role played by TNF-α in the cytopenias associated with HCL—are good indicators of the likely relevant part played by cytokines and growth factors in different human leukemias. We are probably only now starting to recognize the tip of an iceberg that is represented by the complexe cytokine and growth factor network capable of regulating the growth and clinical course of several hematological malignancies.

Although the aforementioned data strongly support the concept that the immunodeficiency in B-CLL is most probably occurring as an event secondary to the neoplastic process, it is also likely that it may play an important contributory role in the development of the infections and second malignancies, and thus in the clinical course of the disease and in the overall prognosis. For these reasons, attempts aimed at improving the immunologic status of the patients, in addition to controlling the neoplastic clone, are warranted. Though the results obtained over the years with treatment do not appear to have modified significantly the natural history of

B-CLL, the new drugs being successfully employed and the different treatment strategies aimed at more intensive courses and contemplating the use, alone or in combination with cytotoxic drugs, of biological response modifiers, will also deserve considerable attention in view of possible modifications within the immune status of the host. In this respect, the example of a closely related chronic B-cell disorder such as HCL is illuminating. The prolonged use of interferon-α alone has not only allowed clinicohematological remissions in the great majority of patients, but has enabled significant improvements within the cytotoxic and T-cell compartment, and has changed the overall natural history of the disease. It is auspicious that in B-CLL, as in other chronic lymphoproliferative disorders, a better understanding of the biology of the neoplastic population and of the accessory cells, as well as of the humoral factors regulating these processes, will allow us to designate new treatment strategies capable of acting on both the leukemic clone and on the residual nonpathological cell populations.

REFERENCES

1. J. E. Ultmann, W. Fish, E. Osserman, and A. Gellhorn, The clinical implications of hypogammaglobulinemia in patients with chronic lymphocytic leukemia and lymphocytic lymphosarcoma, *Ann. Intern. Med., 51*:501 (1959).
2. P. Fiddes, R. Penny, J. V. Wells, and M. C. Rozenberg, Clinical correlation with immunoglobulin levels in chronic lymphocytic leukemia, *Austral. N.Z. J. Med., 4*:346 (1972).
3. R. Foa, D. Catovsky, M. Brozovic, G. Marsh, T. Ooyririlangkumaran, M. Cherchi, and D. A. G. Galton, Clinical staging and immunological findings in chronic lymphocytic leukemia, *Cancer, 44*:483 (1979).
4. I. Ben-Bassat, A. Many, M. Modan, C. Peretz, and B. Ramot, Serum immunoglobulins in chronic lymphocytic leukemia, *Am. J. Med. Sci., 278*:4 (1979).
5. D. Catovsky and R. Foa, *The Lymphoid Leukaemias*, Butterworths, London, p. 133 (1990).
6. J. M. Lang, C. Giron, F. Oberling, M. L. Goetz, and M. L. North, Normal humoral immunity in hairy cell leukemia, *Biomedicine, 25*:41 (1976).
7. F. K. Stevenson, M. Spellerberg, and J. L. Smith, Monoclonal immunoglobulin light chain in urine of patients with B lymphocytic disease: Its source and use as a diagnostic aid, *Br. J. Cancer 47*:607 (1983).
8. M. J. Deegan, J. P. Abraham, M. Sawdyk, and E. J. Van Slyck, High incidence of monoclonal proteins in the serum and urine of chronic lymphocytic leukemia patients, *Blood, 64*:1207 (1984).
9. D. Catovsky, E. Miliani, A. Okos, and D. A. G. Galton, Clinical significance of T cells in chronic lymphocytic leukaemia, *Lancet, ii*:751 (1974).
10. K. R. Rai, A. Sawitsky, E. P. Cronkite, A. D. Chanana, R. M. Levy, and B. C. Pasternack, Clinical staging of chronic lymphocytic leukemia, *Blood, 46*: 219 (1975).

11. N. E. Kay, J. D. Johnson, R. Stanek, and S. D. Douglas, T-cell subpopulations in chronic lymphocytic leukemia: Abnormalities in distribution and in in vitro receptor maturation, *Blood, 54*:540 (1979).

12. F. Lauria, R. Foa, and D. Catovsky, Increase in Tγ lymphocytes in B-cell chronic lymphocytic leukaemia, *Scand. J. Haematol., 24*:187 (1980).

13. C. D. Platsoucas, M. Galinski, S. Kempin, L. Reich, B. Clarkson, and R. A. Good, Abnormal T lymphocyte subpopulations in patients with B cell chronic lymphocytic leukemia: An analysis by monoclonal antibodies, *J. Immunol., 129*:2305 (1982).

14. G. Semenzato, A. Pezzutto, R. Foa, F. Lauria, and R. Raimondi, T lymphocytes in B-cell lymphocytic leukemia: Characterization by monoclonal antibodies and correlation with Fc receptors, *Clin. Immunol. Immunopathol., 26*: 155 (1983).

15. F. Herrmann, A. Lochner, H. Philippen, B. Jauer, and H. Ruhl., Imbalance of T cell subpopulations in patients with chronic lymphocytic leukaemia of the B cell type, *Clin. Exp. Immunol., 49*:157 (1982).

16. G. Pizzolo, M. Chilosi, A. Ambrosetti, G. Semenzato, L. Fiore-Donati, and G. Perona, Immunohistologic study of bone marrow involvement in B-chronic lymphocytic leukemia, *Blood, 62*:1289 (1983).

17. F. Lauria, R. Foa, M. Gobbi, A. Pulvirenti, D. Raspadori, M. C. Giubellino, and S. Tura, Characterization of T-lymphocyte subsets in hairy-cell leukaemia (HCL) by monoclonal antibodies: Comparison with Fcγ, Fcμ receptors and correlation with disease activity, *Br. J. Haematol., 52*:657 (1982).

18. T. H. Totterman, M. Carlsson, B. Simonsson, M. Bengtsson, and K. Nilsson, T-cell activation and subset patterns are altered in B-CLL and correlate with the stage of the disease, *Blood, 74*:786 (1989).

19. A. D. Crockard, H. D. Alexander, C. F. Stephenson, P. McCrea, Z. R. Desai, T. C. M. Morris, and I. A. McNeill, An analysis of circulating CD4 lymphocyte subpopulations in B-cell chronic lymphocytic leukaemia, *Leuk. Lymph., 3*:127 (1990).

20. B. A. Bouroncle, K. P. Klausen, and J. R. Aschenbrand, Studies of the delayed response of phytohemagglutinin (PHA) stimulated lymphocytes in 25 chronic lymphocytic leukemia before and after therapy, *Blood, 34*:166 (1969).

21. J. H. Robbins and W. R. Lewis, Inherent inability of chronic lymphocytic leukaemia lymphocytes to respond to phytohaemagglutinin, *Int. Arch. Allergy, 43*:845 (1972).

22. T. Han, M. L. Bloom, B. Dadey, G. Bennett, J. Minowada, A. A. Sandberg, and H. Ozer, Lack of autologous mixed lymphocyte reaction in patients with chronic lymphocytic leukemia: Evidence for autoreactive T-cell dysfunction not correlated with phenotype, karyotype, or clinical status, *Blood, 60*:1075 (1982).

23. R. Foa and D. Catovsky, T-lymphocyte colonies in normal blood, bone marrow and lymphoproliferative disorders, *Clin. Exp. Immunol., 36*:488 (1979).

24. S. Davis, Characterization of the phytohemagglutinin-induced proliferating lymphocyte subpopulations in chronic lymphocytic leukemia patients using a clonogenic agar technique and monoclonal antibodies, *Blood, 58*:1053 (1981).

25. R. Foa, F. Lauria, D. Catovsky, and D. A. G. Galton, Reduced T-colony

forming capacity in B-chronic lymphocytic leukaemia. II. Correlation with clinical stage and findings in B-prolymphocytic leukaemia, *Leuk. Res., 6*:329 (1982).

26. N. Chiorazzi, S. Fu, M. Ghodrat, H. G. Kunkel, K. Rai, and T. Gee, T cell helper defect in patients with chronic lymphocytic leukemia, *J. Immunol., 122*:1087 (1979).

27. N. E. Kay, Abnormal T-cell subpopulation function in CLL: Excessive suppressor (Tγ) and deficient helper (Tμ) activity with respect to B-cell proliferation, *Blood, 57*:418 (1981).

28. G. Semenzato, A. Pezzutto, C. Agostini, M. Albertini, and G. Gasparotto, T-lymphocyte subpopulations in chronic lymphocytic leukemia: A quantitative and functional study, *Cancer, 48*:2191 (1981).

29. F. Lauria, R. Foa, V. Mantovani, M. T. Fierro, D. Catovsky, and S. Tura, T-cell functional abnormality in B-chronic lymphocytic leukaemia: Evidence of a defect of the T-helper subset, *Br. J. Haematol., 54*:277 (1983).

30. R. Foa and F. Lauria, Reduced T lymphocyte colonies in B chronic lymphocytic leukaemia. III. Evidence of a proliferative abnormality of the T helper cell population, *Clin. Exp. Immunol., 50*:336 (1982).

31. L. J. M. Sabbe, C. J. L. M. Meijer, and J. Jansen, T lymphocyte function in hairy cell leukaemia, *Clin. Exp. Immunol., 42*:336 (1980).

32. R. Foa, F. Lauria, D. Raspadori, P. Lusso, M. L. Ferrando, M. T. Fierro, M. C. Giubellino, and D. Catovsky, Normal helper T-cell function in hairy-cell leukaemia, *Scand. J. Haematol., 31*:322 (1983).

33. R. Foa, D. Catovsky, E. Incarbone, M. Cherchi, A. Wechsler, P. Lusso, M. T. Fierro, M. C. Giubellino, M. G. Bernengo, and G. Semenzato, Chronic T-cell leukaemias. III. T-colonies, PHA response and correlation with membrane phenotype, *Leuk. Res., 6*:809 (1982).

34. H. C. Rumke, F. Miedema, I. J. M. Ten Berge, F. Terpstra, H. J. Van Der Rejden, R. J. Van De Griend, H. G. De Bruin, A. E. G. Kr. Von Dem Borne, J. W. Smit, W. P. Zeijlemaker, and C. J. M. Melief, Functional properties of T cells in patients with chronic Tγ lymphocytosis and chronic T cell neoplasia, *J. Immunol., 129*:419 (1982).

35. S. L. Thien, D. Catovsky, D. Oscier, J. M. Goldman, H. J. Van Der Reijden, C. J. M. Melief, H. C. Rumke, R. J. M. Ten Berge, and A. E. G. Kr. Von Dem Borne, T-chronic lymphocytic leukaemia presenting as primary hypogammaglobulinaemia — evidence of a proliferation of T-suppressor cells, *Clin. Exp. Immunol., 47*:670 (1982).

36. F. Lauria, R. Foa, D. Raspadori, M. R. Motta, P. L. Tazzari, G. Biagini, P. Preda, R. Algeri, and S. Tura, T-cell prolymphocytic leukaemia: A clinical and immunological study, *Scand. J. Haematol., 35*:319 (1985).

37. S. Broder, R. L. Edelson, M. A. Lutzner, D. L. Nelson, R. P. MacDermott, M. E. Durm, C. K. Goldman, B. D. Meade, and T. A. Waldmann, The Sézary syndrome: A malignant proliferation of helper T cells, *J. Clin. Invest., 58*: 1297 (1976).

38. C. L. Berger, D. Warburton, J. Raafat, P. LoGerfo, and R. L. Edelson, Cutaneous T-cell lymphoma: Neoplasm of T cells with helper activity, *Blood, 53*:642 (1979).

39. E. Kansu and S. P. Hauptman, Suppressor cell population in Sézary syndrome, *Clin. Immunol. Immunopathol., 12*:341 (1979).
40. Y. Yamada, Phenotypic and functional analysis of leukemic cells from 16 patients with adult T-cell leukemia/lymphoma, *Blood, 61*:192 (1983).
41. F. Miedema, F. G. Terpstra, J. W. Smit, S. Daenen, W. Gerritz, U. Hedge, E. Matutes, D. Catovsky, M. F. Greaves, and C. J. M. Melief, Functional properties of neoplastic T cells in adult T cell lymphoma/leukemia patients from the Caribbean, *Blood, 63*:477 (1984).
42. C. D. Platsoucas, G. Fernandes, S. L. Gupta, S. Kempin, B. Clarkson, R. A. Good, and S. Gupta, Defective spontaneous and antibody-dependent cytotoxicity mediated by E-rosette-positive and E-rosette-negative cells in untreated patients with chronic lymphocytic leukemia. Augmentation by in vitro treatment with interferon, *J. Immunol., 125*:1216 (1980).
43. R. Foa, F. Lauria, P. Lusso, M. C. Giubellino, M. T. Fierro, M. L. Ferrando, D. Raspadori, and L. Matera, Discrepancy between phenotypic and functional features of natural killer T-lymphocytes in B-cell chronic lymphocytic leukaemia, *Br. J. Haematol., 58*:509 (1984).
44. R. Foa, M. T. Fierro, P. Lusso, D. Raspadori, M. L. Ferrando, L. Matera, F. Malavasi, and F. Lauria, Reduced natural killer T-cells in B-cell chronic lymphocytic leukaemia identified by three monoclonal antibodies: Leu-11, A10, AB8.28, *Br. J. Haematol., 62*:151 (1986).
45. N. E. Kay and J. M. Zarling, Impaired natural killer activity in patients with chronic lymphocytic leukemia is associated with a deficiency of azurophilic granules in putative NK cells, *Blood, 63*:305 (1984).
46. A. Velardi, J. T. Prchal, E. F. Prasthofer, and C. E. Grossi, Expression of NK-lineage markers on peripheral blood lymphocytes with T-helper (Leu3 + / T4 +) phenotype in B cell chronic lymphocytic leukemia, *Blood, 65*:149 (1985).
47. R. Foa, M. T. Fierro, D. Raspadori, M. Bonferroni, S. Cardona, A. Guarini, A. Gillio Tos, P. Francia di Celle, A. Cesano, L. Matera, F. Lauria, and F. Gavosto, Lymphokine-activated killer (LAK) cell activity in B and T chronic lymphoid leukemia: Defective LAK generation and reduced susceptibility of the leukemic cells to allogeneic and autologous LAK effectors, *Blood, 76*:1349 (1990).
48. L. P. Ruco, A. Procopio, V. Maccalini, A. Calogero, S. Uccini, L. Annino, F. Mandelli, and C. D. Baroni, Severe deficiency of natural killer activity in the peripheral blood of patients with hairy cell leukemia, *Blood, 61*:1132 (1983).
49. R. Foa, M. T. Fierro, P. Lusso, M. Bonferroni, D. Raspadori, M. Buzzi, P. L. Zinzani, L. Resegotti, and F. Lauria, Effect of alpha-interferon on the immune system of patients with hairy cell leukemia, *Leukemia, 1*:377 (1987).
50. R. Foa, A. Gillio Tos, P. Francia di Celle, A. Carbone, D. Marchis, F. Vischia, A. Cignetti, and A. Guarini, Cytokines in B-cell chronic lymphocytic leukemia, *Leuk. Lymph., 5*, suppl.:7 (1991).
51. F. Morabito, E. F. Prasthofer, N. E. Dunlap, C. E. Grossi, and A. B. Tilden, Expression of myelomonocytic antigens on chronic lymphocytic leukemia B cells correlates with their ability to produce interleukin 1, *Blood, 70*:1750 (1987).

52. A. Biondi, V. Rossi, R. Bassan, T. Barbui, S. Bettoni, M. Sironi, A. Mantovani, and A. Rambaldi, Constitutive expression of the interleukin-6 gene in chronic lymphocytic leukemia, *Blood, 73*:1279 (1989).

53. S. Karray, T. Defrance, H. Merle-Beral, J. Banchereau, P. Debre, and P. Galanaud, Interleukin 4 counteracts the Interleukin 2-induced proliferation of monoclonal B cells, *J. Exp. Med., 168*:85 (1988).

54. W. Digel, M. Stefanic, W. Schoniger, C. Buck, A. Raghavachar, N. Frickhofen, H. Heimpel, and F. Porzsolt, Tumor necrosis factor induces proliferation of neoplastic B cells from chronic lymphocytic leukemia, *Blood, 73*:1242 (1989).

55. R. Foa, M. Massaia, S. Cardona, A. Gillio Tos, A. Bianchi, C. Attisano, A. Guarini, P. Francia di Celle, and M. T. Fierro, Production of tumor necrosis factor-alpha (TNF) by B-cell chronic lymphocytic leukemia cells: A possible regulatory role of TNF in the progression of the disease, *Blood, 76*:393 (1990).

56. R. Foa, M. Giovarelli, C. Jemma, M. T. Fierro, P. Lusso, M. L. Ferrando, F. Lauria, and G. Forni, Interleukin 2 (IL2) and interferon-γ production by T lymphocytes from patients with B-chronic lymphocytic leukemia: Evidence that normally released IL2 is absorbed by the neoplastic B cell population, *Blood, 66*:614 (1985).

57. O. Ayanlar-Batuman, E. Ebert, and S. P. Hauptman, Defective interleukin-2 production and responsiveness by T cells in patients with chronic lymphocytic leukemia of B cell variety, *Blood, 67*:279 (1986).

58. R. Foa, M. T. Fierro, M. Giovarelli, P. Lusso, G. Benetton, M. Bonferroni, and G. Forni, Immunoregulatory T-cell defects in B-cell chronic lymphocytic leukemia: Cause or consequence of the disease? The contributory role of decreased availability of Interleukin 2 (IL2), *Blood Cells, 12*:399 (1987).

59. M. Alvarez de Mon, J. Casas, R. Laguna, M. L. Toribio, M. O. de Landazuri, and A. Durantez. Lymphokine induction of NK-like cytotoxicity in T cells from B-CLL, *Blood, 67*:228 (1986).

60. O. Lantz, C. Grillot-Courvalin, C. Schmitt, J-P. Fermand, and J-C. Brouet, Interleukin 2-induced proliferation of leukemic human B cells, *J. Exp. Med., 161*:1225 (1985).

61. M. Giovarelli, R. Foa, G. Benetton, P. Lusso, M. T. Fierro, and G. Forni, Release of interleukin-2-like material by B-chronic lymphocytic leukemia cells. An autocrine or paracrine model of production and utilization? *Leuk. Res., 12*:201 (1988).

62. A. Rosolen, M. Nakanishi, D. G. Poplack, D. Cole, R. Quinones, G. Reaman, J. B. Trepel, J. D. Cotelingam, E. A. Sausville, G. E. Marti, E. S. Jaffe, L. M. Neckers, and O. R. Colamonici, Expression of interleukin-2 receptor β subunit in hematopoietic malignancies, *Blood, 73*:1968 (1989).

63. D. Barnett, V. Granger, and J. T. Reilly, Expression of the p75 interleukin-2 receptor (β subunit) in acute and chronic leukaemia, *Br. J. Haematol., 76*:314 (1990).

64. W. C. Greene, W. J. Leonard, and J. M. Depper, Growth of human T lymphocytes: An analysis of interleukin 2 and its cellular receptor, *Progr. Hematol., 14*:283 (1986).

65. L. A. Rubin, C. C. Kurman, M. E. Fritz, W. E. Biddison, B. Boutin, R. Yarchoan, and D. L. Nelson, Soluble interleukin 2 receptors are released from activated human lymphoid cells in vitro, *J. Immunol., 135*:3172 (1985).

66. W. C. Greene, W. J. Leonard, J. M. Depper, D. L. Nelson, and T. A. Waldmann, The human interleukin-2 receptor: Normal and abnormal expression in T cells and in leukemias induced by the human T-lymphotropic retroviruses, *Ann. Intern. Med., 105*:560 (1986).

67. S. J. Korsmeyer, W. C. Greene, J. Cossman, S. M. Hsu, J. P. Jensen, L. M. Neckers, S. L. Marshall, A. Bakhshi, J. M. Depper, W. J. Leonard, E. S. Jaffe, and T. A. Waldmann, Rearrangement and expression of immunoglobulin genes and expression of Tac antigen in hairy cell leukemia, *Proc. Natl. Acad. Sci. USA, 80*:4522 (1983).

68. L. A. Rubin, G. Jay, and D. L. Nelson, The released interleukin 2 receptor binds interleukin 2 efficiently, *J. Immunol., 137*:3841 (1986).

69. W. Domzig, B. M. Stadler, and R. B. Herberman, Interleukin 2 dependence of human natural killer (NK) cell activity, *J. Immunol., 130*:1970 (1983).

70. R. G. Steis, L. Marcon, D. L. Nelson, J. Clark, and A. E. Maluish, Studies of soluble IL-2 (sIL-2R) levels in hairy cell leukemia (HCL) patients, *Proc. Am. Soc. Clin. Oncol., 5*:232 (1986), abstr.

71. P. A. Mackowiak, S. E. Demian, W. L. Sutker, F. K. Murphy, J. W. Smith, R. Tompsett, W. W. Sheehan, and J. P. Luby, Infections in hairy cell leukemia. Clinical evidence of a pronounced defect in cell-mediated immunity, *Am. J. Med., 68*:718 (1980).

72. M. Chilosi, G. Semenzato, G. Cetto, A. Ambrosetti, L. Fiore-Donati, G. Perona, G. Berton, M. Lestani, A. Scarpa, C. Agostini, L. Trentin, R. Zambello, M. Masciarelli, F. Dazzi, F. Vinante, F. Caligaris-Cappio, and G. Pizzolo, Soluble interleukin-2 receptors in the sera of patients with hairy cell leukemia: Relationship with the effect of recombinant α-interferon therapy on clinical parameters and natural killer in vitro activity, *Blood, 70*:1530 (1987).

73. G. Semenzato, R. Foa, C. Agostini, R. Zambello, L. Trentin, F. Vinante, F. Benedetti, M. Chilosi, and G. Pizzolo, High serum levels of soluble interleukin 2 receptor in patients with B chronic lymphocytic leukemia, *Blood, 70*:396 (1987).

74. M. H. Greene and J. Wilson, Second cancer following lymphatic and hematopoietic cancers in Connecticut, *Natl. Cancer Inst. Monogr., 68*:191 (1985).

75. D. Manusow, and B. H. Weinerman, Subsequent neoplasia in chronic lymphocytic leukemia, *J. Am. Med. Assoc., 232*:267 (1975).

76. N. E. Kay, and R. T. Perri, Evidence that large granular lymphocytes from B-CLL patients with hypogammaglobulinemia down-regulate B-cell immunoglobulin synthesis, *Blood, 73*:1016 (1989).

77. T. Wen, H. Mellstedt, and M. Jondal, Presence of clonal T cell populations in chronic B lymphocytic leukemia and smoldering myeloma, *J. Exp. Med., 171*:659 (1990).

78. D. Catovsky, F. Lauria, E. Matutes, R. Foa, V. Mantovani, S. Tura, and D. A. G. Galton, Increase in Tγ lymphocytes in B-cell chronic lymphocytic

leukaemia. II. Correlation with clinical stage and findings in B-prolymphocytic leukaemia, *Br. J. Haematol., 47*:539 (1981).

79. N. E. Kay, R. B. Howe, and S. D. Douglas, Effect of therapy on T cell subpopulations in patients with chronic lymphocytic leukemia, *Leuk. Res., 6*: 345 (1982).

80. S. R. McCann, C. A. Whelan, B. Breslin, and I. J. Temperley, Lymphocyte sub-populations following splenic irradiation in patients with chronic lymphocytic leukaemia, *Br. J. Haematol., 50*:225 (1982).

81. F. Lauria, D. Raspadori, and S. Tura, Effect of a thymic factor on T lymphocytes in B cell chronic lymphocytic leukemia: In vitro and in vivo studies, *Blood, 64*:667 (1984).

82. M. J. Keating, H. Kantarjian, M. Talpaz, J. Redman, C. Koller, B. Barlogie, W. Velasquez, W. Plunkett, E. J. Freireich, and K. B. McCredie, Fludarabine: A new agent with major activity against chronic lymphocytic leukemia, *Blood, 74*:19 (1989).

83. L. D. Piro, C. J. Carrera, E. Beutler, and D. A. Carson, 2-Chlorodeoxyadenosine: An effective new agent for the treatment of chronic lymphocytic leukemia, *Blood, 72*:1069 (1988).

84. B. Jaksic and B. Vitale, Total tumor mass score (TTM): A new parameter in chronic lymphocytic leukaemia, *Br. J. Haematol., 49*:405 (1981).

85. M. Pini and R. Foa, Combined use of alpha 2b interferon and chlorambucil in the management of previously treated B-cell lymphocytic leukemia, *Leuk. Lymph., 5*, suppl.:143 (1991).

86. R. Foa, F. Vischia, M. Pini, F. Lauria, and A. Guarini, Use of the MMT chemosensitivity assay in B-cell chronic lymphocytic leukemia, *Leuk. Lymph., 5*, suppl.:71 (1991).

87. Cooperative Group for the Study of Immunoglobulin in Chronic Lymphocytic Leukemia, Intravenous immunoglobulin for the prevention of infection in chronic lymphocytic leukemia. A randomized, controlled clinical trial, *N. Engl. J. Med., 319*:902 (1988).

8

Hypogammaglobulinemia and Disordered Immunity in CLL

Guillaume Dighiero
Institut Pasteur, Paris, France

INTRODUCTION

Chronic lymphocytic leukemia (CLL) is a hematological neoplasm characterized by proliferation and accumulation of mature-appearing small lymphocytes. In Western countries, it corresponds in most cases (95%) to expansion of a single B-cell clone. During recent years, there have been important advances in our understanding of the biology of CLL. Considerable progress has been made in the characterization of the cell that proliferates in CLL, which displays peculiar phenotypic characteristics when compared to other B-cell malignancies. Another interesting feature of CLL, which distinguishes it from the other B-cell malignancies, is the high frequency with which hypogammaglobulinemia and autoimmune-associated phenomena are observed. In this chapter we shall review these topics.

THE B-CLL LYMPHOCYTE

Phenotypic Characteristics

In the early 1970s, several reports based on the presence of surface membrane Ig (SmIg) (1–4) C3dR complement receptors (5,6) and receptors for the Fc fraction of Ig (7) clearly established that CLL usually corresponds to expansion of a B-cell clone. The clonal nature of the proliferating cell initially suggested by the expression of a single immunoglobulin light chain, κ or λ, on the cell membrane was confirmed by showing that CLL B cells from a given patient expressed a unique immunoglobulin-idiotype specificity (8–10), a single pattern of glucose 6-phosphate dehydrogenase activity (11), and clonal chromosomal abnormalities (12). Moreover, unique immunoglobulin gene rearrangements were almost invariably observed, although in some cases, heterogeneity of the hybridization patterns was observed when probes for the heavy-chain J segment were used (13).

SmIgs are constantly restricted to a single light chain, and frequently express IgM or both IgM and IgD. In the latter case, IgM and IgD have been shown to share idiotypic and antigenic specificities (9). There is controversy, however, as to whether the CLL B lymphocyte displays μ, δ, and γ chains. Some studies have indicated that a heavy-chain switch can occur in B-CLL (14); hence, those authors have suggested that there is a certain degree of maturation of malignant cells. Other studies have suggested that it is extrinsic and not synthesized by the cell (15). CLL B cells also express several antigens, including D-related human leukocyte antigens and antigens related to B cells. Most cases of B-CLL appear to react with CD19, CD20, CD24, CD37, and CD21 monoclonal antibodies (16–19). About 60% of CLL are positive for CD23 (20), whereas membrane positivity with CD22 is infrequent (17). CLL B cells and hairy cell leukemia B cells have been found to express a 69-kD glycoprotein that is not expressed by normal blood T and B lymphocytes, thymocyte-cultured T- and B-cell lymphoblastoid cell lines, or acute lymphoblastic leukemia cells (21,22). In contrast to B-cell prolymphocytic leukemia, which constantly binds the FMC7 antibody, the reactivity of CLL B cells is not frequent (23). CALLA (CD10) is almost constantly negative, whereas reactivities with subepitopes of CD1 (24–27) and CD11 (28), as well as with CD6, CD7, and the TQ1 antigen (24,29), have been reported in some cases of B-CLL. Interestingly, myelomonocytic antigens have also been found to be expressed by CLL B cells (30). Moreover, CLL B cells frequently express activation antigens such as CD23 (20), CD25, and Blast 1, whereas BB1 and CD71 are rarely observed (24).

Contrary to most other B-cell malignancies, CLL B lymphocytes are characterized by three particular phenotypic patterns: (a) B-CLL lymphocytes almost always express low amounts of SmIg (31,32), although increased amounts of intracytoplasmic Ig have been observed (15); (b) 31–95% of CLL-B lymphocytes frequently form rosettes with mouse erythrocytes (33,34); (c) they also express the CD5 antigen, a 67-kD antigenic determinant initially described as a pan-T-cell marker (35–37).

The normal counterpart of the CD5 B cells that proliferate in CLL was initially found by Caligaris-Capio et al. (38) to be located at the edge of the germinal center in human lymph nodes. Furthermore, a substantial number of B cells in 20-week-old fetal lymph nodes and spleen express the CD5 marker as well as μ and δ chains on their membrane (39,40). These fetal cells also appeared to share lectin nonresponsiveness and the inability to cap SIg with CLL B lymphocytes, supporting the idea that they were normal counterparts of B-CLL lymphocytes (41). With the advent of double-labeling cytofluorometry techniques, it is presently clear that about 15% of normal B cells express CD5 markers (42,43).

Does the CD5 + B Lymphocyte Constitute a Different B-Cell Subset?

A high prevalence of CD5 cells during early ontogeny led some authors to assume that the CD5 + CLL B lymphocyte corresponds to expansion of an immature B-cell clone arrested at an immature stage between pre-B and mature B cell (44). This hypothesis, however, does not provide a satisfactory explanation for the difficulty of B-cell differentiation pathways to integrate CD5 antigen expression (45,46). Alternatively, it has been postulated that CD5 B cells could correspond to a separate B-cell lineage.

The expectation of a murine counterpart to the human CD5 + B cells observed in B-CLL led to the discovery in mice of the Ly1-B (CD5 + -B)-cell subset. The advent of more sensitive methods in flow cytometry allowed the definition of a small B-cell subpopulation bearing the Ly-1 marker, which could be differentiated from the majority of normal B cells, which do not express this marker (47–49). This subset constitutes about 5% of B lymphocytes in BALB/c mice, 20% in autoimmune NZB mice, and most B cells in autoimmune Motheaten Viable (MeV) mice (50). Interestingly, Ly1 + B cells are particularly enriched in the peritoneal cavity compartment, where they represent 40% of B cells in normal mice, and 80% in NZB mice (48). The facts that Ly1 + B cells secrete and continue to secrete IgM during several weeks of culture, whereas Ly1 − B cells do not survive more than a few days, and that this Ly1 + B subset could not be reconstituted by reinjecting bone marrow cells to lethally irradiated mice, led Herzenberg and other groups to postulate that they constitute a separate B-cell lineage (51,52). In addition, results obtained with purified Ly1 + B cells indicated that this subpopulation could be mainly involved in the production of autoantibodies (48,49). Development of this subset occurs before and only shortly after birth. At this time, the CD5 + subpopulation expresses a random selection of germline genes. However, after the first weeks of life, skewing of this repertoire to overexpression of the paucigenic VH11 and VH12 families occurs through a driven clonal selection by predominantly thymus-independent class 2 self-antigens such as phosphatidyl choline (53).

Although these results consistently favor the hypothesis that CD5+ B cells constitute a separate lineage, some discrepancies concerning this assumption and its exclusive involvement in the production of autoantibodies exist (45,46): (a) Despite increased frequency of this subset in autoimmune NZB and MeV mice, this subpopulation is not augmented in other autoimmune strains (45); (b) Xid mice, which are known because they do not express the Ly-1 marker on B cells, display a frequency of autoantibody precursors similar to that observed in non-Xid mice (54); (c) Conger et al. have shown that both Ly1+ and Ly1− B-cell subsets were involved in production of autoantibodies (55); (d) a study based on detection of the mRNA transcript of the Ly-1 gene by Northern blotting among hybridomas with autoantibody specificity derived from several mouse strains indicated that natural autoantibodies arise from both Ly-1+ and Ly-1− B-lymphocyte subsets (56); and (e) CD5 expression could be induced in CD5− B cells upon stimulation with phorbolesters (57), suggesting that this marker may constitute a differentiation and/or an activation marker.

B-Cell Differentiation, Antibody Activity, and Gene Expression of the B-CLL Lymphocyte

Although earlier studies postulated that B-CLL lymphocytes were frozen at an early stage of differentiation, considerable evidence has accumulated indicating that these cells are able to differentiate. Stevenson et al. (58), using anti-idiotypic reagents, have shown that the pentameric form of SmIg was present in CLL serum. Some studies have shown that heavy-chain switch can occur in B-CLL, and hence, some authors have suggested that there is a certain degree of maturation of malignant cells. In-vitro experiments with different mitogens such as pokeweed, nocardia, or phorbol esters have succeeded in inducing differentiation of CLL B lymphocytes (59). With phorbol esters, increased presence of RNA coding for secretory IgM was observed (59–64). Interestingly, upon phorbol ester stimulation, normal CD5− B cells expressed CD5 markers (57), and B-CLL cells developed tartrate-resistant phosphatase activity and resembled hairy cells, whereas with LPS they were found to express increased levels of SmIg and the FMC7 marker (65). A variable pattern in the response to different cytokines such as IL-2, B-cell growth factors (BCGF, IFN-α, and) and IL-4 has been reported in B-CLL; this may be indicative of discrete stages of maturation and activation in B-CLL patients. Among these cytokines, IL-2 appears to be the most consistent activator, whereas IL-4 downregulates CLL B lymphocytes in contrast to its effect on normal B cells (66–71).

One of the main difficulties in working with CLL B lymphocytes arises from the fact that these cells are highly resistant to transformation by Epstein-Barr virus (EBV), and only a few EBV cell lines have so far been obtained (72,73). Given this difficulty, the antibody activity of CLL was only recently assessed by studying the antibody activity of Ig-containing supernatants obtained after stimulation of B-CLL lymphocytes with phorbol esters (74,75) or by studying the antibody activity of hybridomas derived from B-CLL lymphocytes (76). All reports succeeded in demonstrating a high proportion of CLL B cells displaying natural autoantibody activity. Indeed, about half of the CLL B cells displayed rheumatoid factor activity and about 20% showed multispecific activity against autoantigens such as DNA and cytoskeleton proteins (76).

In a recent work, Kipps et al. (77) found that a high proportion of B-CLL cells expressing κ at the membrane reacted with a murine anti-idiotypic antibody raised against a monoclonal IgM rheumatoid factor expressing the Wa idiotype (major cross-reactive idiotype expressed by cryoglobulins). Analysis of κ light-chain variable region genes expressed by leukemic cells from different patients sharing the Wa idiotype enabled these authors to demonstrate that they all employed the unmutated germinal Hum Kv 325 gene. Similar restriction was found when VH genes were analyzed (78). These results confirm that CD5 + B-CLL lymphocytes are frequently committed to the production of natural autoantibodies. Furthermore, results from Kipps et al. (77,78) strongly suggested the use of a restricted set of genes by CLL B lymphocytes, and this was confirmed by the high frequency of natural autoantibody activity found among CLL B lymphocytes (76). Interestingly, similar results indicating a high restriction in gene usage were found in the case of CD5 + murine lymphomas (79).

The antibody activity found for CLL B lymphocytes was in aid to the hypothesis that CD5 + B cells are mainly involved in autoantibody secretion. However, in a recent work we have studied 31 hybridomas obtained in the laboratories of R. A. Miller and R. Levy, from CD5 − B-cell follicular lymphomas. Our results showed a high frequency of autoantibody activity among these hybrids, which was close to that observed for CD5 + CLL cells. These results indicate that the CD5 − B-cell subset is also involved in the production of natural autoantibodies (80).

HYPOGAMMAGLOBULINEMIA IN B-CLL

Hypogammaglobulinemia occurs in 10–60% of B-CLL cases, depending on the values used as the lower limit (81–83). This is the major cause of infection in CLL (82). Patients with early forms of the disease tend to have defective specific antibody responses to infection or immunization (83).

Hypogammaglobulinemia is probably a consequence of accumulation of these individual defects. The pathogenesis of hypogammaglobulinemia in B-CLL is poorly understood, as this phenomenon is rare in other B-cell malignancies, including acute lymphoblastic leukemia, nodular and diffuse lymphomas, hairy cell leukemia, etc., though it is frequently observed in the case of Kähler's disease (46). Although regulatory abnormalities in T cells may play a role in the induction of hypogammaglobulinemia, data concerning helper, suppressive, NK, and ADCC are contradictory, and fail to firmly establish their contribution to the development of hypogammaglobulinemia (45,46,84).

Leukemic B-CLL lymphocytes have been shown to frequently express CD25 and also, weakly, receptors for B-cell growth factor (24,86). As CLL leukemia cells are present in very large numbers, the possibility that they could soak up such growth factors, essential for adequate immune function, cannot be excluded. Mechanical perturbations of normal communication within the immune system, due to important infiltration by leukemic cells leading to important alterations in the normal interplay, could also play a role in the genesis of hypogammaglobulinemia. However, these last abnormalities are also observed in other B-cell malignancies, in which hypogammaglobulinemia is only rarely observed (46,84).

Based on the information presently available, it appears logical to assume that hypogammaglobulinemia in B-CLL is probably the result of dysfunction of nonclonal B cells. Thus, hypogammaglobulinemia in B-CLL could be a consequence of progressive dilution or inhibition of normal CD5 − B cells. This decrease in or inhibition of normal CD5 − B cells could also explain the classical inability of B-CLL to respond to new antigenic challenges, since Ly1 − B cells (the murine counterpart of human CD5 B cells) have been claimed to be unable to respond to exogenous antigens (85,87).

The fact that hypogammaglobulinemia was the major cause of the increased risk of sepsis in CLL prompted the use of intravenous immunoglobulins to prevent infection. In a double-blind randomized study, intravenous immunoglobulins (400 mg/kg of body weight given every 3 weeks) was found to reduce the overall incidence of bacterial infections. However, survival was not modified, and the number of severe bacterial infections, viral or fungal infections was unaffected (88).

A prominent monoclonal immunoglobulin peak, usually of the IgM type, is found in 5% of CLL patients. However, with high-resolution agarose gel electophoresis and immunofixation, a small amount of a monoclonal component can be identified in the serum or urine of 60% of patients (89).

AUTOIMMUNE PHENOMENA IN B-CLL

Autoimmune-associated phenomena are frequently observed in B-CLL. These autotoxic manifestations are directed mainly against hematopoietic cells (46,90). A positive direct antiglobulin test has been reported to be as high as 7.7% to 35% of B-CLL patients, depending on the series and stage of disease (46,84,90). In the French Cooperative Group series (CLL 1980 and 1985), positive Coombs test was found at diagnosis in only 1.8%. This lower prevalence is probably explained by the fact that the French Cooperative Group series included higher numbers of initial forms than previous series. Nevertheless, autoimmune hemolytic anemia occurs in 10–25% of patients at some time during the course of the disease. Although Feizi et al. (91) described one case of cold agglutinin disease in which autoantibodies were the product of CLL B cells, in most cases, autoantibodies against red blood cells are warm reactive polyclonal IgG and display activity against monomorphic antigens of the rhesus system (46,90). Immune thrombocytopenia is observed in about 2% of cases, but higher frequencies of increased platelet-associated Igs have been reported (90). Pure red cell aplasia and autoantibodies against neutrophils are only rarely observed, and there is conflicting evidence concerning the frequency of other autoantibodies. This pattern is similar to that observed in primary immunodeficiency syndromes, in which immune thrombocytopenia, autoimmune hemolytic anemia, and pure red cell aplasia are frequently observed (45,84). Since, in B-CLL, autoantibodies, in most cases, are not secreted by the malignant clone, it can be postulated that hypogammaglobulinemia could induce a disturbance in the idiotypic network, in such a way that anti-idiotypic antibodies designed to antagonize autoimmune clones are not made (46). Recently, Sultan et al. succeeded in suppressing production of anti-VIII autoantibodies by injecting intravenous Ig and speculated that anti-idiotypic suppression mediated by injected Igs could occur (92). However, no conclusive evidence concerning the role of intravenous Ig in the treatment of autoimmune-associated phenomena in B-CLL has so far been reported.

CONCLUSIONS

One of the main questions in B-CLL biology is to determine whether CLL B lymphocytes, which, in contrast to most other B-cell malignancies, express CD5, correspond to an immature clone arrested at an intermediate stage of maturation or correspond to a different B-cell subset. Whether the CD5 marker defines a discrete lineage or is a maturation marker is one of the main issues that may be solved in the near future. Another important advance was the discovery that the CLL B lymphocyte is frequently involved in the production of natural autoantibodies and that it expresses a restricted set of germinal genes. These results may provide a basis for passive immunotherapy with anti-idiotypic antibodies.

Hypogammaglobulinemia may result as a consequence of impaired function of residual normal B cells. This could occur as a consequence of progressive dilution of normal nonclonal B cells, or because normal B cells are downregulated by an unknown mechanism. The fact that hypogammaglobulinemia was the major risk factor in CLL prompted the prophylactic usage of intravenous immunoglobulins. Although its use in severe hypogammaglobulinemic patients appears logical, present results failed to demonstrate a significant decrease of severe infections.

Autoimmune-associated phenomena are an important complication in CLL. They are related to the presence of autoantibodies directed mainly against blood components, which in most cases are not a product of the malignant clone. The relationship between autoimmune phenomena and hypogammaglobulinemia is not definitively substantiated. Whether hypogammaglobulinemia could determine the loss of some anti-idiotypic antibodies designed to antagonize autoimmune clones is an attractive hypothesis that needs to be demonstrated.

REFERENCES

1. T. Eskeland, E. Klein, M. Inoue, and B. Johansson, Characterization of immunoglobulin structures from the surface of chronic lymphocytic leukemia cells, *J. Exp. Med., 134*:265 (1971).
2. H. M. Grey, E. Rabellino, and B. Pirofsky, Immunoglobulins on the surface of lymphocytes. IV. Distribution of hypogammaglobulinemia cellular immune deficiency and chronic lymphocytic leukemia, *J. Clin. Invest., 50*: 2368 (1971).
3. J. L. Preud'homme and M. Seligmann, Surface bound immunoglobulins as a cell marker in human proliferative diseases, *Blood, 40*:777 (1972).
4. T. Ternynck, G. Dighiero, J. Y. Follezou, and J. L. Binet, Comparison of normal and CLL lymphocytes surface Ig determinants using peroxidase labelled antibodies. I. Detection and quantitation of light chain determinants, *Blood, 43*:789 (1974).
5. S. Pincus, C. Bianco, and V. Nussenweig, Increased proportion of complement receptor lymphocytes in the peripheral blood of patients with chronic lymphocytic leukemia, *Blood, 40*:303 (1972).
6. A. S. Freedman, A. W. Boyd, F. R. Bieber, J. F. Daley, K. J. Rosen, J. C. Horowitz, D. N. Levy, and L. M. Nadler, Normal cellular counterparts of B cell chronic lymphocytic leukemia, *Blood, 70*:418 (1987).

7. H. B. Dickler and H. G. Kunkel, Interaction of aggregated gammaglobulins with B lymphocytes, *J. Exp. Med., 136*:191 (1972).

8. S. M. Fu, R. J. Winchester, and H. G. Kunkel, Similar idiotype specificity for the membrane IgD and IgM of human B lymphocytes, *J. Immunol., 114*: 250 (1975).

9. B. Pernis, J. C. Brouet, and M. Seligmann, IgD and IgM on the membrane of lymphoid cells in macroglobulinemia. Evidence for identity of membrane IgD and IgM antibody activity in a case with IgG receptors, *Eur. J. Immunol., 4*: 776 (1974).

10. K. R. Schoer, D. E. Briles, A. VanBonel, and J. M. David, Idiotypic uniformity of cell surface immunoglobulin in chronic lymphocytic leukemia: Evidence for monoclonal proliferation, *J. Exp. Med., 140*:1416 (1974).

11. P. J. Fialkow, V. Najfeld, A. Lashka Reddy, L. Singer, and L. Steinmann, Chronic lymphocytic leukemia: Clonal origin in a committed B-lymphocyte progenitor, *Lancet, ii*:444 (1978).

12. G. Juliusson, D. Oscier, M. Fitchett, M. Fiona, F. Ross, G. Stockdil, M. Mackie, A. Parker, G. Castoldi, A. Cuneo, S. Knuutila, E. Elonen, and G. Gahrton, Prognostic subgroups in B cell chronic lymphocytic leukemia defined by specific chromosomal abnormalities, *N. Engl. J. Med., 323*:720 (1990).

13. S. J. Korsmeyer, Hierarchy of immunoglobulin gene rearrangements in B-cell leukemias, in Molecular genetic analyses of human lymphoid neoplasms: Immunoglobulin genes and the c-myc oncogene (T. A. Waldmann, moderator), *Ann. Intern. Med., 102*:497 (1985).

14. F. Liegler, J. Kettman, and R. Smith, Immunoglobulin phenotype of B cells correlated with clinical stage of chronic lymphocytic leukemia, *Blood, 62*:256 (1983).

15. A. P. Johnstone, Chronic lymphocytic leukaemia and its relationship to normal B lymphopoiesis, *Immunol. Today, 3*:343 (1982).

16. C. S. Abramson, J. H. Kersey, and T. W. LeBien, A monoclonal antibody (BA-1) reactive with cells of B lymphocyte lineage, *J. Immunol., 126*:83 (1981).

17. L. M. Nadler, B Cell/leukemia panel workshop: summary and comments, in *Leucocyte Typing II*, Springer-Verlag, Berlin, p. 3 (1986).

18. L. M. Nadler, K. C. Anderson, G. Marti, M. Bates, E. Park, J. F. Daley, and S. F. Schlossman, B4, a human B lymphocyte-associated antigen expressed in normal, mitogen-activated, and malignant B lymphocytes, *J. Immunol., 131*: 244 (1983).

19. L. M. Nadler, P. Stashenko, R. Hardy, A. Vangthoven, C. Terhorst, and S. F. Schlossmann, Characterization of a human B cell-specific antigen (B2) distinct from B1, *J. Immunol., 126*:1941 (1981).

20. M. Sarfati, D. Bron, L. Lagneaux, C. Fonteyn, H. Frost, and G. Delespesse, Elevation of IgE binding factors in serum of patients with B cell derived chronic lymphocytic leukemia, *Blood, 71*:94 (1988).

21. J. F. Agee, F. A. Garver, and G. B. Faguet, An antigen common to chronic lymphocytic and hairy cell leukemia cells not shared by normal lymphocytes or by other leukemic cells, *Blood, 68*:62 (1986).

22. G. B. Faguet and J. F. Agee, Modulation, shedding and serum titers of the chronic lymphatic leukemia-associated antigen: Characterization and clinical correlations, *Blood, 74*:2493 (1989).

23. D. Catovsky, M. Cherchi, and D. Brooks, Heterogeneity of B cell leukemias demonstrated by the monoclonal antibody FMC7, *Blood, 58*:406 (1981).

24. H. Merle-Béral, C. Blanc, C. Chastang, and P. Debré, Phenotypic heterogeneity of B and T cell differentiation antigens in B CLL, *Eur. J. Haematol., 41*: 197 (1988).

25. D. Delia, G. Cattoretti, N. Polli, E. Fontanella, A. Aiello, R. Giardini, F. Rilke, and G. Della Porta, CD1c but neither CD1a nor CD1b are expressed on normal activated and malignant human B cells: Identification of a new B cell subset, *Blood, 72*:241 (1988).

26. H. Merle-Béral, L. Boumsell, A. Michel, and P. Debré, CD1 expression on B CLL lymphocytes, *Br. J. Haematol., 71*:209 (1989).

27. T. N. Small, R. W. Knowles, C. Keever, N. A. Kernan, N. Collins, R. J. O'Reilly, B. Dupont, and N. Flomenberg, M241 (CD1) expression on B lymphocytes, *J. Immunol., 138*:2864 (1987).

28. S. B. Wormsley, S. M. Baird, N. Gadol, K. R. Rai, and R. E. Sobol, Characteristics of CD11c + CD5 + chronic B-cell leukemias and the identification of novel peripheral blood B-cell subsets with chronic lymphoid leukemia immunophenotypes, *Blood, 76*:123 (1990).

29. R. H. Keller, J. A. Libnoch, G. Kallas, L. C. Patrick, and C. W. Patrick, Sequential T-cell immunoregulatory subsets and function in B-CLL, in *Chronic Lymphocytic Leukemia: Recent Progress and Future Direction*, Alan R. Liss, New York, p. 147 (1987).

30. F. Morabito, E. F. Prasthofer, N. E. Dunlap, C. E. Grossi, and A. B. Tilden, Expression of myelomonocytic antigens on chronic lymphocytic leukemia B cells correlates with their ability to produce interleukin 1, *Blood, 70*:1750 (1987).

31. G. Dighiero, J. Y. Follezou, J. P. Roisin, T. Ternynck, and J. L. Binet, Comparison of normal and CLL lymphocyte surface Ig determinants using peroxidase labelled antibodies. II. Quantitation of light chain determinants in atypical lymphoid leukemia, *Blood, 48*:559 (1976).

32. G. Dighiero, E. Bodega, R. Mayzner, and J. L. Binet, Individual cell-by-cell quantitation of lymphocyte surface membrane Ig in normal and CLL lymphocytes and during ontogeny of mouse B lymphocytes by immunoperoxidase assay, *Blood, 55*:93 (1980).

33. G. Stathopoulos and E. V. Elliot, Formation of mouse or sheep red blood cell rosette by lymphocytes from normal and leukemic individuals, *Lancet, i*:229 (1974).

34. D. Catovsky, M. Cherchi, and A. Okas, Mouse red-cell rosettes in B lymphoproliferative disorders, *Br. J. Haematol., 33*:173 (1976).

35. L. Boumsell, A. Bernard, V. Lepage, L. Degos, J. Lemerle, and J. Dausset, Some chronic lymphocytic leukemia cells bearing surface immunoglobulins share determinants with T cells, *Eur. J. Immunol., 8*:900 (1978).

36. I. Royston, J. A. Majda, S. M. Baird, B. E. Mierserve, and E. C. Griffiths,

Human T-cell antigens defined by monoclonal antibodies: The 65000 dalton antigen of T cells (T65) is also found on chronic lymphocytic leukemia cells bearing surface immunoglobulin, *J. Immunol., 125*:275 (1980).

37. Ch. Wang, R. A. Good, P. Ammirak, G. Dymbore, and R. E. Evans, Identification of a p69, 71 complex expressed on human T cells sharing determinants with B type chronic lymphatic leukemic cells, *J. Exp. Med., 151*:1539 (1980).

38. E. Caligaris-Cappio, M. Gobbi, M. Bofill, and G. Janossy, Unfrequent normal B lymphocytes express features of B-chronic lymphocytic leukemia, *J. Exp. Med., 155*:623 (1985).

39. M. Bofil, G. Janossy, M. Janossa, G. D. Burford, G. J. Seymour, P. Wernet, and E. Kelemen, Human B cell development. H. Subpopulations in the human fetus, *J. Immunol., 134*:1531 (1985).

40. J. H. Antin, S. P. Emerson, P. Martin, N. Gaddol, and K. A. Ault, Leu 1 (CD5) B cells, a major lymphoid subpopulation in human fetal spleen: phenotypic and functional studies, *J. Immunol., 136*:505 (1986).

41. F. Caligaris-Cappio and G. Janossy, Surface markers in chronic lymphoid leukemias of B cell type, *Semin. Hematol., 22*:1 (1985).

42. N. Gadol and K. A. Ault, Phenotypic and functional characterization of human Leu 1 (CD5) B cells, *Immunol. Rev., 93*:23 (1986).

43. A. S. Freedman, G. Freeman, J. Whitman, J. Segil, J. Daley, and L. M. Nadler, Studies of in vitro activated CD5+ B cells, *Blood, 73*:202 (1989).

44. S. E. Salmon and M. Seligmann, B-cell neoplasia in man, *Lancet, ii*:1230 (1974).

45. G. Dighiero, Relevance of murine models in elucidating the origin of B-CLL lymphocytes and related immune associated phenomena, *Semin. Hematol., 24*:240 (1987).

46. G. Dighiero, An attempt to explain disordered immunity and hypogammaglobulinemia in CLL, *Nouv. Rev. Franc. Hematol., 30*:283 (1988).

47. V. Manohar, E. Brown, W. M. Leiserson, and T. M. Chused, Expression of Ly-1 by a subset of B lymphocytes, *J. Immun., 129*:532 (1982).

48. K. Hayakawa, R. R. Hardy, D. R. Parks, and L. A. Herzenberg, The "Ly-1 B" cell subpopulation in normal immunodefective and autoimmune mice. *J. Exp. Med., 157*:202–218 (1983).

49. K. Hayakawa, R. R. Hardy, and L. A. Herzenberg, Peritoneal Ly-1B cells: Genetic control, autoantibody production, increased lambda light chain expression, *Eur. J. Immunol., 16*:450 (1986).

50. L. A. Herzenberg, A. M. Stall, P. A. Lalor, C. Sidman, W. A. Moore, and D. R. Pards, The Ly1-B cell lineage, *Immunol. Rev., 93*:81–102 (1986).

51. K. Hayakawa, R. R. Hardy, L. A. Herzenberg, and L. A. Herzenberg, Progenitors for Ly-1 B cells are distinct from progenitors for other B cells, *J. Exp. Med., 161*:1554, (1985).

52. I. Förster and K. Rajewsky, Expansion and functional activity of Ly-1+ B cells upon transfer of peritoneal cells into allotype-congenic newborn mice, *Eur. J. Immunol., 17*:521 (1987).

53. T. J. Mercolino, A. L. Locke, A. Afshari, D. Sasser, W. W. Travis, L. W. Arnold, and G. Haughton, Restricted immunoglobulin variable region gene

usage by normal Ly-1 (CD5+) B cells that recognize phosphatidyl choline. *J. Exp. Med., 169*:1869 (1989).

54. G. Dighiero, P. Poncet, S. Rouyre, and J. C. Mazié, New-born Xid mice carry the genetic information for the production of natural autoantibodies, *J. Immunol., 136*:4000–4005 (1986).

55. J. D. Conger, B. L. Pike, and G. J. V. Nossal, Clonal analysis of the anti-DNA repertoire of murine B lymphocytes, *Proc. Natl. Acad. Sci. USA, 84*: 2931 (1987).

56. A. Kaushik, R. Meyer, V. Fidanza, A. Lim, C. Bona, and G. Dighiero, Ly1 and V-gene expression among hybridomas secreting natural autoantibody. *J. Autoimmun., 3*:687–700 (1991).

57. R. A. Miller and J. Gralow, The induction of Leu-1 antigen expression in human malignant and normal B cells by phorbol myristic acetate (PMA), *J. Immunol., 133*:3408–3412 (1984).

58. F. K. Stevenson, T. J. Hamblin, G. T. Stevenson, and A. L. Tuh, Extracellular idiotypic immunoglobulin arising from human leukemia B lymphocytes, *J. Exp. Med., 152*:1484 (1980).

59. T. H. Tötterman, K. Nilsson, and C. Sundström, Phorbol ester-induced differentiation of chronic lymphocytic leukaemia cells, *Nature, 288*:176 (1980).

60. J. Okamura, E. W. Gelfand, and M. Letarte, Heterogeneity of the response of chronic lymphocytic leukemia cells to phorbol ester, *Blood, 60*:1082 (1982).

61. J. Okamura, M. Letarte, L. D. Stein, N. J. Segal, and E. W. Gelfand, Modulation of chronic lymphocytic leukemia cells by phorbol esters: Increase in Ia expression. IgM secretion and MLR stimulatory capacity, *J. Immunol., 128*: 2276 (1982).

62. P. Guglielmi, J. L. Preud'homme, M. F. Gourdin, F. Reyes, and M. T. Daniel, Unusual intracytoplasmic immunolglobulin inclusions in chronic lymphocytic leukaemia, *Br. J. Haematol., 50*:123 (1982).

63. A. Rubartelli, R. Sitia, A. Zicca, C. E. Grossi, and M. Ferrarini, Differentiation of chronic lymphocytic leukemia cells: Correlation between the synthesis and secretion of immunoglobulins and the ultrastructure of the malignant cells, *Blood, 62*:495 (1983).

64. J. Gordon, H. Mellstedt, P. Aman, P. Biberfeld, and G. Klein, Phenotypic modulation of chronic lymphocytic leukemia cells by phorbol ester: Induction of IgM secretion and changes in the expression of B-cell associated surface antigens, *J. Immunol., 132*:541 (1984).

65. F. Caligaris-Cappio, G. Janossy, and D. Campana, Lineage relationship of chronic lymphocytic leukaemia and hairy cell leukaemia: Studies with TPA, *Leuk. Res., 8*:567 (1984).

66. S. Karray, H. Merle-Beral, A. Vazquez, J. P. Gérard, P. Debré, and P. Galanaud, Functional heterogeneity of B-CLL lymphocytes: Dissociated responsiveness to growth factors and distinct requirements for a first activation signal, *Blood, 70*:1105 (1987).

67. S. Karray, J. F. Delfraissy, H. Merle-Béral, C. Wallon, P. Debré, and P. Galanaud, Positive effect of interferon alpha on B cell-type chronic lymphocytic leukemia proliferative response, *J. Immunol., 140*:774 (1988).

68. S. Karray, A. Vazquez, H. Merle-Béral, D. Olive, P. Debré, and P. Galanaud, Synergistic effect of recombinant IL2 and interferon gamma on the proliferation of human monoclonal lymphocytes, *J. Immunol., 138*:2824 (1987).
69. S. Karray, T. DeFrance, H. Merle-Béral, J. Banchereau, P. Debré, and P. Galanaud, Interleukin 4 counteracts the interleukin 2-induced proliferation of monoclonal B cells, *J. Exp. Med., 168*:85 (1988).
70. C. Hivroz, C. Grillot-Courvalin, J. C. Brouet, and M. Seligmann, Heterogeneity of responsiveness of chronic lymphocytic leukemic B cells to B cell growth factor or interleukin 2, *Eur. J. Immunol., 16*:1001 (1986).
71. O. Lantz, C. Grillot-Courvalin, C. Schmitt, J. P. Fermand, and J. C. Brouet, Interleukin-2 induced proliferation of leukemic human B cells, *J. Exp. Med., 161*:1225 (1985).
72. M. L. Levitt, W. E. Barry, M. K. Helfrich, B. Kaiser McCaw Hecht, and E. E. Henderson, Characterization of Epstein-Barr virus carrying cell lines established from chronic lymphocytic leukemia, *Cancer Res., 43*:1195 (1983).
73. M. Crescenzi, M. Napolitano, M. Carbonari, A. Antonelli, P. Petrinelli, C. Gaetano, and M. Fiorilli, Establishment of a new Epstein-Barr virus immortalized cell line from chronic lymphocytic leukemia with trisomy of chromosome 12 that produces monoclonal IgM against sheep RBC antigen, *Blood, 71*:9–12 (1988).
74. B. M. Bröker, A. Klajman, P. Youinou, J. Jouquan, C. P. Worman, J. Murphy, L. Mackenzie, R. Quartey-Papafio, M. Blaschek, P. Collins, S. Lal, and P. M. Lydyard, Chronic lymphocytic leukemic (CLL) cells secrete multispecific autoantibodies, *J. Autoimmun., 1*:469 (1988).
75. Z. M. Sthoeger, M. Wakai, D. B. Tse, V. P. Vinciguerra, S. L. Allen, D. R. Budman, S. M. Lichtman, P. Schulman, L. R. Weiselbert, and N. Chiorazzi, Production of autoantibodies by CD5-expressing B lymphocytes from patients which chronic lymphocytic leukemia, *J. Exp. Med., 169*:255 (1989).
76. L. Borche, A. Lim, J. L. Binet, and G. Dighiero, Evidence that chronic lymphocytic leukemia B lymphocytes are frequently committed to production of natural autoantibodies, *Blood, 76*:562 (1990).
77. T. J. Kipps, E. Tomhave, P. P. Chen, and D. A. Carson, Autoantibody associated k-light chain variable region gene expressed in chronic lymphocytic leukemia with little or no somatic mutation, implications for etiology and immunotherapy, *J. Exp. Med., 167*:840 (1988).
78. T. J. Kipps, E. Tomhave, L. F. Pratt, S. Duffy, P. P. Chen, and D. A. Carson, Developmentally restricted immunoglobulin heavy chain variable region gene expressed at high frequency in chronic lymphocytic leukemia. *Proc. Natl. Acad. Sci. USA, 86*:5913 (1989).
79. C. A. Pennell, L. W. Arnold, G. Haughton, and S. H. Clark, Restricted immunoglobulin variable region gene expression among Ly-1 cell lymphomas, *J. Immunol., 141*:2788 (1988).
80. G. Dighiero, S. Hart, A. Lim, L. Borche, R. Levy, and R. A. Miller, Autoantibody activity of immunoglobulins isolated from B-cell follicular lymphomas, *Blood, 78*:581 (1991).
81. G. H. Fairley and R. B. Scott, Hypogammaglobulinemia in chronic lymphocytic leukemia, *Br. Med. J., 4*:920 (1961).

82. H. Chapel and C. Buch, Mechanisms of infection in chronic lymphocytic leukemia, *Semin. Hematol., 24*:291 (1987).

83. M. H. Chapel, Hypogammaglobulinemia and chronic lymphocytic leukemia, in *Chronic Lymphocytic Leukemia: Recent Progress, Future Directions* (R. P. Gale and K. Rai, eds.), Alan R. Liss, New York, p. 383 (1987).

84. G. Dighiero, P. Travade, S. Chevret, P. Fenaux, C. Chastang, J. L. Binet and the French Cooperative Group on CLL B-cell chronic lymphocytic leukemia: Present status and future directions, *Blood, 78*:1901 (1991).

85. R. R. Hardy and K. Hayakawa, Development and physiology of Ly-1 B and its human homolog, Leu-1 B, *Immunol. Rev., 93*:53 (1986).

86. R. Foa, M. Giovanelli, M. T. Fierro, M. Bonferroni, and G. Forni, Autocrine or paracrine models of cytokine production and utilization in B-cell chronic lymphocytic leukemia, *Nouv. Rev. Fr. Hematol., 30*:339–341 (1988).

87. L. A. Herzenberg, A. M. Stall, P. A. Lalor, C. Sidman, W. A. Moore, and D. R. Parks, The Ly-1 B cell lineage, *Immunol. Rev., 93*:81 (1986).

88. Cooperative Group for the Study of Immunoglobulin in Chronic Lymphocytic Leukemia, Intravenous immunoglobulin for the prevention of infection in chronic lymphocytic leukemia. A randomized control trial, *N. Engl. J. Med., 319*:902 (1988).

89. M. J. Deegan, High incidence of monoclonal proteins in the serum and urine of chronic lymphocytic leukemia patients, *Blood, 64*:1207 (1984).

90. T. J. Hamblin, D. J. Oscier, and B. J. Young, Autoimmunity in chronic lymphocytic leukemia, *J. Clin. Pathol., 39*:713 (1986).

91. T. Feizi, P. Wernet, H. G. Kunkel, and S. D. Douglas, Lymphocytes forming red cell rosettes in the cold in patients with chronic cold agglutinin disease, *Blood, 42*:753 (1983).

92. Y. Sultan, P. Maisonneuve, M. D. Kazatchkine, and U. Nydegger, Anti-idiotypic suppression of autoantibodies to factor VIII (anti-hemophilic factor) by high-dose intravenous gammaglobulin, *Lancet, ii*:765 (1984).

9

Clonal Evolution in Chronic Lymphocytic Leukemia

LoAnn Peterson
Northwestern University Medical School, Chicago, Illinois

Mark Blackstadt
Veterans Affairs Medical Center, Minneapolis, Minnesota

Neil Kay
Hybritech, Inc. and University of California, San Diego, San Diego, California

In this chapter we present evidence for clonal evolution in B-cell chronic lymphocytic leukemia (B-CLL). Clonal evolution may involve alterations in surface phenotype, cell function, karyotype, or immunoglobulin (Ig) gene rearrangement patterns in the B-cell clone. To date, most investigations have suggested that there is little or no clonal evolution in B-CLL (reviewed below). These previous findings correlate well with the "usual" clinical history of most patients with this B-cell malignancy. However, rapid clinical evolution into a more aggressive malignancy occurs in some patients. In addition, many B-CLL patients develop secondary lymphoid malignancies with a more acute clinical course. We have recently evaluated a cohort of Midwestern B-CLL patients who demonstrated rapid clonal evolution as characterized by both cytogenetic and immunoglobulin gene rearrangement alterations. This chapter will first describe, in brief, previous investigations of clonal evolution in B-CLL. Then we will describe the cytogenetic and gene rearrangement data, which indicates that clonal evolution occurs in B-CLL.

CLONAL EVOLUTION—THE CLINICAL ISSUE

Patients with B-CLL are frequently informed about the relatively "benign" nature of this leukemia. However, the median life span of 5–7 years is counterbalanced by several morbid clinical features including concomitant hypogammaglobulinemia, autoimmune syndromes, and the diagnosis of second tumors (skin tumors, adenocarcinoma) (5). More life-threatening clinical alterations include stage progression or (rarely) acute transformation events (5). The former is much more common than the latter, but both are associated with significant mortality and/or therapeutic difficulties. Patients who have more advanced stage (i.e., Rai stage 3 or 4) survive less than 2 or 3 years (6–7). The acute transformation events include development of large cell lymphoma (Richter's syndrome), prolymphocytic transformation, and acute blast crisis. These entities have been reviewed in detail elsewhere (5–6), but are uniformly associated with poor response to therapy and shortened survival.

Because of the clinical severity of the latter clinical syndromes, insight into events responsible may be helpful. The most obvious explanation for development of the aggressive clinical B-CLL syndromes, over the usual indolent disease, is the emergence of B-cell clone(s) with enhanced proliferative and infiltrative abilities. This aggressive B-cell clone would develop from an alternative B-cell clone, within an oligoclonal population or through clonal evolution. Thus the presence of multiple B-cell clones in B-CLL may permit selection of one clone with predominant growth characteristics. Alternatively, clonal evolution of the sole B-cell clone may result in alteration of cellular parameters that result in transformation to a more aggressive B-cell disease.

In order to gain insight into the latter possibilities, we have initiated sequential studies of B-cell clones from CLL patients. Specifically, we have evaluated both cytogenetic and Ig gene rearrangement status of individual CLL B-cell clones over a $2\frac{1}{2}$-year follow-up. These biologic parameters were used to determine if single or multiple B-cell clones were present on initial evaluation. In addition, follow-up studies of these parameters were used to detect clonal stability or evolution. The remainder of this chapter will detail both cytogenetic and Ig gene rearrangement studies in previously published reports and in the cohort of B-CLL patients that we studied. We believe that these data indicate that clonal evolution is a more common feature of B-CLL than is currently reported.

CLONAL EVOLUTION BY GENE REARRANGEMENT— PREVIOUS STUDIES

The analysis of Ig gene rearrangement with cDNA probes for the J region or the constant region of kappa or lambda light chains documented the clonal B-cell derivation of CLL (1–3). In addition, the hierarchy of rearrangement for kappa and lambda light chains in B-CLL was consistent with the ordered process believed to occur in normal ontogeny. These studies did not report detection of either multiple bands on Southern, indicative of oligoclonality, or alteration of heavy- or light-chain patterns (1–4). Thus, stability of Ig gene rearrangement appeared to correlate with the usual, stable clinical course. These early studies, however, did not report on the Ig gene rearrangement patterns of CLL B-cell clones studied over the disease course, and several recent investigations suggest that CLL B-cell clones may be subject to clonal evolution over time.

Evidence for clonal evolution in B-CLL has been studied primarily in B-CLL patients with subsequent transformation to a large-cell lymphoma (Richter's syndrome) (8). Analysis of surface Ig isotypes and light chain phenotype has generated conflicting data in these patients. Thus, clones with similar and dissimilar Ig isotypes and/or light chains have been found (9–13). The difficulty of using surface Ig as proof of clonal similarities (i.e., because of isotype switch or somatic mutation) prompted the use of anti-idiotypic antibodies. These antibodies detect unique idiotypic determinants of the variable (V) heavy- and V light-chain domains (14–16). An anti-idiotype reactive for a CLL patient's B cells was found to react with a diffuse large-cell lymphoma diagnosed 6 years later in this patient (14). Ig gene rearrangement patterns on Southern blot were identical for the CLL cells and the new lymphoma (14). This case clearly documented the potential for a given B-cell clone to differentiate into a more aggressive type of lymphoma. Anti-idiotype antibodies have documented that multiple myeloma clones (N = 2) were probably related to chronic lymphocytic leukemia clones (7). Unfortunately, there have been very few additional cases of B-CLL with transformation to lymphoma that were studied by anti-idiotype reagents. In addition, Ig gene rearrangement studies have shown that evolution to lymphoma in some patients with B-CLL may result from emergence of an alternative clone (9,13). Most recently, a study of 38 B-CLL patients was conducted to correlate clinical stage with Ig gene rearrangement patterns (17). This study detected multiple clonal bands using J_H or C_μ cDNA probes in the DNA of CLL B cells. Importantly, several patients had more than two clonal bands, implying that there were several circulating clones (17). Patients with more advanced stage had multiple C_{MU} bands or loss of germline J_H bands. These investigators speculated that in more advanced B-CLL, unstable B-cell clones may exist. This latter characteristic could predispose a B-cell clone to clonal evolution.

In summary, prior Ig gene rearrangement studies have generated data suggesting that B-CLL patients may possess multiple clones. In addition, the use of anti-idiotype sera has shown that B-CLL clones may undergo clonal evolution related to clinical stage or disease transformation. We reasoned that the evidence for either multiple clones or clonal evolution would be detected through a prospective and sequential evaluation of individual B-cell clones. The following section details our Southern blot results of sequential Ig gene rearrangement patterns from our CLL patient cohort.

DETECTION OF CLONAL EVOLUTION USING BASELINE AND SEQUENTIAL Ig GENE REARRANGEMENT

The analysis of rearranged Ig genes by the Southern blot method has convincingly demonstrated that CLL B cells are (a) clonal and (b) capable of extensive and intricate Ig gene segment shuffling (1-5). The latter parameter was helpful in proving that CLL B cells possess a relatively mature and active Ig recombination potential. The clonal nature of CLL B cells is also potentially subject to subsequent modification through clonal evolution. In normal B cells, alteration of Ig genes during maturation is believed to generate a diverse repertoire of antibody-producing cells. However, the same mechanisms, if operative in B-CLL, might be a mechanism whereby this B-cell tumor generates a more aggressive or malignant course. Indeed, clonal evolution has been described for certain lymphomas and related to their clinical transformation (reviewed below). However, until recently, clonal evolution in CLL was not believed to be a frequent occurrence. We believe that this process may be an important and relatively frequent event in B-CLL.

The strategy we used for definition of B-cell multiclonality and/or clonal evolution was to sequentially assess Ig gene rearrangement patterns of purified B-CLL clones. DNA was isolated from blood B-cell clones, digested with restriction nucleases, electrophoresed on agarose gel, blotted on nitrocellulose, and hybridized to three separate radiolabeled Ig cDNA probes. We used a J_H, C_κ, and C_λ cDNA probe to assess the Ig gene rearrangement status of the B cell clone. Sixty-one B-CLL patients representing all four stages of B-CLL were evaluated by Southern blot upon entry to the study and subsequently on a 3- to 6-month basis over a 30-month period. Twenty-four of the original cohort had at least three repetitive studies with all three Ig cDNA probes. The data presented here are from these 24 B-CLL patients. The patients had a mean follow-up of 11.5 months with a range of 8 to 21 months. Table 1 summarizes the sequential gene rearrangement data. The major findings from this analysis include the following: (a) The light-chain alleles (kappa and lambda) were uniformly stable; however, and in contrast, (b) J_H alleles showed considerable lability in 8 of 24 (33%) CLL patients. These CLL patients had either gain (N = 4) or loss (N = 4) of a J_H allele. Because of possible variable migration rates of Ig DNA on different Southern blots, we reassessed all patients with loss or acquisition of

Table 1 Clone Stability: Evaluation of Ig Gene Rearrangement Using cDNA Probes for J_H, C_κ or C_λ[a]

	J_H Allele	C_κ Allele	C_λ Allele
Stable clones	15	24	24
Unstable clone	8	0	0
Gain of allele	4	—	—
Loss of allele	4	—	—

[a]Estimate of unstable clones was based on sequential evaluation of J_H alleles on Southern blot.

rearranged alleles on the same Southern blot. This allowed hybridization patterns to the respective Ig cDNA probes to be compared for more precise size determination on all sequential DNA samples.

Four patients developed an additional J_H allele, while four patients lost one rearranged allele. In two cases with gain of an allele, an original rearranged allele was retained and a single new rearranged allele was detected (Fig. 1, PT D). One patient had loss of two original alleles and acquisition of one additional allele (Fig. 2, PT E), and one patient lost a single allele and gained a single, new rearranged allele (Fig. 3, PT A). All four patients with a single allele loss had retention of the remaining original J_H allele (Fig. 3, PT B). The mean follow-up time for these seven B-CLL patients was 14 months with a range of 9 to 21 months. Three of the seven B-CLL patients had previously been on chemotherapy, while the other four had never been treated for B-CLL. Two patients who lost a J_H allele had been on chemotherapy, while one patient who gained a new J_H allele had been previously treated.

The mechanism for gain or loss of the J_H alleles in these B-cell clones appears to be as a result of clonal evolution. The major evidence for this is our sequential evaluation of the Ig light-chain genotype in these B-cell clones. All seven B-CLL patients, despite alteration of J_H alleles, retained their baseline original light-chain gene rearrangement clonal band. To ensure that the light-chain gene rearrangements were identical, we evaluated the DNA obtained from sequential samples on the same Southern blot. Thus, we were able to compare the light-chain Ig gene rearrangement fragments directly. This method of analysis confirmed the constancy of the light-chain gene rearrangements (data not shown). More definitive proof for retention of the original light-chain rearrangement will require nucleotide sequencing. Nevertheless, the frequent alteration of J_H alleles seen in our patient population suggests a relatively high rate of clonal evolution in B-CLL. We believe our frequent sequential analysis, using both heavy- and

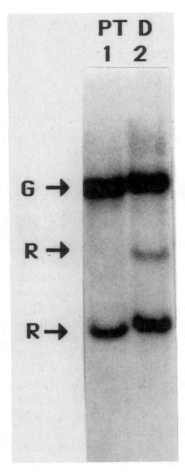

Figure 1   Ig gene rearrangement studies on blood B cells of patient (PT) D using a cDNA probe for J_H. A germline (G) fragment and a single rearranged (R) fragment are detected on study 1 (lane 1). Study 2 (lane 2) shows the original R and G fragment as well as a new, fainter R fragment.

light-chain Ig cDNA probes, has permitted detection of this event. To date, follicular lymphomas are the only B-cell tumor that have been shown to undergo frequent clonal evolution. These studies were prompted by the relatively frequent histologic conversion of follicular lymphoma to an aggressive diffuse histology (18,19). In some of these cases, Southern blot

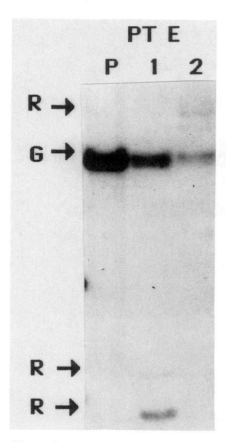

Figure 2 Ig gene rearrangement studies on blood B cells of PT E using a cDNA probe for J_H. Control lane is placenta (P) DNA. Study 1 (lane 1) shows a G fragment and two clonal R fragments. Study 2 (lane 2) now detects a new, larger R fragment and a G fragment with disappearance of the original two R fragments.

studies showed that no concordant bands were observed in the two lymphoma types from the same individual (20). This could be interpreted as biclonal tumors, i.e., two separate malignant transformations. However, if mutations reside within restriction nuclease sites, these discordant bands would not have to be of bi- or multiclonal origin. In addition, nucleotide sequencing of these clonal bands has frequently shown a nonrandom pattern indicating common rearrangement origins (21). Finally, analysis of idiotype expression in patients with both follicular and diffuse lymphoma

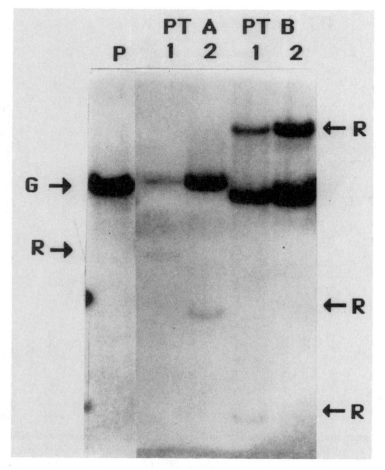

Figure 3 PT A and PT B. Sequential study times for immunoglobulin (Ig) gene rearrangement are shown for two patients. PT A has a germline fragment (G) and a rearranged clonal (R) fragment at the first study (lane 1). The second study (lane 2) shows an increased germline fragment (G) and a new rearranged (R) fragment with disappearance of the original (R) fragment. PT B has a G fragment and two R clonal fragments at baseline study (lane 1). The second, follow-up study (lane 2) shows only the G and one R fragment. Placental (P) DNA is control lane for the germline (G) fragment.

has shown retention of idiotype in both lymphomas (22). This helps to confirm the common clonal origin of both tumors in these patients. In sum, the follicular lymphomas have been shown to have B cells capable of nonrandom, somatic mutations that may relate to clonal evolution and histologic transformation (23,24). While previous studies have suggested other B-cell tumors are less likely to undergo somatic mutation and clonal evolution (25,26), our data indicate that B-CLL clones are also capable of clonal evolution. This predisposition apparently resides to a large extent in the J region of the heavy chain, since light-chain gene rearrangement was identical in all cases.

CLONAL EVOLUTION BY CYTOGENETIC ANALYSIS—PREVIOUS STUDIES

The introduction of B-cell mitogens into cytogenetic techniques has made it possible to karyotype the lymphocytes in B-CLL and to define the cytogenetic abnormalities in this disease. Clonal cytogenetic abnormalities occur in about 50–65% of patients with B-CLL (27,28). Trisomy 12, either as a sole abnormality or with other abnormalities, appears to be the most common clonal alteration in B-CLL (27,29–34). Other recurring abnormalities include structural alterations of the long arm of chromosome 13 (13q), chromosome 14 (14q), chromosome 6 (6q) and 11 (11q) (27,28,35–37). For a more detailed discussion of chromosomal abnormalities of B-CLL, see Chapter 4.

The karyotypic profile in B-CLL appears to provide prognostic information. Patients with normal karyotypes survive longer than those with clonal abnormalities, and patients with single abnormalities do better than those with complex karyotypes. Among patients with single abnormalities, those with trisomy 12 appear to have the shortest survivals (34). Alterations of 14q have also been associated with shortened survivals (34,35).

Karyotypic evolution is common in some hematologic malignancies, especially chronic myeloid leukemia (CML), where chromosomal changes in addition to the Philadelphia chromosome occur in more than 75% of patients studied. Most of the additional changes in CML occur shortly before or during blast crisis and therefore can be used as predictive indicators of this aggressive phase of the disease (38). Although the issue of karyotypic or clonal evolution and its correlation with clinical course is of great importance in B-CLL, only a few sequential karyotypic studies have been reported thus far. Most studies have argued for karyotypic stability in B-CLL, with the same karyotype being detected in some patients over a period of months or years (39–41). However, changes in the karyotype indicating clonal or karyotypic evolution have also been reported. No karyotypic evolution was identified in 21 B-CLL patients followed with serial cytogenetic studies for 2 to 16 years; karyotypic changes, however, were demonstrated in 4 of 12 (33%) patients studied for less than 2 years (40). Forty-one B-CLL patients were studied cytogenetically for 1.5 to 8.5 years, and additional or new clonal aberrations were found in three, or 7% of the patients (39). In another report, two, or 25%, of eight patients who initially had trisomy 12 as the sole chromosomal abnormality developed additional clonal alterations in from 1 to 2 years (42). More recently, serial chromosomal analysis was performed on 112 B-CLL patients over a mean interval of 2.9 years. Karyotypic evolution was found in 18, or 16% of the patients. In addition, in complex karyotypic abnormalities were found in 17% of the patients on initial analysis, indicating that karyotypic evolution had already occurred. The secondary karyotypic changes were similar to those detected as single abnormalities (41). These studies show that most patients with B-CLL exhibit stable karyotypes. They also document karyotypic evolution in a subpopulation of patients, although the reported incidence is relatively low.

KARYOTYPIC EVOLUTION—
RELATION TO CLINICAL COURSE

The relationship of karyotypic evolution to clinical course is a question that has not been completely answered. Most authors, however, agree that disease progression occurs in many patients who do not exhibit karyotypic evolution but who maintain a stable karyotype. In a series of 112 B-CLL patients, the incidence of progressive disease was no different between patients with a stable karyotype and those with karyotypic evolution (41). Occasional patients, however, are reported in whom detection of additional chromosomal abnormalities appears to correlate with disease progression and shortened survival (40–42). In some patients karyotypic evolution and clinical deterioration has also been associated with change in lymphocyte morphology or development of a large-cell lymphoma (Richter's syndrome) (41,42). In summary, prior reports suggest that many B-CLL patients who exhibit clinical deterioration have stable karyotypes, suggesting that disease progression may be more dependent on other factors. However, karyotypic evolution in some B-CLL patients appears to correlate with clinical aggressiveness of the disease, leading some authors to suggest that its occurrence indicates a poor prognosis (40). The correlation of karyotypic evolution with disease progression is supported by the observation that patients with complex karyotypes have more advanced disease than those with single aberrations (43,44).

DETECTION OF CLONAL EVOLUTION BY BASELINE AND SEQUENTIAL CYTOGENETIC ANALYSIS

We have recently karyotyped 79 Midwestern patients with B-CLL. This patient population represented all clinical stages and included both treated and untreated patients. Twenty-eight of these patients had repeat cytogenetic analysis. At baseline, 50, or 63%, of the 79 patients analyzed had clonal chromosomal abnormalities. Structural alterations of chromosome band 13q14, site of the retinoblastoma gene, were the most common abnormalities detected, identified in 22 (28%) patients. Structural alterations of 6q were found in nine (13%) of patients, trisomy 12 in eight (10%) patients, and structural alterations of 14q in four (5%). Twelve (15%) patients had clonal abnormalities other than those mentioned above (45).

Many of the patients at baseline had complex karyotypes with more than one chromosomal aberration. Nineteen (38%) of the 50 patients with clonal chromosomal abnormalities had a single abnormality, while 31 (62%) had more complex abnormalities. In addition, 19 (38%) patients with clonal abnormalities had more than one clone or subclone. In 9 of the 19 patients, the clones had abnormalities in common and appeared to result from clonal evolution within a single neoplastic clone. In contrast, the multiple clones in seven patients appeared to be unrelated. Three patients had some related subclones that shared abnormalities and other cytogenetically unrelated clones (46). The presence of unrelated clones could imply a multiclonal disease; however, they could also be the result of karyotypic evolution along two separate pathways in which the primary abnormality is not detected (41). The presence of complex karyotypes, including many patients with multiple clones, suggests that karyotypic evolution had already taken place in a high percentage of cases by the time the baseline karyotypic analysis was performed. Thus we missed the opportunity to observe progression in these patients.

Repeat cytogenetic analysis was performed on cells from 28 patients ranging from 4 to 19 months from baseline. Seven were cytogenetically normal at baseline; only three of these patients remained normal, while four developed clonal abnormalities (Table 2). Twenty-one patients had chromosomal abnormalities at baseline; three of these patients developed additional abnormalities indicating clonal evolution (Table 3); four developed additional clones that appeared unrelated to the original clones. Therefore, new or additional clonal abnormalities were identified in 11 of 28 (39%) patients. In addition, three patients who originally had clonal abnormalities had loss of previously detected normal metaphase cells, and six had loss of previously identified clonal aberrations.

Both the complex karyotypes at baseline and the results of the sequential

Table 2 Sequential Chromosome Analysis of a B-CLL Patient Who Had a Normal Karyotype at Baseline but Who Developed a Clonal Abnormality over Time

| Date of study | Number of metaphase cells | | Karyotype |
	Total	Normal and Abnormal	
5–88	20	20	46,XY
11–88	20	20	46,XY
1–90	25	25	46,XY
11–90	20	8	46,XY/
		7	46,XY,del(13)(q14q22)/
		3	46,XY,t(3;13)(p26;q14)/
		2	46,XY,del(13)(q14q22),t(7;18)(q22;p11)

Table 3 Sequential Chromosome Analysis of a B-CLL Patient Who Developed Additional Clonal Abnormalities Indicating Karyoptypic Evolution

| Date of study | Number of metaphase cells | | Karyotype |
	Total	Normal and Abnormal	
5–88	20	5	46,XY/
		15	46,XY,del(13)(q13q22)
7–90	20	4	46,XY/
		16	46,XY,del(13)(q13q22)
1–90	21	1	46,XY/
		15	46,XY,del(13)(q13q22)/
		5	46,XY,del(6)(q15q24),del(13)(q13q22)

chromosomal analysis in our patient population suggests that clonal evolution may be more frequent in B-CLL than is currently appreciated. Sequential karyotypic changes were identified in patients with disease length ranging from 2 to 15 years. They also occurred in both treated and untreated patients. This suggests that these changes are inherent to the disease process and that B-CLL may be more cytogenetically unstable than previously recognized.

CONCLUSION

The fate of clonal B cells during the clinical progression of B-cell chronic lymphocytic leukemia is more diverse than originally predicted. The biologic parameters that originally characterized this clonal B cell indicated a relatively stable and inert cell. These immunobiologic features were and are mimicked by a relatively long, stable clinical course. However, prior cytogenetic and membrane idiotype evaluation did suggest that these cells may be subject to a more active alteration of their clonal status. Our immunoglobulin gene rearrangement and cytogenetic laboratory studies have uncovered that approximately a third of our patients exhibit an array of immunoglobulin gene rearrangement and/or cytogenetic changes that highly suggest clonal evolution. Since this concept of clonal evolution appears to be valid in B-CLL, several important issues remain to be answered. These include the mechanisms for generation of alternative clonal forms and their relationship to clinical progression. Future studies aimed at elucidating answers to these questions will provide an important area of research into this disease.

REFERENCES

1. L. Foroni, D. Catovsky, and L. Luzzatto, Immunoglobulin gene rearrangements in hairy cell leukemia and other chronic B cell lymphoproliferative disorders, *Leukemia, 1*:389 (1987).
2. R. P. Gale and K. A. Foon, Chronic lymphocytic leukemia. Recent advances in biology and treatment, *Ann. Intern. Med., 103*:101 (1985).
3. R. Foa, N. Migone, G. Basso, G. Cattoretti, G. Pizzolo, F. Lauria, G. Casoreti, M. C. Guibellino, F. Capuzzo, A. Cantu-Rajnoldi, P. Lusso, A. O. Carbonar, and F. Gavosto, Molecular and immunological evidence of B-cell committment in "null" acute lymphoblastic leukemia, *Int. J. Cancer, 38*:317 (1986).
4. L. Luzzatto and L. Foronia, DNA rearrangements of cell lineage specific genes in lymphoproliferative disorders, *Prog. Hematol., 14*:303 (1986).
5. N. E. Kay, R. Suen, and B. Van Ness, Analysis of kappa gene rearrangements in lambda-expressing B-chronic lymphocytic leukemia, *Blood, 76*:356a (1990).
6. K. A. Foon and R. P. Gale, Chronic lymphocytic leukemia: New insights into biology and therapy, *Ann. Intern. Med., 113*:525 (1990).
7. K. A. Foon and R. P. Gale, Clinical transformation of chronic lymphocytic leukemia, *Nouv. Rev. Fr. Haematol., 30*:385 (1988).
8. J. C. Brouet, J. L. Preud'homme, G. Flandrin, N. Chelloul, and M. Seligmann, Membrane markers in "histiocytic" lymphoma (reticulum cell sarcomas), *J. Natl. Cancer Inst., 56*:631 (1976).
9. T. A. W. Splinger, A. Bom-van Noorloos, and P. van Heerde, CLL and diffuse histiocytic lymphoma in one patient: Clonal proliferation of two different B cells, *Scand J. Haematol., 20*:29 (1978).
10. G. Delsol, G. Laurent, E. Kuhlein, J. Farmiliades, F. Rigal, and J. Pris, Richter's syndrome. Evidence for the clonal origin of the two proliferations, *Am. J. Clin. Pathol., 76*:308 (1981).

11. J. L. Harousseau, G. Flandrin, G. Tricot, J. C. Brouet, M. Seligmann, and J. Bernard, Malignant lymphoma supervening in chronic lymphocytic leukemia and related disorders – Richter's syndrome: A study of 25 cases, *Cancer, 48*: 1302 (1981).
12. P. Moller, G. E. Feichter, D. Fritze, D. Hagg, and B. Schule, J-chain producing immunoblastic lymphoma in a case of Richter's syndrome, *Virchow's Arch. [Pathol. Anat.], 396*:213 (1982).
13. J. J. M. van Dongen, H. Hooijkass, J. J. Michiels, G. Grosveld, A. de Klein, Th. H. van der Kwast, M. E. F. Prins, J. Abels, and A. Hagemeijer, Richter's syndrome with different immunoglobulin light chains and different heavy chain gene rearrangements, *Blood, 64*:571 (1984).
14. L. F. Bertoli, H. Kubagawa, G. V. Borzillo, M. Mayumi, J. T. Prehal, J. F. Kearney, J. R. Durant, and M. D. Cooper, Analysis with anti-idiotype antibody of a patient with chronic lymphocytic leukemia and a large cell lymphoma (Richter's syndrome), *Blood, 70*:45 (1987).
15. S. J. Korsmeyer, A. Arnold, A. Bakshi, J. V. Ravetch, and U. Siebeinlist, Immunoglobulin gene rearrangement and cell surface antigen expression in acute lymphocytic leukemia of T cell and B cell precursor origins, *J. Clin. Invest., 71*:301 (1983).
16. K. Thielemus, D. G. Maloney, T. Meeker, C. Fujimoto, R. A. Doss, R. A. Warnke, J. Bindl, J. Gralow, R. A. Miller, and R. Levy, Strategies for production of monoclonal anti-idiotype antibodies against human B cell lymphomas, *J. Immunol., 133*:495 (1984).
17. G. Rechari, M. Mandel, N. Katzen, F. Brok-Simoni, I. Hakim, F. Holtzman, M. Biniaminor, D. Girol, I. Ben-Bassat, and B. Ramot, Immunoglobulin heavy chain gene rearrangements in chronic lymphocytic leukemia: Correlation with clinical stage, *Br. J. Haematol., 72*:524 (1989).
18. S. M. Hubbard, B. A. Chabner, V. T. DeVita, R. Simon, C. W. Berard, R. B. Jones, A. J. Garvin, G. P. Canellos, C. K. Osborne, and R. C. Young, Histologic progression in non-Hodgkin's lymphoma, *Blood, 59*:258 (1982).
19. B. Acker, R. T. Hoppe, T. V. Colby, R. S. Cox, H. S. Kaplan, and S. A. Rosenberg, Histologic conversion in the non-Hodgkin's lymphomas, *J. Clin. Oncol., 1*:11 (1983).
20. M. H. Siegelman, M. L. Cleary, R. Warnke, and J. Sklar, Frequent biclonality and Ig gene alterations among B cell lymphomas that show multiple histologic forms, *J. Exp. Med., 161*:850 (1985).
21. M. L. Cleary, N. Galili, M. Trela, R. Levy, and J. Sklar, Single cell origin of bigenotypic and biphenotypic B cell proliferation in human follicular lymphomas, *J. Exp. Med., 167*:582 (1985).
22. A. D. Zelenetz, T. T. Chen, and R. Levy, Histologic transformation of follicular lymphoma to diffuse lymphoma represents tumor progression by a single malignant B cell, *J. Exp. Med., 173*:197 (1991).
23. R. Levy, S. Levy, M. L. Cleary, W. Carroll, S. Kon, J. Bird, and J. Sklar, Somatic mutation in human B-cell tumors, *Immunol. Rev., 96*:43 (1987).
24. M. L. Clary, T. C. Meeker, S. Levy, E. Lee, M. Trela, J. Sklar, and R. Levy, Clustering of extensive somatic mutations in the variable region of an

immunoglobulin heavy chain gene from a human B cell lymphoma, *Cell, 44*: 97 (1986).

25. T. J. Kipps, E. Tomhave, P. P. Chen, and D. A. Carson, Autoantibody-associated kappa light chain variable region gene expressed in chronic lymphocytic leukemia with little or no somatic mutation. Implications for etiology and immunotherapy, *J. Exp. Med., 167*:840 (1988).

26. T. C. Meeker, J. C. Grimaldi, R. O'Rourke, J. Loeb, G. Juliusson, and S. Einhorn, Lack of detectable somatic hypermutation in the V region of the Ig H chain gene of a human chronic B lymphocytic leukemia, *J. Immunol., 141*: 3994 (1988).

27. P. E. Crossen, Cytogenetic and molecular changes in chronic-B-cell leukemia, *Cancer Genet. Cytogenet., 43*:143 (1989).

28. L. Peterson, L. Lindquist, and N. Kay, A subset of B-chronic lymphocytic leukemia with chromosomal changes at 13q14, site of the retinoblastoma (Rb) locus, *Lab. Invest., 62*:78A (1989).

29. N. Sadamori, T. Han, J. Minowada, and A. A. Sandberg, Chromosomes and causation of human cancer and leukemia LII. Chromosome findings in treated patients with B-cell chronic lymphocytic leukemia, *Cancer Genet. Cytogenet., 11*:161 (1984).

30. G. Juliusson, K-H. Robert, A. Ost, K. Friberg, P. Biberfeld, B. Nilsson, L. Zech, and G. Gahrton, Prognostic information from cytogenetic analysis in chronic B-lymphocytic leukemia and leukemic immunocytoma, *Blood, 65*:134 (1985).

31. T. Han, E. S. Henderson, L. J. Emrich, and A. A. Sandberg, Prognostic significance of karyotypic abnormalities in B cell chronic lymphocytic leukemia: An update (1987), *Semin. Hematol., 24*:257 (1987).

32. M. L. Bird, Y. Ueshima, J. D. Rowley, J. M. Haren, and J. W. Vardiman, Chromosome abnormalities in B cell chronic lymphocytic leukemia and their clinical correlations, *Leukemia, 3*:182 (1989).

33. G. Juliusson and G. Gahrton, Chromosome aberrations in B-cell chronic lymphocytic leukemia: Pathogenetic and clinical implications, *Cancer Genet. Cytogenet., 45*:143 (1990).

34. G. Juliusson, D. G. Oscier, M. Fitchett, F. M. Ross, G. Stocdill, M. J. Mackie, A. C. Parker, G. L. Castoldi, A. Cuneo, S. Knuutila, E. Elonen, and G. Gahrton, Prognostic subgroups in B-cell chronic lymphocytic leukemia defined by specific chromosomal abnormalities, *N. Engl. J. Med., 323*:720 (1990).

35. S. Pittman and D. Catovsky, Prognostic significance of chromosome abnormalities in chronic lymphocytic leukaemia, *Br. J. Haematol., 58*:649 (1984).

36. Y. Ueshima, M. L. Bird, J. W. Vardiman, and J. D. Rowley, A 14;19 translocation in B-cell chronic lymphocytic leukemia: A new recurring chromosome aberration, *Int. J. Cancer, 36*:287 (1985).

37. P. C. Nowell, E. C. Vonderheid, E. Besa, J. A. Hoxie, L. Moreau, and J. B. Finan, The most common chromosome change in 86 chronic B cell or T cell tumors: A 14q32 translocation, *Cancer Genet. Cytogenet., 19*:219 (1986).

38. N. Sadamori, M. Matsunaga, E. Yao, M. Ichimaru, and A. A. Sandberg,

Chromosomal characteristics of chronic and blastic phases of Ph-positive chronic myeloid leukemia, *Cancer Genet. Cytogenet., 15*:17 (1985).

39. G. Juliusson, K. Friberg, and G. Gahrton, Consistency of chromosomal aberrations in chronic B-lymphocytic leukemia: A longitudinal cytogenetic study of 41 patients, *Cancer, 62*:500 (1988).

40. P. C. Nowell, L. Moreau, P. Growney, and E. C. Besa, Karyotypic stability in chronic B-cell leukemia, *Cancer Genet. Cytogenet., 33*:155 (1988).

41. D. Oscier, M. Fitchett, T. Herbert, and R. Lambert, Karyotypic evolution in B-cell chronic lymphocytic leukaemia, *Genes Chromosomes Cancer, 3*:16 (1991).

42. T. Han, K. Ohtaki, N. Sadamori, A. W. Block, B. Dadey, H. Ozer, and A. A. Sandberg, Cytogenetic evidence for clonal evolution in B-cell chronic lymphocytic leukemia, *Cancer Genet. Cytogenet., 23*:321 (1986).

43. T. Han, H. Ozer, N. Sadamori, L. Emrich, G. A. Gomez, E. S. Henderson, M. L. Bloom, and A. A. Sandberg, Prognostic importance of cytogenetic abnormalities in patients with chronic lymphocytic leukemia, *N. Engl. J. Med., 310*:288 (1984).

44. G. Juliusson, K-H. Robert, A. Ost, K. Friberg, P. Biberfeld, B. Nilsson, L. Zech, and G. Gahrton, Prognostic information from cytogenetic analysis in chronic B-lymphocytic leukemia and leukemic immunocytoma, *Blood, 65*:134 (1985).

45. L. C. Peterson, L. L. Lindquist, S. Church, and N. E. Kay, Frequent clonal abnormalities of chromosome band 13q14 in B-cell chronic lymphocytic leukemia: Multiple clones, subclones, and nonclonal alterations in 82 Midwestern patients, *Genes Chromosomes Cancer*, in press.

46. L. C. Peterson, L. Lindquist, and N. E. Kay, Loss of tumor suppressor genes (13q14), clonal and nonclonal cytogenetic abnormalities, and karyotypic evolution in B-chronic lymphocytic leukemia (CLL), *Blood, 76*:1223A (1991).

10

Cellular Metabolism of Nucleoside Analogs in CLL: Implications for Drug Development

William Plunkett and Varsha Gandhi

The University of Texas M. D. Anderson Cancer Center, Houston, Texas

INTRODUCTION

In recent years, three adenine nucleoside analogs have been found to exhibit major clinical activity in the management of chronic lymphocytic leukemia (CLL) and other indolent lymphocytic diseases. Pentostatin, 2-chlorodeoxyadenosine, and fludarabine share structural similarities, aspects of their metabolism, and elements of their mechanisms of action. However, there are also substantial differences in the pharmacology and pharmacodynamics of these drugs that may contribute to the heterogeneity that has been observed in their clinical activities. In order to discover how each acts and how they differ, it is necessary to understand where they go in the body, what they become, and what processes are affected by their presence. To answer these questions, approaches utilizing classical plasma pharmacology, cellular pharmacokinetics, and molecular pharmacodynamics have been employed.

ADENINE NUCLEOSIDE ANALOGS

Structural Characteristics

The structures of pentostatin, chlorodeoxyadenosine, and fludarabine are shown in Fig. 1. Pentostatin was originally isolated from cultures of *Strep-*

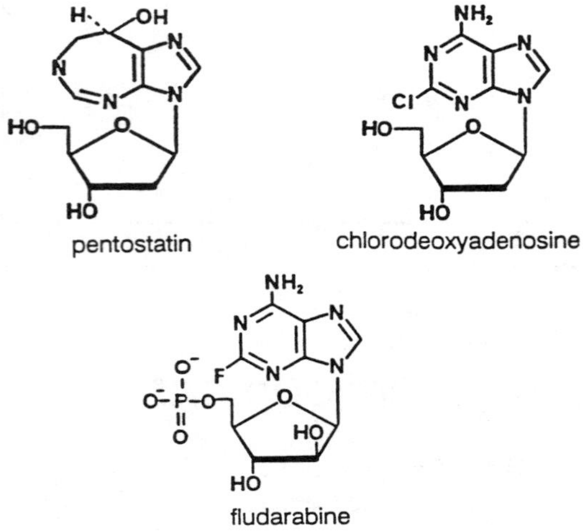

Figure 1   Structures of pentostatin, chlorodeoxyadenosine, and fludarabine.

tomyces antibioticus by a group at Parke-Davis; after solution of its structure, it was chemically synthesized by Woo et al. (1). The 2'-deoxyribose as the carbohydrate moiety distinguishes it from the ribosyl congener, which was named coformycin in recognition of the fact that it markedly potentiated the toxicity of the adenine nucleoside analog, formycin A (2). Hence, 2'-deoxycoformycin was the early name for pentostatin, the designation that will be used hereafter. It was soon understood that these compounds were extremely potent inhibitors of adenosine deaminase (3). The potency of deaminase-sensitive adenine nucleoside analogs such as arabinosyladenine (4,5), xylosyladenine (6), and 3'-deoxyadenosine (cordycepin) (7) was greatly increased by coadministration with inhibitors of adenosine deaminase.

It is clear from the work of Agarwal et al. (8,9) that the seven-membered diazapin ring of the aglycone enables both coformycin and pentostatin to function in a pseudo-irreversible manner as transition-state analogs of the reaction intermediates during deamination of adenosine and deoxyadenosine and their monophosphates. Pentostatin exhibits a K_i for erythrocyte adenosine deaminase of 2×10^{-12} M, and was until recently (10) the most potent inhibitor of this enzyme known. The high potency and relative availability of pentostatin were major factors in its selection for clinical trials.

Montgomery and Hewson (11) first demonstrated that placement of a halogen atom on the 2-carbon on adenine nucleosides essentially rendered the resulting analogs inert to adenosine deaminase, although they are not very effective inhibitors of the enzyme (12). This modification of adenosine and 2′-deoxyadenosine resulted in compounds that were extremely cyto-toxic, but without demonstrable therapeutic promise in experimental sys-tems (13). Nevertheless, this experience inspired Montgomery and Hewson to synthesize 2-fluoro-substituted nucleosides of adenine nucleoside analogs as a strategy to protect the molecule from inactivation by deamination (14). Because it was appreciated that the therapeutic activity of arabinosylade-nine was limited by the action of adenosine deaminase (15), modification of this molecule was of priority; their successful efforts resulted in the synthesis of arabinosyl-2-fluoroadenine (F-ara-A). The dosing of arabino-syladenine had been restricted by the relative insolubility of this drug; how-ever, this problem was circumvented by formulating the drug as the soluble 5′-monophosphate, ara-AMP (16). Therefore, F-ara-A was also formu-lated as its very soluble 5′-monophosphate, fludarabine (Fig. 1) (sometimes referred to as fludarabine phosphate), to assure flexibility for dosing sched-ules in clinical trials.

2-Chlorodeoxyadenosine (CldAdo, Fig. 1) was first synthesized chemi-cally and shown to be a fair inhibitor of L1210 leukemia in mice (17). Subsequently, two groups have detailed methods utilizing a stereospecific enzymatic transfer of a deoxyribosyl moiety from a deoxynucleoside to 2-chloroadenine or other purine analogs (18,19) to produce deoxyribosyl-nucleosides. CldAdo is a poor substrate for adenosine deaminase and is only a relatively weak inhibitor of the enzyme ($K_i = 2 \times 10^{-5}$ M, Ref. 20). Analogous to the action of the fluorine in fludarabine, the chlorine atom on the 2-carbon of the purine ring of CldAdo acts as an electrophilic center to withdraw electrons from the 6-amino group, thus decreasing its reactivity with adenosine deaminase. When administered in clinically active protocols, the steady-state plasma concentrations achieved are below 5×10^{-8} M (21). Thus, it may be assumed that CldAdo is unlikely to be acting by a mechanism that involves the direct inhibition of adenosine deaminase.

Clinical Use of Adenine Nucleoside Analogs

The relatively limited availability of all of these drugs to clinical investiga-tors has generally curtailed the expansion of investigations of the anticancer activities of each agent. In particular, efforts to develop strategies for com-binations with other active drugs have been hampered by lack of drug supplies. At the present time, pentostatin is approved for treatment of hairy cell leukemia and has demonstrable activity in CLL. Fludarabine has been approved for treatment of CLL, and its activity in low-grade lymphomas is being investigated. Preliminary studies suggest that fludarabine may also be active in hairy cell leukemia. Initial reports of remarkable activity of CldAdo against hairy cell leukemia (22) have been confirmed (23), and approval for treatment of this disease is currently being evaluated. Activity of CldAdo has been reported for CLL (24), and these investigations are being extended at several centers. Thus, the three adenine nucleoside analogs exhibit interrelated clinical activities in the indolent B-cell lymphocytic diseases. Whether each drug acts in a particular disease by the same or similar mechanisms, or if a single agent is active in each disease by the same mechanism(s), remains to be determined.

The most widely used clinical schedules for the adenine nucleoside analogs will be considered as a means of introducing the pharmacologic characteristics of these drugs. Pentostatin is generally administered for the treatment of hairy cell leukemia at doses of 4–5 mg/m^2 infused i.v. over 30 min at biweekly intervals for several months (25,26). CldAdo is given at similar daily doses, but as an i.v. continuous infusion that extends over 7 days. In contrast, treatment of CLL with fludarabine is usually conducted with 30-min infusions of 20–30 mg/m^2 daily for 3–5 days (27–29). Courses are repeated at monthly intervals, and may be extended for more than a year. Thus, despite similarities in the molecular weights of these drugs, the variations in the doses and schedules of administration predict differences in their plasma pharmacology.

Plasma Pharmacokinetics
Administered as a bolus of 4 mg/m^2, pentostatin plasma concentrations were close to 1 μM an hour after injection (30). Considering that the terminal elimination phase has a half-life of about 8 h (31) and that the plasma level at 1 h exceeded the K_i value for adenosine deaminase by roughly 10^6, it is not surprising that deaminase activities are suppressed for long times. Such a pharmacodynamic profile supports the use of an intermittent infusion schedule with a 14-day interval between doses.

When CldAdo, 5.6 mg/m^2, was administered as a continuous infusion over 24 h, a steady-state plasma level of only 20 nM was achieved (21). Because this concentration is unlikely to inhibit adenosine deaminase, it appears that both hairy cells and CLL cells have remarkable abilities to salvage the parent nucleoside to the putative active nucleotide forms. When studied after a 2-h i.v. infusion of 5.6 mg/m^2, CldAdo achieved a peak plasma concentration of 0.2 μM, which was eliminated with triphasic kinetics, exhibiting a terminal half-life of 8 h (21).

Fludarabine is rapidly and quantitatively dephosphorylated to its nucleoside F-ara-A upon infusion (32). Because of its short residence time and the inpenetrability of fludarabine to cells, it can be assumed that F-ara-A is the metabolite that is taken into cells to be phosphorylated to the active nucleotide. During infusion of fludarabine, 30 mg/m² over 30 min, plasma F-ara-A concentrations reach 2–5 μM (33). The most sensitive determinations of F-ara-A elimination have found this to be a triphasic process with a terminal half-life of up to 30 h (33–35). Most F-ara-A is excreted in the urine, with no evidence of additional metabolites (35). Thus, it is expected that the relatively slow elimination of the F-ara-A would be available to support continued accumulation of fludarabine nucleotides in cells. A phase I study of a fludarabine bolus followed by a 96-h continuous infusion demonstrated proportionality between the dose and steady-state F-ara-A levels in plasma (36). Given the slow terminal elimination of F-ara-A, steady-state levels in plasma would not have been expected for several days without a loading bolus dose. This study documented the value of the loading dose for reaching steady-state plasma F-ara-A levels within 2 h. A phase II investigation of a similar dosing schedule demonstrated its effectiveness in refractory advanced CLL, and that it was well tolerated in most patients (37).

Bioavailability

Administration of these adenine nucleoside analogs intravenously necessarily commits the patient to hospital visits that extend for up to a week. Although gastric acidity precludes use of pentostatin by the oral route, chlorodeoxyadenosine and fludarabine are more stable in an acid environment. Therefore, the possible use of alternative routes of administration of these drugs has been evaluated in recent studies that have investigated their pharmacokinetics after oral dosing as well as subcutaneous injections. Liliemark et al. (38) report a 90% bioavailability of CldAdo after subcutaneous injection of 5.6 mg/m² in six patients. When the same dose was given as a capsule to three of these patients, a median bioavailability of 41% was observed, whereas the median bioavailability was 51% when CldAdo was swallowed as a solution. These preliminary findings suggest the likelihood that formulations of CldAdo in addition to intravenous injection will be possible.

Kemena et al. (34) have studied the bioavailability of F-ara-A in plasma and that of the active triphosphate F-ara-ATP in circulating CLL cells after oral dosing with fludarabine in solution. F-ara-A was 78% bioavailable in plasma in this study of 12 patients. Parallel investigation of the area under the accumulation and elimination curve of F-ara-ATP in circulating CLL lymphocytes showed a 68% bioavailability. Subcutaneous injections of fludarabine have not been investigated. Nevertheless, these preliminary results indicate a favorable bioavailability for each drug after dosing by these routes. If efficacy studies are positive, it is likely that both patients and physicians will benefit from increased flexibility in the use of these drugs.

METABOLISM AND ACTIONS OF
ADENINE NUCLEOSIDE ANALOGS

Pentostatin

The major activity of pentostatin is the potent and long-lived inhibition of adenosine deaminase. Although this enzyme is capable of deaminating both adenosine and deoxyadenosine, it is principally deoxyadenosine that increases in plasma after pentostatin dosing, whereas the normally low levels of adenosine remain unperturbed (39). An explanation for this was provided by the work of Bagnara and Hershfield (40) and of Barankiewicz and Cohen (41), who demonstrated that the major route for deamination of adenosine is at the monophosphate level, whereas deoxyadenosine deamination is dependent on adenosine deaminase. Adenosine monophosphate is an excellent substrate for AMP deaminase. Thus, when adenosine deaminase is inhibited, AMP is deaminated by this alternative route and there is no buildup of adenosine. In contrast, dAMP is a poor substrate for AMP deaminase. Therefore, when adenosine deaminase is inhibited, there is no effective alternative route for catabolism of deoxyadenosine and its nucleotides to deoxyinosine and subsequently to uric acid (Fig. 2). This provides an explanation for the observed increase in deoxyadenosine in plasma after pentostatin infusions and in severe combined immunodeficiency disease

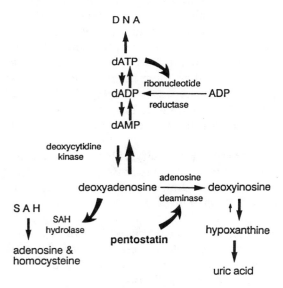

Figure 2   Mechanism of action of pentostatin.

associated with congenital deficiency of adenosine deaminase. It may be assumed that a major source of deoxyadenosine is the turnover of ortho-chromatic erythroblast nuclei in normal hematopoiesis, which occurs at the rate of 5×10^{11} cells per day in a 70-kg individual. It can be calculated that this alone would generate the equivalent to 260 mg of deoxyadenosine each day.

Deoxyadenosine itself is an inhibitor of S-adenosylhomocysteine (SAH) hydrolase, the enzyme needed for elimination of S-adenosylhomocysteine and regeneration of adenosine and homocysteine (42). Increased cellular levels of S-adenosylhomocysteine may disrupt reactions that require S-ade-nosylmethionine as a carbon donor. In particular, inhibition of the methyl-ation reactions involved in RNA metabolism provides a mechanism by which pentostatin may act on quiescent cells by routes other than those requiring active DNA replication or repair.

The initial step in the accumulation of deoxyadenosine nucleotides is phosphorylation by deoxycytidine kinase (43), although adenosine kinase is likely to contribute to this conversion, particularly in erythrocytes, which lack deoxycytidine kinase. Low concentrations of dAMP and dADP in cells suggests that the equilibrium of this pathway is toward dATP synthesis and that phosphorylation of deoxyadenosine is rate limiting. Following pentostatin infusion, dATP accumulates to relatively high levels in erythro-cytes, an action associated with toxicity in early clinical studies that em-ployed relatively high pentostatin doses (44). dATP also accumulates in circulating leukemia cells, and in leukemic lymphoblasts (45), from which it is eliminated slowly.

The major mechanism of action of pentostatin is thought to be mediated through the abnormally high levels of dATP. Because dATP is a global negative regulator of the activity of ribonucleotide reductase (46), this is likely to cause an imbalance of deoxynucleotide pools. This activity may have a direct action on DNA replication and repair, leading to the observed inhibition of DNA synthesis and breaks in DNA. As discussed in detail below, DNA replication and repair are at very low activities in the indolent B-cell malignancies in which pentostatin has clinical activity. Therefore, it may be necessary to postulate other mechanisms by which pentostatin af-fects its clinical activity in hairy cell leukemia and CLL.

Chlorodeoxyadenosine

Chlorodeoxyadenosine must be phosphorylated to its triphosphate CldATP to exhibit biological activity (18). Phosphorylation of the nucleoside ap-pears to be conducted exclusively by deoxycytidine kinase (Fig. 3). How-ever, unlike deoxyadenosine and pentostatin, this step is not rate limiting

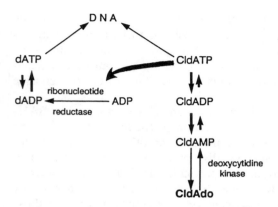

Figure 3   Metabolism and actions of chlorodeoxyadenosine.

to triphosphate accumulation. Rather, the monophosphate CldAMP accumulates to cellular concentrations that greatly exceed that of either CldAdo or the diphosphate, suggesting that phosphorylation of CldAMP is limiting to CldATP accumulation (47,48). Cells accumulate relatively low levels of CldATP (< 10 μM) compared to the cellular concentrations of adenine nucleoside analog triphosphates such as F-ara-ATP or ara-ATP achieved with similar incubation conditions. Both CldATP and CldAMP were eliminated rapidly after washing cell into drug-free medium; the half-lives of retention were generally less than 1 h in 11 cell lines that were tested (48). The rapid elimination of the triphosphate is consistent with both the findings that optimal therapeutic activity against murine tumors was achieved by schedules of frequent drug administration (18) and the utility of a continuous infusion schedule in the clinic (22,24).

DNA synthesis is inhibited in growing cells during treatment with CldAdo (47,49), and the evidence suggests that this effect is brought about by at least two mechanisms. First, extending earlier investigations that suggested CldAdo is incorporated into DNA, Parker et al. (50) demonstrated that CldATP is an inhibitor of mammalian DNA polymerases and is incorporated into elongating primers in the M13 system. Using gapped duplex DNA as a substrate, inhibition of DNA synthesis by CldATP was competitive with dATP. The apparent K_i values were 3.5 μM, 4.2 μM, and 21 μM for DNA polymerases α, β, and γ, respectively. In studies, utilizing the M13 assay system, Hentosh et al. (51) demonstrated that CldATP substituted effectively for dATP during primer extension over an M13 single-strand template by purified human DNA polymerase α or β. DNA synthesis was interrupted, however, when either polymerase was forced to incorporate two or more analog molecules in sequence, with polymerase β being the more sensitive enzyme. This observation provides a possible mechanism by which the incorporation of CldAdo into DNA may inhibit further DNA synthesis.

Second, CldAdo is one of the most potent inhibitors of ribonucleotide reductase that has been identified. Studies of the partially purified enzyme showed IC_{50} values of 65–100 nM (50,52). Studies in intact cells treated with CldAdo show a depletion of the deoxynucleoside triphosphates (52). Depletion of dCTP, which normally has the lowest concentration of the four deoxynucleotides in exponentially growing cultures of CCRF-CEM cells, appeared to be limiting to DNA synthesis. Although the mechanism of this inhibition has not been clearly elucidated, it is reasonable to speculate that CldATP may be interacting with the dATP regulatory site on the enzyme (46) as an alternative global inhibitor. Incubation of CldAdo-inhibited cells with deoxycytidine repletes dCTP levels, but only partially restores DNA synthesis, consistent with incorporation being an additional mechanism for DNA synthesis inhibition (52).

Fludarabine

The clinical formulation of fludarabine is as the 5'-monophosphate of F-ara-A. This is quantitatively dephosphorylated to F-ara-A virtually immediately upon intravenous infusion (32), presumably by the 5'-nucleotidase activity in erythrocytes, endothelial cells, and large organs (Fig. 4). As such, F-ara-A may be considered as identical to the parent drug in pharmacokinetic considerations of the metabolism, and actions of F-ara-A in cells in culture may be taken as a reflection of the pharmacodynamics of clinical fludarabine.

F-ara-A is taken into cells by nucleoside-transport systems of varying affinities (53,54). Studies with mutants have provided strong evidence that

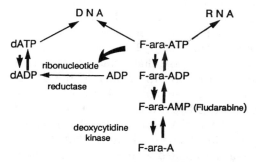

Figure 4 Metabolism and actions of fludarabine.

deoxycytidine kinase is the dominant, if not the exclusive, kinase for phosphorylation to the monophosphate (18,55). The relatively low levels of fludarabine mono- and diphosphate in cells suggest that the activity of deoxycytidine kinase is rate limiting to triphosphate formation (56). Although not formally identified, the kinase that phosphorylates F-ara-AMP to the diphosphate (adenylic kinase) and triphosphate (nucleoside diphosphate kinase) may be assumed to have higher activities for their respective substrates than does deoxycytidine kinase for F-ara-A.

Every demonstrably cytotoxic mechanism of action of fludarabine requires the presence of F-ara-ATP. The principal action of F-ara-ATP is the inhibition of DNA synthesis (57,58). Nevertheless, this arabinosyl nucleotide is unique in its ability to inhibit RNA synthesis as well (59,60). Considered as general mechanisms, F-ara-ATP can inhibit DNA polymerases directly as an alternative substrate that competes with dATP. Thus, the ratio of the cellular concentrations of dATP and F-ara-ATP may be an important determinant of the extent of this activity (61). In addition, the survival of cells incubated with F-ara-A is strongly correlated with the extent of incorporation of the analog into DNA (59,62). It is now clear that several specific enzymes involved with DNA synthesis are targets for inhibition by F-ara-ATP (63).

Human DNA polymerases α, β, γ, and ϵ have all been shown to be sensitive to inhibition by F-ara-ATP (62,64–66). This action is competitive with the normal substrate, dATP, for incorporation into sites complementary to thymidylate in the DNA template (62). F-ara-ATP is capable of inhibiting DNA primase, an accessory protein that synthesizes an RNA primer required for initiation of lagging-strand synthesis by DNA polymerase α (66,67). Once incorporated into DNA, F-ara-AMP is a poor substrate for addition of further nucleotides (50,62,68). This property makes it an unusually effective chain terminator, in contrast to incorporated CldAMP, which is a rather good substrate for addition of subsequent nucleotides (51,68). Consistent with its properties as a DNA chain terminator in cell-free systems, it was observed that 95% of F-ara-AMP was at terminal positions in DNA extracted from cells incubated with ^{3}H-F-ara-A (62). In addition to being a poor substrate for elongation by DNA polymerases, the stability of F-ara-AMP in the 3'-termini suggests that it may be resistant to removal by proofreading activities. Therefore, the ability of the $3' \rightarrow 5'$ exonuclease of human DNA polymerase ϵ to remove F-ara-AMP from DNA was evaluated. Consistent with this hypothesis, incubation of DNA extracted from cells incubated with ^{3}H-F-ara-A with human DNA polymerase ϵ failed to remove the analog (62). Molecular analysis of DNA duplexes in which the 3'-end of the DNA was terminated with F-ara-AMP demonstrated altered excision patterns by DNA polymerase ϵ compared to those of normal DNA (62). In contrast, similar experiments resulted in the excision of the incorporated nucleotides of ara-C (69) and zidovudine (70).

DNA ligase I is essential for the joining of pieces of DNA by catalyzing the formation of a phosphodiester linkage from the 3'-hydroxyl and the 5'-phosphate of adjacent deoxynucleotides (71). Recent studies have demonstrated that human DNA ligase I is inhibited in two modes by F-ara-ATP (72). First, the free triphosphate interacts with the enzyme to block AMP binding and ligation of single strands. Second, when F-ara-AMP is incorporated at the 3'-terminus, as has been reported above to occur both in intact cells and in cell-free systems, DNA ligase I is unable to join it to an adjacent piece of DNA. These actions on DNA ligase I have important implications for the actions of the drug on the function of this enzyme in DNA replication and repair. Together, these findings suggest that effective termination of DNA extension and ligation are the mechanisms by which incorporated F-ara-AMP can function as a DNA chain terminator to produce DNA deletions and mutations (73).

KILLING QUIESCENT CELLS

Although these mechanisms account satisfactorily for the killing of actively dividing cells by purine nucleoside analogs, alternatives must be sought to explain the toxicity of the drug to quiescent lymphocytes. Early studies demonstrated that resting human lymphocytes were lysed after exposure to deoxyadenosine and pentostatin (74-76). Subsequently, it was observed that resting lymphocytes accumulated DNA strand breaks during treatment with deoxyadenosine plus pentostatin (77). This work was extended by Seto et al. (78), who used a DNA-unwinding assay to measure DNA strand breaks in quiescent lymphocytes treated with either pentostatin and deoxyadenosine or CldAdo. This group also demonstrated that RNA synthesis was reduced, and that this was paralleled by a decrease in the cellular content of NAD and ATP. Toxicity was partially spared by incubating lymphocytes simultaneously with the nucleosides and either the NAD precursor nicotinamide, which maintained NAD pools, or by co-incubation with 3-aminobenzamide an inhibitor of poly(ADP-ribose) synthetase. In the light of these results, the authors interpreted the toxicity of deoxyadenosine and CldAdo toward resting lymphocytes in the contest of a process of programmed cell death (79,80).

Resting lymphocytes are thought to contain single-strand breaks in DNA (81,82), which are repaired once cells are stimulated to proliferate. This is envisioned as a process that is balanced by a proportional consumption of NAD for poly(ADP-ribose) synthesis associated with the cellular response to DNA damage. High cellular concentrations of dATP and the presence of CldAdo nucleotides are thought to interfere with the DNA repair processes, thus triggering a disproportionate utilization of NAD for poly-(ADP-ribosyl)ation of nuclear proteins; subsequently, ATP is depleted in an attempt to replenish diminished NAD^+ levels (78–80).

Additional experimental evidence is needed to substantiate this hypothesis more fully and to distinguish the proposed actions in quiescent cells such as normal and leukemic lymphocytes in peripheral blood from those observed in proliferating cells. For instance, the condition of DNA in these lymphocytes needs to be characterized further, because recent studies using the more sensitive alkaline and neutral filter elution procedures have failed to detect strand breaks in the DNA of resting lymphocytes (83,84). If normal and leukemic lymphocytes lack DNA strand breaks, it is unclear how increased cellular concentrations of dATP or the presence of either CldATP or F-ara-ATP could initiate the poly(ADP-ribosyl)ation response.

Nevertheless, recent reports have indicated that DNA isolated from CldAdo-treated leukemic lymphocytes from patients with chronic lymphocytic leukemia has been degraded into multimers of nucleosomal size (190 base pairs) (85–87). This is consistent with the onset of programmed cell death, since the production of such DNA fragments is a hallmark of this process (88). Inhibitors of RNA and protein synthesis did not affect this process, although it was inhibited by calcium chelators and phorbol esters. These findings suggest that fludarabine and CldAdo either activate or release an apoptotic program involving a calcium-dependent endonuclease. The challenge for the future is to elucidate the steps involved between nucleotide-analog accumulation and DNA fragmentation.

Evidence has been presented for increased strand breaks in DNA from lymphocytes treated with CldAdo, shown by an alkaline unwinding assay (78). However, as argued before (83,84), this procedure is not capable of differentiating between single breaks and the formation of double-strand fragments that are associated with programmed cell death. Large (100–200 kilobase pair) pieces of DNA were observed by pulse gel electrophoresis in proliferating mouse mammary tumor cells treated with CldAdo (89). Tanabe et al. (90) used neutral elution procedures to demonstrate that CldAdo treatment was associated with the formation of double-strand breaks in the DNA of exponentially growing Chinese hamster V79 cells. Incubation of these cells with 5-μM CldAdo for 15 min partially inhibited repair of X-ray-induced double-strand DNA breaks (91). These findings gave rise to the suggestion that a drug-induced imbalance of deoxynucleotides may be a stimulus to DNA fragmentation in proliferative cells. There is at present no direct evidence for the accumulation of poly(ADP-ribosyl)ated nuclear proteins in response to CldAdo treatment. Considering a different approach, CldATP has been demonstrated to be an inhibitor of human DNA polymerase β (51,68), which has been considered integral to DNA repair. However, recent studies have cast doubt on the contribution of this enzyme to DNA repair, because other DNA polymerases are now thought to participate in this process (92,93). Thus, considerable information is required before the proposed mechanism(s) by which dATP, F-ara-ATP, and CldATP, generated secondarily to treatment with pentostatin, CldAdo, and fludarabine, respectively, are toxic to chronic lymphocytic leukemia cells can be understood in detail.

FUTURE DIRECTIONS

The remarkable activities of pentostatin, CldAdo, and fludarabine in indolent lymphocytic disease in general, and in CLL in particular, clearly demonstrate the promise of ostensibly cycle-active drugs in these diseases. The clinical responses in these low-growth-fraction tumors have forced us to reevaluate our approaches to understanding the mechanisms by which adenine nucleoside analogs may be exerting selective actions. It will be important to understand if the activity of each drug against CLL is affected by the same mechanism. Similarly, because these adenine nucleoside analogs are active in the same malignancies, an understanding of whether there are commonalities in the mechanisms of actions among the drugs will be of interest. Understanding the activities and interactions of pathways involved in initiating an apparent program of cell death will prepare us for devising strategies to combat the emergence of resistance to these drugs. Clinical crossover studies of the adenine nucleoside analogs will likely provide some indication of the level of cross-resistance among these drugs.

The remarkable activity of these purine nucleoside analogs against B-cell malignancies leads to the expectation that pyrimidines with similar or related mechanisms of action may also be effective drugs in these diseases. Thus, arabinosylcytosine (ara-C), a mainstay in the treatment of adult acute leukemia, should be evaluated for activity in CLL. Although ara-C has been combined with other agents for CLL therapy, a single-drug study of ara-C has not been reported in this disease. As is the case for dATP and F-ara-ATP, the pharmacokinetics of its active 5'-triphosphate ara-CTP can be readily evaluated in circulating leukemic lymphocytes. This poses the opportunity to use cellular pharmacology to guide the design of clinical infusion schedules. Indeed, it has already been determined that intermittent doses of 0.25 g/m^2/h produce plasma levels of ara-C that saturate the ability of leukemic lymphocytes to accumulate ara-CTP (94,95). These studies should be extended to determine the optimum dose and duration for continuous-infusion administration schedules.

This approach has recently been reported for a new pyrimidine analog,

2′,2′-difluorodeoxycytidine (dFdC, gemcitabine), in patients with CLL (96) and acute leukemia (97). Like the purine analogs and ara-C, the triphosphate of dFdC is incorporated into DNA and this action inhibits further replication (69). In addition, the diphosphate of dFdC is a potent inhibitor of ribonucleotide reductase (98). The deoxynucleotide pools of cells treated with dFdC are disrupted in a manner similar to the action of fludarabine and CldAdo. Like CldAdo and fludarabine, dFdC also induces apoptosis in CLL cells in vitro. The similarities in the actions of dFdC and the purine analogs suggest that clinical trials, which are underway in adults with relapsed acute leukemia (97), should be extended to CLL.

Finally, cellular pharmacokinetics of nucleotide analogs should be employed to provide guidance for the design of combination chemotherapy for CLL. This is being done for the combination of fludarabine and ara-C (99,100). Based on their laboratory studies in leukemia cell lines (101,102), Gandhi et al. (103) designed in vitro investigations that demonstrated that prior treatment with F-ara-A enhanced the rate of ara-CTP accumulation by two- to threefold in CLL cells treated with ara-C. Application of this pharmacologically guided design to clinical trials has recently resulted in a similar biochemical modulation of ara-CTP metabolism in circulating leukemic lymphocytes during therapy (99,100). Thus, intermittent doses of ara-C that would otherwise produce maximal ara-CTP levels in leukemic lymphocytes have been potentiated by fludarabine to significantly increase the area under the ara-CTP concentration-times-time curve in circulating leukemic lymphocytes of CLL patients. Extensions of these pilot trials of the combination of fludarabine and ara-C, which has substantial activity in acute leukemia (104), should be pursued to evaluate the clinical efficacy of this regimen against CLL.

Finally, a knowledge of the cellular pharmacology of a nucleoside analog may also be employed in the design of combinations with frank DNA-damaging agents. For instance, studies of ara-CTP metabolism in ficoll/hypaque bouyant marrow cells from patients treated with high-dose ara-C for non-marrow-involved malignancies showed mean cellular ara-CTP concentrations of 86 μM and 46 μM at the end of infusion of 3 g/m^2 (2 h) and at 12 h, respectively (105). In contrast, CLL patients who received identical treatment had peak ara-CTP levels of 625 μM in circulating leukemic lymphocytes. By 24 h after the infusion, ara-CTP concentrations were calculated to be 102 μM in CLL cells, but only 20 μM in normal marrow. These data suggest that there is differential metabolism of ara-CTP in normal marrow and leukemic lymphocytes, which may be used as the basis for the design of a treatment strategy.

Thus, 24 h after ara-C infusion, the relatively high concentrations of ara-CTP in leukemic cells should be sufficient to inhibit repair of DNA damage inflicted by a frankly DNA-damaging drug administered at that time. The DNA damaging drug could be an alkylating agent such as chlorambucil or cisplatin, or a topoisomerase-active drug such as etoposide (topoisomerase II) or topotecan (topoisomerase I). In contrast, the low levels of ara-CTP predicted to be present in normal marrow should not be sufficient to block repair of DNA damage.

The positive therapeutic index should be derived from first, the higher levels of ara-CTP that are retained more effectively in leukemic cells. When ara-C is administered on an intermittent schedule, this should maintain a strong inhibition of DNA synthesis in leukemic cells throughout the duration of therapy. Normal cells, on the other hand, may be able to recover DNA synthesis as ara-CTP is eliminated; this action is associated with lower toxicity. Second, the differential ability of normal cells to eliminate ara-CTP should allow them to repair DNA damage caused by the DNA-reactive drug. Because leukemic cells would contain levels of ara-CTP that would be inhibitory to DNA repair, they would be selectively affected by this pharmacologically guided treatment strategy. The cellular pharmacokinetics of clinically active nucleotide analogs are clearly amenable to this type of analysis. New procedures for evaluating the pharmacodynamics of DNA-reactive drugs will contribute important information for the design of future protocols (106).

ACKNOWLEDGMENTS

Studies conducted in the authors' laboratories were supported by grants CA28596, CA32839, and CA53311 from the National Cancer Institute, Department of Health and Human Services, and by grant CH-130 from the American Cancer Society.

REFERENCES

1. P. K. W. Woo, H. W. Dion, S. M. Lange, L. F. Duhl, and L. J. Durham, A novel adenosine and ara-A deaminase inhibitor, (R)-3-(2-deoxy-β-D-erythro-pentofuranosyl)-3,6,7,8-tetrahydroimidazo[4,5][1,3]-diazapin-8-ol, *J. Heterocyclic Chem., 11*:641–643 (1974).
2. H. Nakamura, G. Koyama, Y. Iitaka, M. Ohno, N. Yagisawa, S. Kondo, K. Maeda, and H. Umezawa, Structure of coformycin, an unusual nucleoside of microbial origin, *J. Am. Chem. Soc., 96*:4327–4328 (1974).
3. R. P. Agarwal, Inhibitors of adenosine deaminase, *Pharmacol. Ther., 17*: 399–429 (1982).
4. C. E. Cass and T. Au-Yeung, Enhancement of 9-β-D-arabinofuranosyladenine toxicity to mouse leukemia L1210 in vitro by 2′-deoxycoformycin, *Cancer Res., 36*:1508–1513 (1976).

5. G. A. LePage, L. S. Worth, and A. P. Kimball, Enhancement of the antitumor activity of arabinofuranosyladenine by 2'-deoxycoformycin, *Cancer Res., 36*:1481–1485 (1976).

6. B. A. Harris and W. Plunkett, Biochemical basis for the cytotoxicity of 9-β-D-xyolofuranosyladenine in Chinese hamster ovary cells, *Cancer Res., 41*: 1039–1044 (1981).

7. D. G. Johns and R. H. Adamson, Enhancement of the biological activity of cordycepin (3'-deoxyadenosine) by the adenosine deaminase inhibitor 2'-deoxycoformycin, *Biochem. Pharmacol., 25*:1441–1444 (1979).

8. R. P. Agarwal, T. Spector, and R. E. Parks, Jr., Tight-binding inhibitors IV. Inhibition of adenosine deaminase by various inhibitors, *Biochem. Pharmacol., 26*:359–367 (1977).

9. R. P. Agarwal and R. E. Parks, Jr., Potent inhibition of muscle 5'-AMP deaminase by the nucleoside antibiotics coformycin and deoxycoformycin, *Biochem. Pharmacol., 26*:663–666 (1977).

10. D. K. Wilson, F. B. Rudolph, and F. A. Quiocho, Atomic structure of adenosine deaminase complexed with transition-state analog: Understanding catalysis and immunodeficiency mutations, *Science, 252*:1278–1284 (1991).

11. J. A. Montgomery and K. Hewson, Synthesis of potential anticancer agents. XX. 2-fluoropurines, *J. Am. Chem. Soc., 82*:463–468 (1960).

12. L. L. Bennett, Jr., C.-H. Chang, P. W. Allan, J. J. Adamson, L. M. Rose, R. W. Brockman, J. A. Secrist, III, A. Shortnacy, and J. A. Montgomery, Metabolism and metabolic effects of halopurine nucleosides in tumor cells in culture, *Nucleosides Nucleotides, 4*:107–116 (1985).

13. H. E. Skipper, J. A. Montgomery, J. R. Thompson, and F. M. Schabel, Jr., Structure-activity relationships and cross-resistance observed on evaluation of a series of purine analogs against experimental neoplasms, *Cancer Res., 19*:425–437 (1959).

14. J. A. Montgomery and K. Hewson, Nucleosides of 2-fluoroadenine, *J. Med. Chem., 12*:498–504 (1969).

15. G. A. LePage, A. Khaliq, and J. A. Gottlieb, Studies of 9-β-D-arabinofuranosyladenine in man, *Drug Metab. Dispos., 1*:756–759 (1973).

16. G. A. LePage, Y. T. Lin, R. E. Orth, and J. A. Gottlieb, 5'-Nucleotides as potential formulations for administering nucleoside analogs in man, *Cancer Res., 32*:2441–2444 (1972).

17. L. F. Christensen, A. D. Broom, M. J. Robins, and A. Bloch, Synthesis and biological activity of selected 2,6,-disubstituted-(2-deoxy-α- and β-D-erythro-pentofuranosyl)purines, *J. Med. Chem., 15*:735–739 (1972).

18. D. A. Carson, D. B. Wasson, J. Kaye, B. Ullman, D. W. Martin, Jr., R. K. Robins, and J. A. Montgomery, Deoxycytidine kinase-mediated toxicity of deoxyadenosine analogs toward human lymphoblasts in vitro and toward murine L1210 leukemia in vivo, *Proc. Natl. Acad. Sci. USA, 77*:6865–6869 (1980).

19. M.-C. Huang, K. Hatfield, A. W. Roetker, J. A. Montgomery, and R. L. Blakley, Effects of cytotoxicity of 2-chloro-2'-deoxyadenosine: Facile enzymatic preparation and growth inhibitory effects on human cell lines, *Biochem. Pharmacol., 30*:2663–2671 (1981).

20. L. N. Simon, R. J. Bauer, R. L. Tolman, and R. K. Robins, Calf intestine adenosine deaminase. Substrate specificity, *Biochemistry, 9*:573–577 (1970).
21. J. O. Liliemark and G. Juliusson, On the pharmacokinetics of 2-chloro-2'-deoxyadenosine in humans, *Cancer Res., 51*:5570–5572 (1991).
22. L. D. Piro, C. J. Carrera, D. A. Carson, and E. Beutler, Lasting remissions in hairy-cell leukemia induced by a single infusion of 2-chlorodeoxyadenosine, *N. Engl. J. Med., 322*:1117–1121 (1990).
23. E. H. Estey, R. Kurzrock, H. M. Kantarjian, S. M. O'Brien, K. B. McCredie, M. Beran, C. Koller, M. J. Keating, C. Hirsch-Ginsberg, Y. O. Huh, S. Stass, and E. J. Freireich, Treatment of hairy cell leukemia with 2-chlorodeoxyadenosine (2-CdA), *Blood, 79*:882–887 (1992).
24. L. D. Piro, C. J. Carrera, D. A. Carson, and E. Beutler, 2-Chlorodeoxyadenosine: An effective new agent for the treatment of chronic lymphocytic leukemia, *Blood, 72*:1069–1073 (1989).
25. M. R. Grever, J. M. Leiby, E. H. Kraut, H. E. Wilson, J. A. Neidhart, R. I. Wall, and S. P. Balcerzak, Low-dose deoxycoformycin in lymphoid malignancy, *J. Clin. Oncol., 3*:1196–1201 (1985).
26. A. S. Spiers, D. Moore, P. A. Cassileth, D. P. Harrington, F. J. Cummings, R. S. Neiman, J. M. Bennett, and M. J. O'Connell, Remissions in hairy-cell leukemia with pentostatin (2'-deoxycoformycin), *N. Engl. J. Med., 316*:825–830 (1987).
27. M. J. Keating, H. Kantarjian, M. Talpaz, J. Redman, C. Koller, B. Barlogie, W. Velasquez, W. Plunkett, E. J. Freireich, and K. B. McCredie, Fludarabine: A new agent with major activity against chronic lymphocytic leukemia, *Blood, 74*:19–25 (1989).
28. M. Grever, J. Leiby, E. Kraut, E. Metz, J. Neidhart, S. P. Balcerzak, and L. Malspeis, A comprehensive phase I and phase II clinical investigation of fludarabine, *Sem. Oncol., 17*(Suppl. 8):39–48 (1990).
29. M. J. Keating, H. Kantarjian, S. O'Brien, C. Koller, M. Talpaz, J. Schachner, C. C. Childs, E. J. Freiriech, and K. B. McCredie, Fludarabine: A new agent with marked cytoreductive activity in untreated chronic lymphocytic leukemia, *J. Clin. Oncol., 9*:44–49 (1991).
30. J. F. Smyth, R. M. Paine, A. L. Jackman, K. R. Harrap, M. M. Chassin, R. H. Adamson, and D. G. Johns, The clinical pharmacology of the adenosine deaminase inhibitor 2'-deoxycoformycin, *Cancer Chemother. Pharmacol., 5*:93–101 (1980).
31. L. Malspeis, A. B. Weinrib, A. E. Staubus, M. Grever, S. P. Balcerzak, and J. A. Neidhart, Clinical pharmacokinetics of 2'-deoxycoformycin, *Cancer Treatment Symp., 2*:7–15 (1984).
32. L. Danhauser, W. Plunkett, M. Keating, and F. Cabanillas, 9-β-D-Arabinofuranosyl-2-fluoroadenine 5'-monophosphate pharmacokinetics in plasma and tumor cells of patients with relapsed leukemia and lymphoma, *Cancer Chemother. Pharmacol., 18*:145–152 (1986).
33. A. Kemena, M. Fernandez, J. Baumann, M. Keating, and W. Plunkett, A sensitive fluorescence assay for quantitation of fludarabine and metabolites in biological fluids, *Clin. Chim. Acta, 200*:95–106 (1991).

34. A. Kemena, M. J. Keating, and W. Plunkett, Plasma and cellular bioavailability of oral fludarabine, *Blood, 78*(Suppl. 1):52a (1991).

35. L. Malspeis, M. R. Grever, A. E. Staubus, and D. Young, Pharmacokinetics of 2-F-ara-A (9-β-D-arabinofuranosyl-2-fluoroadenine) in cancer patients during the phase I clinical investigations of fludarabine phosphate, *Sem. Oncol., 17*(Suppl. 8):18–32 (1990).

36. V. I. Avramis, J. Champagne, J. Sato, M. Krailo, L. J. Ettinger, D. G. Poplack, J. Finkelstein, G. Reaman, G. D. Hammond, and J. S. Holcenberg, Pharmacology of fludarabine phosphate after a phase I/II trial by a loading bolus and continuous infusion in pediatric patients, *Cancer Res., 50*:7226–7231 (1990).

37. C. A. Puccio, A. Mittelman, S. M. Lichtman, R. T. Silver, D. R. Budman, T. Ahmed, E. J. Feldman, M. Coleman, P. M. Arnold, Z. A. Arlin, and H. G. Chun, A loading dose/continuous infusion schedule of fludarabine phosphate in chronic lymphocytic leukemia, *J. Clin. Oncol., 9*:1562–1569 (1991).

38. J. O. Liliemark, F. Albertioni, B. Pettersson, and G. Juliusson, Bioavailability of oral and subcutaneous 2-chloro-2'-deoxyadenosine (CdA), *Proc. Am. Soc. Clin. Oncol.*, in press (1992).

39. P. P. Major, R. P. Agarwal, and D. W. Kufe, Clinical pharmacology of deoxycoformycin, *Blood, 58*:91–96 (1981).

40. A. S. Bagnara and M. S. Hershfield. Mechanism of deoxyadenosine-induced catabolism of adenine ribonucleotides in adenosine deaminase-inhibited human T lymphoblastoid cells, *Proc. Natl. Acad. Sci. USA, 79*:2673–2677 (1982).

41. J. Barankiewicz and A. Cohen, Evidence for distinct catabolic pathways of adenine ribonucleotides and deoxyribonucleotides in human T lymphoblastoid cells, *J. Biol. Chem., 259*:15178–15181 (1984).

42. M. S. Hershfield, N. M. Kredich, D. R. Ownby, and R. Buckley, In vivo inactivation of S-adenosyl homocysteine hydrolase by 2'-deoxyadenosine in adenosine deaminase deficient patients, *J. Clin. Invest., 63*:807–811 (1979).

43. M. S. Hershfield, J. E. Fetter, M. C. Small, A. S. Bagnara, S. R. Williams, B. Ullman, D. W. Martin, Jr., D. B. Wasson, and D. A. Carson, Effects of mutational loss of adenosine kinase and deoxycytidine kinase on deoxyATP accumulation and deoxyadenosine toxicity in cultured CEM human T-lymphoblastoid cells, *J. Biol., Chem., 257*:6380–6386 (1982).

44. M. R. Grever, M. F. E. Siaw, W. F. Jacob, J. A. Neidhart, J. S. Miser, M. S. Coleman, J. J. Hutton, and S. P. Balcerzak, The biochemical and clinical consequences of 2'-deoxycoformycin in refractory lymphoproliferative malignancy, *Blood, 57*:406–417 (1981).

45. W. Plunkett, R. S. Benjamin, M. J. Keating, and E. J. Freireich, Modulation of 9-β-D-arabinofuranosyladenine 5'-triphosphate and deoxyadenosine triphosphate in leukemic cells by 2'-deoxycoformycin during therapy with 9-β-D-arabinofuranosyladenine, *Cancer Res., 42*:2092–2096 (1982).

46. L. Thelander and P. Reichard, Reduction of ribonucleotides, *Ann. Rev. Biochem., 48*:133–158 (1979).

47. D. A. Carson, D. B. Wasson, R. Taetle, and A. Yu, Specific toxicity of

2-chlorodeoxyadenosine toward resting and proliferating human lymphocytes, *Blood, 62*:737–743 (1983).

48. T. L. Avery, J. E. Rehg, W. C. Lumm, F. C. Harwood, V. M. Santana, and R. L. Blakley, Biochemical pharmacology of 2-chlorodeoxyadenosine in malignant human hematopoietic cell lines and therapeutic effects of 2-bromo-deoxyadenosine in drug combinations in mice, *Cancer Res., 49*:4972–4978 (1989).

49. M.-C. Huang, R. A. Ashmun, T. L. Avery, M. Kuehl, and R. L. Blakley, Effects of cytotoxicity of 2-chloro-2'-deoxyadenosine and 2-bromo-2'-deoxyadenosine on cell growth, clonogenicity, DNA synthesis and cell cycle kinetics, *Cancer Res., 46*:2363–2368 (1986).

50. W. B. Parker, A. R. Bapat, J.-X. Shen, A. J. Townsend, and Y.-C. Cheng, Interaction of 2-halogenated dATP analogs (F, Cl, and Br) with human DNA polymerases, DNA primase and ribonucleotide reductase, *Molec. Pharmacol., 34*:485–491 (1988).

51. P. Hentosh, R. Koob, and R. L. Blakley, Incorporation of 2-halogeno-2'-deoxyadenosine 5'-triphosphates into DNA during replication by human DNA polymerases α and β, *J. Biol. Chem., 265*:4033–4040 (1990).

52. J. Griffig, R. Koob, and R. L. Blakley, Mechanisms of inhibition of DNA synthesis by 2-chlorodeoxyadenosine in human lymphoblastoid cells, *Cancer Res., 49*:6923–6928 (1989).

53. F. M. Sirotnak, P. L. Chello, D. M. Dorick, and J. A. Montgomery, Specificity of systems mediating transport of adenosine, 9-β-D-arabinofuranosyl-2-fluoroadenine, and other purine nucleoside analogous in L1210 cells, *Cancer Res., 43*:104–109 (1983).

54. J. R. Barrueco, D. M. Jacobsen, C.-H. Chang, R. W. Brockman, and F. M. Sirotnak, Proposed mechanism of therapeutic selectivity of 9-β-D-arabino-furanosyl-2-fluoroadenine against murine leukemia based upon lower capacities for transport and phosphorylation in proliferative intestinal epithelium compared to tumor cells, *Cancer Res., 47*:700–706 (1987).

55. L. W. Dow, D. E. Bell, L. Poulakos, and A. Fridland, Difference in metabolism and cytotoxicity between 9-β-D-arabinofuranosyladenine and 9-β-D-arabinofuranosyl-2-fluoroadenine in human leukemic lymphoblasts, *Cancer Res., 40*:1405–1410 (1980).

56. V. I. Avramis and W. Plunkett, Metabolism and therapeutic efficacy of 9-β-D-arabinofuranosyl-2-fluoroadenine against murine leukemia P388, *Cancer Res., 42*:2587–2591 (1982).

57. R. W. Brockman, F. M. Schabel, Jr., and J. A. Montgomery, Biologic activity of 9-β-D-arabinofuranosyl-2-fluoroadenine, a metabolically stable analog of 9-β-D-arabinofuranosyladenine, *Biochem. Pharmacol., 26*:2193–2196 (1977).

58. W. Plunkett, L. Alexander, S. Chubb, and J. A. Montgomery, Comparison of the toxicity and metabolism of 9-β-D-arabinofuranosyl-2-fluoroadenine and 9-β-D-arabinofuranosyladenine in human lymphoblastoid cells, *Cancer Res., 40*:2349–2355 (1980).

59. D. Spriggs, G. Robbins, T. Mitchell, and D. Kufe, Incorporation of 9-β-D-

arabinofuranosyl-2-fluoroadenine into HL-60 cellular RNA and DNA, *Biochem. Pharmacol.*, *35*:247–252 (1986).

60. P. Huang and W. Plunkett, Action of 9-β-D-arabinofuranosyl-2-fluoroadenine on RNA metabolism, *Molec. Pharmacol.*, *39*:449–455 (1991).

61. W. Plunkett, P. Huang, and V. Gandhi, Metabolism and action of fludarabine phosphate, *Sem. Oncol.* *17*(Suppl. 8):3–17 (1990).

62. P. Huang, S. Chubb, and W. Plunkett, Termination of DNA synthesis by 9-β-D-arabinofuranosyl-2-fluoroadenine. A mechanism for cytotoxicity, *J. Biol. Chem.*, *265*:16617–16625 (1990).

63. W. Plunkett and P. P. Saunders, Metabolism and action of purine nucleoside analogs, *Pharmacol. Ther.*, *49*:239–268 (1991).

64. L. White, S. C. Shaddix, R. W. Brockman, and L. L. Bennett, Jr., Comparison of the actions of 9-β-D-arabinofuranosyl-2-fluoroadenine and 9-β-D-arabinofuranosyladenine on target enzymes from mouse tumor cells, *Cancer Res.*, *42*:2260–2264 (1982).

65. W. C. Tseng, D. Derse, Y.-C. Cheng, R. W. Brockman, and L. L. Bennett, Jr., In vitro activity of 9-β-D-arabinofuranosyl-2-fluoroadenine and the biochemical actions of its triphosphate on DNA polymerases and ribonucleotide reductase from HeLa cells, *Molec. Pharmacol.*, *21*:474–477 (1982).

66. W. Parker and Y.-C. Cheng, Inhibition of DNA primase by nucleoside triphosphates and their arabinofuranosyl analogs, *Molec. Pharmacol.*, *31*:146–151 (1987).

67. C. V. Catapano, K. B. Chandler, and D. J. Fernandes, Inhibitions of primer RNA formation in CCRF-CEM leukemia cells by fludarabine triphosphate, *Cancer Res.*, *51*:1829–1835 (1991).

68. W. B. Parker, S. C. Shaddix, C.-H. Chang, E. L. White, L. M. Rose, R. W. Brockman, A. T. Shortnacy, J. A. Montgomery, J. A. Secrist, III, and L. L. Bennett, Jr., Effects of 2-chloro-9-(2-deoxy-2-fluoro-β-D-arabinofuranosyl) adenine on K562 cellular metabolism and the inhibition of human ribonucleotide reductase and DNA polymerases by its 5′-triphosphate, *Cancer Res.*, *51*:2386–2394 (1991).

69. P. Huang, S. Chubb, L. W. Hertel, G. B. Grindey, and W. Plunkett, Action of 2′,2′-difluorodeoxycytidine on DNA synthesis, *Cancer Res.*, *51*:6110–6117 (1991).

70. P. Huang, D. Farquhar, and W. Plunkett, Selective action of 2′,3′-didehydro-2′,3′-dideoxythymidine triphosphate on HIV reverse transcriptase and human DNA polymerases, *J. Biol. Chem.*, *267*:2817–2822, (1992).

71. D. D. Lasko, A. E. Tomkinson, and T. Lindahl, Eukaryotic DNA ligases, *Mutation Res.*, *236*:277–287 (1990).

72. S.-W. Yang, P. Huang, W. Plunkett, F. F. Becker, and J. Y. H. Chan, Dual mode of inhibition of purified DNA ligase I from human cells by 9-β-D-arabinofuranosyl-2-fluoroadenine triphosphate, *J. Biol. Chem.*, *267*:2345–2349, (1992).

73. P. Huang, M. J. Siciliano, and W. Plunkett, Gene deletion, a mechanism of induced mutation by arabinofuranosyl-2-fluoroadenine, *Mutation Res.*, *210*: 291–301 (1989).

74. R. F. Kefford and R. M. Fox, Deoxycoformycin-induced response in chronic lymphocytic leukemia: Deoxyadenosine toxicity in non-replicating lymphocytes, *Br. J. Haematol., 50*:627–636 (1982).

75. R. F. Kefford and R. M. Fox, Purine deoxynucleoside toxicity in non-dividing human lymphoid cells, *Cancer Res., 42*:324–330 (1982).

76. D. A. Carson, D. B. Wasson, E. Lakow, and N. Kamatani, Possible metabolic basis for the different immunodeficient states associated with genetic deficiencies of adenosine deaminase and purine nucleoside phosphorylase, *Proc. Natl. Acad. Sci. USA, 79*:3848–3852 (1982).

77. L. Brox, A. Ng, E. Pollock, and A. Belch, DNA strand breaks induced in human T-lymphocytes by the combination of deoxyadenosine and deoxycoformycin, *Cancer Res., 44*:934–937 (1984).

78. S. Seto, C. J. Carrera, M. Kubota, D. B. Wasson, and D. A. Carson, Mechanism of deoxyadenosine and 2-chlorodeoxyadenosine toxicity to nondividing human lymphocytes, *J. Clin. Invest., 75*:377–383 (1985).

79. D. A. Carson, S. Seto, D. B. Wasson, and C. J. Carrera, DNA strand breaks, NAD metabolism, and programmed cell death, *Exp. Cell Res., 164*: 273–281 (1986).

80. D. A. Carson, C. J. Carrera, D. B. Wasson, and H. Yamanaka, Programmed cell death and adenine deoxynucleotide metabolism in human lymphocytes, *Adv. Enzyme Reg., 27*:395–404 (1987).

81. A. P. Johnstone and G. T. Williams, Role of DNA breaks and ADP-ribosyl transferase in eukaryotic differentiation demonstrated in human lymphocytes, *Nature, 300*:368–370 (1982).

82. W. L. Greer and J. G. Kaplan, Early nuclear events in lymphocyte proliferation. The role of DNA strand break repair and ADP ribosylation, *Exp. Cell Res., 166*:399–415 (1986).

83. R. Jostes, J. A. Reese, J. E. Cleaver, M. Molero, and W. F. Morgan, Quiescent human lymphocytes do not contain DNA strand breaks detectable by alkaline elution, *Exp. Cell Res., 182*:513–520 (1989).

84. M. E. T. I. Boerrigter, DNA strand break metabolism in human lymphocytes: A reevaluation, *Exp. Cell Res., 196*:1–5 (1991).

85. L. E. Robertson, S. Chubb, M. Story, R. Meyn, and W. Plunkett, Induction of DNA cleavage in chronic lymphocytic leukemia cells by chlorodeoxyadenosine and fludarabine, *Proc. Am. Assoc. Cancer Res., 32*:415 (1991).

86. L. E. Robertson, S. Chubb, W. N. Hittelman, A. Sandoval, and W. Plunkett, Programmed cell death (apoptosis) in chronic lymphocytic leukemia cells after fludarabine and chlorodeoxyadenosine, *Blood, 78*(Suppl. 1):173a (1991).

87. C. J. Carrera, C. Terai, L. D. Piro, A. Saven, E. Beutler, and D. A. Carson, 2-Chlorodeoxyadenosine chemotherapy triggers programmed cell death in normal and malignant lymphocytes, *Int. J. Purine Pyrimidine Res., 2*(Suppl. 1):38 (1991).

88. W. J. Arrends, R. G. Morris, and A. H. Wyllie, Apoptosis. The role of the endonuclease, *Am. J. Pathol., 136*:593–608 (1990).

89. Y. Hirota, A. Yosioka, S. Tanaka, K. Watanabe, T. Otani, J. Minowada,

A. Matuda, T. Ueda, and Y. Wataya, Imbalance of deoxyribonucleoside triphosphates, DNA double strand breaks, and cell death caused by 2-chloro-deoxyadenosine in mouse FM3A cells, *Cancer Res., 49*:915–919 (1989).

90. K. Tanabe, W. Hiraoka, M. Kuwabara, F. Sato, A. Matsucda, and T. Ueda, Induction of DNA double-strand breaks in Chinese hamster V79 cells by 2-chlorodeoxyadenosine, *Chem.-Biol. Interact., 71*:167–175 (1989).

91. M. Kuwabara, K. Tanabe, W. Hiraoka, Y. Tamura, F. Sato, A. Matsuda, and T. Ueda, 2-Chlorodeoxyadenosine inhibits the repair of DNA double-strand breaks and does not inhibit the repair of DNA single-strand breaks in X-irradiated Chinese hamster V79 cells, *Chem.-Biol. Interact., 79*:349–358 (1991).

92. S. L. Dresler, B. J. Gowans, R. M. Robinson-Hill, and D. J. Hunting, Involvement of DNA polymerase δ in DNA repair synthesis in human fibro-blasts at late times after ultraviolet irradiation, *Biochemistry, 27*:6379–6383 (1988).

93. R. A. Hammond, J. K. McClung, and M. R. Miller, Effect of DNA polymer-ase inhibitors on DNA repair in intact and permeable human fibroblasts evidence that DNA polymerase δ and β are involved in DNA repair synthesis induced by N-methyl-N'-nitro-N-nitrosoguanidine, *Biochemistry, 29*:286–291.

94. W. Plunkett, J. O. Liliemark, T. M. Adams, B. Nowak, E. Estey, H. Kantar-jian, and M. J. Keating, Saturation of 1-β-D-arabinofuranosylcytosine 5'-tri-phosphate accumulation in leukemia cells during high-dose 1-β-D-arabino-furanosylcytosine therapy, *Cancer Res., 47*:3005–3011 (1987).

95. W. Plunkett, J. O. Liliemark, E. Estey, and M. J. Keating, Saturation of ara-CTP accumulation during high-dose ara-C therapy: Pharmacologic ra-tionale for intermediate-dose ara-C, *Sem. Oncol. 14*(Suppl. 1):159–166 (1987).

96. R. Grunewald, H. Kantarjian, M. J. Keating, J. Abbruzzese, P. Tarassoff, and W. Plunkett, Pharmacologically directed design of the dose rate and schedule of 2',2'-difluorodeoxycytidine (gemcitabine) administration in leu-kemia, *Cancer Res., 50*:6823–6826 (1990).

97. R. Grunewald, H. Kantarjian, M. Du, K. Faucher, P. Tarassoff, and W. Plunkett, Gemcitabine in leukemia: A phase I clinical, plasma, and cellular pharmacology study, *J. Clin. Oncol., 10*:406–413 (1992).

98. V. Heinemann, Y.-Z. Xu, S. Chubb, A. Sen, L. W. Hertel, G. B. Grindey, and W. Plunkett, Inhibition of ribonucleotide reduction in CCRF-CEM cells by 2',2'-difluorodeoxycytidine, *Molec. Pharmacol., 38*:567–572 (1990).

99. V. Gandhi, M. J. Keating, K. B. McCredie, and W. Plunkett, Fludarabine infusion enhances ara-C triphosphate (ara-CTP) metabolism in CLL cells during therapy, *Blood, 76*(Suppl. 1):273a, (1990).

100. V. Gandhi, A. Kemena, M. J. Keating, and W. Plunkett, Fludarabine infu-sion potentiates arabinosylcytosine metabolism in lymphocytes of patients with chronic lymphocytic leukemia, *Cancer Res., 52*:897–903 (1992).

101. V. Gandhi and W. Plunkett, Modulation of arabinosyl nucleoside metabo-

lism by arabinosyl nucleotides in human leukemia cells, *Cancer Res.,* *48*:329–334 (1988).

102. V. Gandhi and W. Plunkett, Interaction of arabinosyl nucleotides in K562 human leukemia cells, *Biochem. Pharmacol., 38*:4115–4121 (1989).
103. V. Gandhi, B. Nowak, M. J. Keating, and W. Plunkett, Modulation of arabinosylcytosine metabolism by arabinosyl-2-fluoroadenine in lymphocytes from patients with chronic lymphocytic leukemia: Implications for combination therapy, *Blood, 74*:2070–2075 (1989).
104. V. Gandhi, E. Estey, M. J. Keating, and W. Plunkett, Synergistic combination of fludarabine and ara-C for AML therapy, *Blood, 78*(Suppl. 1):52a (1991).
105. W. Plunkett, T. Adams, and M. J. Keating, Pharmacologic basis for the therapeutic index of high-dose ara-C: Implications for combinations, *Proc. Am. Assoc. Cancer Res., 17*:174 (1986).
106. A. Ellis, B. Nowak, W. Plunkett, and L. Zwelling, Drug-induced DNA-protein crosslinks in non-radiolabeled cells: Potential application to patient material, *Proc. Am. Assoc. Cancer Res.*, in press (1992).

11

Drug Resistance in Chronic Lymphocytic Leukemia

Robert Silber and Milan Potmesil
New York University Medical Center, New York, New York

B-Chronic lymphocytic leukemia (CLL), the most common leukemia in the Western world, remains an incurable disease. Following standard alkylating agent therapy with or without corticosteroids, most patients achieve partial remissions. Complete remissions, however, are seen in fewer than one-third of cases (1). Since complete remissions are a prerequisite for the cure of leukemia, their scarcity in CLL is consistent with the marginal effectiveness of treatment on survival. Moreover, all patients eventually relapse, and meaningful responses to subsequent therapy are uncommon. As in most malignancies, the occurrence of de-novo drug resistance and the development of resistance during therapy are major obstacles to a cure. Recently, three purine analogs, 2′-deoxycoformycin (pentostatin) (2), 2-chlorodeoxy-adenosine (3), and fludarabine (4), have shown activity against CLL. In previously untreated patients, fludarabine achieves remission rates of >70% (with 30% complete remissions), according to the National Cancer Institute Working Group criteria. No long-term survival figures are yet available; however, no cures are expected for this leukemia using the new agents.

CLL has been defined as an "accumulative" disease (5), with the vast majority of leukemic cells arrested in the G_0/G_1 phase of the cell cycle. The quiescent state of CLL lymphocytes may contribute to drug resistance. This chapter reviews available information on known mechanisms underlying this therapeutically unfavorable event and possible approaches on how to circumvent it.

ALKYLATING AGENTS

Alkylating agents were the first nonhormonal drugs used in cancer chemotherapy (6). Following the administration of radioactive nitrogen mustard (7), covalent binding of the labeled compound was found in many types of cellular molecules. Interaction with its principal target, DNA, accounts for cytotoxic, mutagenic, and ultimately carcinogenic properties. The N-7 position of guanine may be the most common alkylation site; this reaction results in intrastrand and interstrand cross-linking of DNA (8). It is the production of the latter lesion that may explain why bifunctional alkylating agents are more effective than the monofunctional alkylating agents. There is abundant evidence for the importance of DNA cross-link formation as a cause of cytotoxicity in vivo (9–16). Various alkylating agents differ markedly in terms of intestinal absorption, cellular uptake, activation or inactivation, DNA damage and repair. Their diverse pharmacokinetics may be responsible for the partial cross-resistance among them.

Chlorambucil

Chlorambucil (CLB), with or without prednisone, remains the standard treatment for CLL. Like other aklylating agents, CLB binds to DNA, RNA, and proteins (8). The drug's effectiveness is probably related to the formation of DNA interstrand cross-links (17). Most patients respond to CLB when first treated, but become resistant during subsequent treatment courses.

CLB is readily absorbed from the gut (18,19), and is detected in plasma within 1 h of ingestion. The cellular pharmacokinetics and some possible mechanisms of drug resistance are shown in Fig. 1. These include decreased CLB uptake, inactivation by nonenzymatic or enzymatic hydrolysis, thioether formation by interaction of CLB molecules with sulfhydryl (SH) groups, and a failure to form and/or efficiently repair DNA cross-links. The effects of temperature on the interaction between CLB and DNA suggests an energy-dependent activation process (17).

Uptake

Begleiter and Goldenberg (20) in a lymphoblast L5178Y cell line, Harrap and Hill (21) in Yoshida ascites sarcoma cells, and Hill and Harrap in CLL lymphocytes (22), showed that CLB uptake occurs by simple passive diffusion. Combining radiometric and HPLC techniques, Bank et al. (17) also concluded that CLB enters and exits CLL lymphocytes by this process. Drug accumulation is immediate, unsaturable over a > 100-fold concentra-

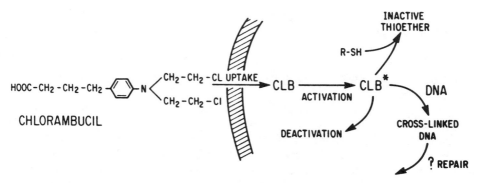

Figure 1 A summary of chlorambucil uptake, interactions, and sites of drug resistance. (Modified from T. A. Connors in *Antitumor Drug Resistance*, B. W. Fox and M. Fox (Eds.), Springer Verlag, 1984.)

tion range, temperature independent, and is not altered by sodium azide or 2-deoxyglucose. CLB uptake is also unaffected by hemicholium-3, an inhibitor of the choline transport system that carries nitrogen mustard into the cell. The different modes of cell entry by CLB and nitrogen mustard are consistent with their individual resistance patterns: Decreased cellular uptake of nitrogen mustard by the choline transport system may cause drug resistance (23–25). However, as anticipated from the passive-diffusion pattern, the drug uptake by lymphocytes from CLB-resistant or untreated CLL patients was similar. No heterogeneity was found in peak cell-associated CLB among 17 patients with all stages of CLL, including three with CLB-resistant disease (17).

Metabolism

The suggestion that lymphocytes from resistant patients degraded CLB at the benzene ring (22) was not supported by a more recent report (17). The later study indicates that the resistance of CLL lymphocytes is not explained by altered intracellular drug metabolism. Following incubation with labeled CLB, two metabolites (probably mono- and bishydroxyethyl compounds) were formed rapidly in lymphocytes from untreated as well as from resistant patients. Oxidation of the butyric acid side chains yields phenyl acetic acid, a product that retains alkylating properties but has an uncertain role in drug resistance (26).

Interaction with Sulfhydryl Groups

For over two decades data have been accumulating that indicate a relationship between intracellular SH groups and resistance to aklylating agents (27,28). SH groups may prevent CLB from forming DNA cross-links, either by direct binding to the drug forming a thioether, or by quenching DNA-CLB mono-adducts, precursors of more toxic CLB-DNA bifunctional adducts (29). Correlation between CLB resistance and an increased content of metallothionein (MT), an SH-rich protein, was reported recently (30): The introduction of an MT gene into cells of a CLB-sensitive line led to CLB resistance.

Other studies of cell lines show an association between resistance, glutathione (GSH) levels, and glutathione-S-transferase (GST) activity (31). For example, high levels of GSH are found in L-phenylalanine mustard-resistant L1210 cells (32). In contrast, the GSH level in CLL lymphocytes cannot be correlated with the patient's prior treatment with alkylating agents or clinical onset of resistance (33,34). GSTs are a multigene family of proteins, which catalyze many metabolic detoxication processes (35–38). Altered expression of these enzymes enhances resistance to several cytotoxic drugs, including alkylating agents. The GST activity and GST-mRNA in a Chinese hamster ovary (CHO) cell line resistant to nitrogen mustard and CLB was two- to three-fold higher than in drug-sensitive cells (39,40). The resistant line also had decreased drug-induced DNA cross-linking. Resistance to alkylating agents has been associated with elevations of the π or α form of GST in leukemia cells (28). Reversal of the α-form-GST resistance in cell lines by indomethacin or ethacrynic acid was also reported (41). A similar effect of ethacrynic acid was found in lymphocytes from patients with CLL exposed to nitrogen mustard using a dye diffusion viability assay (42). Upregulation of the GST π mRNA occurs in a variety of hematologic malignancies, but no clear relationship to drug resistance was demonstrated (42–45). Only a modest increase of GST was observed in lymphocytes from CLB-resistant patients as compared to those from untreated patients (46). While this enzyme may be of relevance to the resistant phenotype, its precise clinical importance in CLB-unresponsive patients remains to be clarified.

DNA Cross-linking

Since the majority of studies have been unable to detect differences in either alkylating agent uptake or metabolism in lymphocytes between untreated or drug-resistant patients, a number of investigators have evaluated the CLB- or melphalan-induced DNA interstrand cross-links. Using an ethidium bromide fluorescence assay, Panasci et al. found a significantly lower percentage of DNA cross-links in lymphocytes from CLB-treated than in lymphocytes from untreated CLL patients (33). In a recent study of the kinetics of cross-link formation, enhanced removal of melphalan-induced DNA cross-links was observed in lymphocytes from resistant patients (47). So far, no studies on the removal of CLB-induced DNA cross-links in CLL lymphocytes have appeared.

The extensive information on DNA repair processes in bacteria and eukaryotes provided a framework for studies with the aim of identifying the enzyme(s) responsible for repair of alkylator-induced DNA lesions. It appears that enzymes encoded in the gene implicated in the repair of ultraviolet-light damage also play a role in repair of DNA lesions induced by mitomycin and cisplatinum. Recent cloning of these and other genes provides appropriate probes to study their putative role in CLB resistance. The possibility that the ERCC-1 gene is involved in alkylator resistance in CLL is supported by the finding of a two- to three-fold increase in expression in CLB-resistant as compared to untreated patients. The CLL-resistant lymphocytes also had increased 3-methyl adenine DNA glycosidase, which can release altered bases at the N-7 position of guanine (48).

Several studies have demonstrated that decreased formation of DNA cross-links, or the presence of cross-link excision, may be involved in the resistance to nitrogen mustard and melphalan (49–51). Following CLB exposure, a significantly lower number of cross-links was found in a CLB-resistant CHO line than in the parental cells (52). It is likely that in the resistant line the elevated GST activity modulates responses to CLB by inactivating the drug. No correlation was found between prior clinical exposure to alkylating agents and GSH content or GST activity in lymphocytes from 12 patients with CLL. DNA cross-linking induced by CLB, however, showed an inverse correlation to GST activity (34).

ANTIMETABOLITES

Purine Analogs

Fludarabine Phosphate (53)

Since its first clinical trials in the early 1980s, fludarabine phosphate (F-ara-A-PO_4) has undergone extensive evaluation. While its therapeutic value is considerable (see elsewhere in this volume), patients treated with F-ara-A-PO_4 eventually become resistant. Review of the drug's metabolism (Fig. 2) reveals several targets for resistance to develop (54). Following cleavage of the PO_4 group, cells accumulate F-ara-A against a concentration gradient. L1210 cells have a seven- to eight-fold greater uptake than mouse intestinal cells, thereby establishing a favorable therapeutic index (55). While this is a potential mechanism of resistance, no transport mutants have been identified so far.

The drug's sequential phosphorylation to a triphosphate form is essential for cytotoxic activity. Three enzymes catalyze these reactions: deoxycytidine kinase, adenylate kinase, and nucleoside diphosphate kinase (54). In mutant cell lines the loss of the enzyme deoxycytidine kinase, which cata-

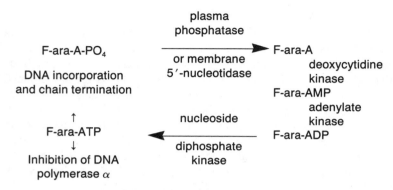

Figure 2 Metabolism of fludarabine (F-ara-A-MP).

lyzes the initial phosphorylation step, makes the cell resistant to F-ara-A (56,57). Clinical studies of this enzyme in CLL would be of utmost interest. Loss of the enzymes that catalyze the phosphorylation of F-ara-A to F-ara-ATP may also make cells resistant.

While the presence of the F in the 2-position substantially decreases the affinity of adenosine deaminase for the drug, and makes deamination a less likely mechanism for F-ara-A resistance, metabolic studies have identified arabinosyl-2-fluorohypoxanthine in the urine of dogs, mice, and monkeys treated with the drug (58–61). It therefore seems possible that some deamination to an inert metabolite occurs. Increased deamination, or generation of the free base 2-fluoroadenine, would provide other mechanisms of resistance. Nevertheless, the precise mechanism of resistance to fludarabine remains uncertain.

2'-Deoxycoformycin

2'-Deoxycoformycin (DCF) is a potent inhibitor of adenosine deaminse (ADA); however, there is no apparent correlation between the level of reduction of ADA and responsiveness in chronic B-cell leukemias (62). Therefore, its mechanism of action in CLL is unknown.

2-Chlorodeoxyadenosine

2-Chlorodeoxyadenosine (CDA) is believed to induce lymphocytotoxicity and monocytotoxicity through an induction of DNA strand breaks (63). However, it is unclear whether this mechanism of action is relevant to nonproliferating lymphocytes such as in CLL.

GLUCOCORTICOIDS (64)

Pharmacologic doses of corticosteroids cause lymphocytopenia in experimental animals and kill some human lymphoid lineage cells. The importance of glucocorticoids in the treatment of many lymphoproliferative disorders has stimulated much work aimed at determining the mechanism(s) responsible for glucocorticoid resistance. Despite numerous studies, the actual mechanism is not known.

Since drug resistance ultimately develops during steroid therapy of CLL, a better understanding of this phenomenon is important. Much is known about the hormone's action. Corticosteroid resistance may occur naturally in the course of lymphopoiesis. Unlike mature T cells and B cells, the immature T cells are lysed by an unknown mechanism when exposed to glucocorticoids. Corticosteroids may influence some of the growth factors that regulate lymphoproliferation. For example, glucocorticoids inhibit IL-2 production, thereby reducing the growth of T cells (65). Glucocorticoid hormones enter cells by passive diffusion and bind to a cytosol receptor (66), a transcriptional regulator protein. This 95-kD phosphorylated protein has specific DNA-binding and steroid-binding domains. The activated ligand-hormone complex is translocated into the nucleus and bound to specific enhancer DNA sequences. RNA transcription is initiated, proteins synthesized, and responses elicited.

The concept that the receptors mediate steroid effects on leukemia and lymphoma lines is based on the following evidence: (a) Receptor occupancy by the hormone correlate well with cell kill in the sensitive mouse-lymphoma cell lines S49 and WEH17, and in the P1798 transplantable lymphoma (64). (b) Cells not killed by the steroids had reduced numbers and/or abnormal receptors.

Three types of resistant sublines were isolated from a CCRF-CEM, human lymphoblastic leukemia line, which was cloned under the selective pressures of glucocorticoids: (a) receptor-deficient mutants, with 10% or less of the glucocorticoid bound to the wild-type cells; (b) activation-deficient mutants, which bound glucocorticoids with normal affinity but did not retain them when the steroid-receptor complex was activated; and (c) receptor-positive mutants, which bound and activated the steroid, but in which the cells still resisted lysis by the hormone. The most common defect in resistant cells is the lack of corticosteroid receptor. No defect of intracellular transport mechanism was reported.

Early studies suggested that, in the absence of a cytoplasmic receptor for the hormone, human leukemia cells become resistant to steroids (67). A longer remission duration was reported in receptor-positive than in receptor-negative ALL patients. In six of seven subsequent studies, "high" glucocorticoid receptor levels generally predicted a response to therapy, while only half of patients with a "low" receptor level responded (64). More recent studies show that glucocorticoid receptors are present on most leukemic cells, but their level does not correlate with in-vitro sensitivity to glucocorticoid cytotoxicity as measured by inhibition of uridine, thymidine, or leucine uptake. Relatively low numbers of glucocorticoid receptors are found on CLL lymphocytes (68,69,70). Their presence seems to be without prognostic significance.

In general, the receptor may be required for the responsiveness to glucocorticoid treatment, but the receptor's presence does not guarantee a response. The question as to why some leukemic cells containing glucocorticoid receptors are glucocorticoid resistant remains unanswered. The suggestion (71) that corticosteroid resistance of patients with systemic lupus erythematosus is related to a higher rate of hormone degradation deserves further evaluation in lymphoid malignancies.

DNA TOPOISOMERASE-DIRECTED AGENTS

DNA topoisomerases are enzymes that resolve topological problems arising during semiconservative replication of DNA, and participate in other cellular functions such as transcription, recombination, and chromosomal organization. They act via two different mechanisms: Topoisomerase I introduces breaks in one strand of DNA, whereas topoisomerase II cleaves both strands of the helix and passes a double-strand DNA segment through the opening. In either case, the breaks are transient (72).

Topoisomerase inhibitors block the rejoining of broken DNA and reversibly trap a covalent enzyme-DNA complex. Studies of mammalian cells have suggested that the collision between the trapped complex and the DNA-replication fork is responsible for the S- and G_2-phase arrest of cells treated with these drugs. This, and additional not fully understood events, result in cell death. Trapped complexes can be detected by various techniques, and their quantity correlates well with the cytotoxicity of topoisomerase-targeted drugs.

While anthracyclines and epipodophyllotoxins, inhibitors of topoisomerase II (73), are widely used in chemotherapy, a plant alkaloid, camptothecin (74), and its semisynthetic or totally synthetic analogs, are the only well-studied inhibitors of topoisomerase I (75,76). Drugs such as doxorubicin and etoposide have found wide use in the management of some solid tumors, lymphomas, and acute leukemia, but have been, at best, only marginally effective in the treatment of CLL. Two possible explanations can be provided for this relative ineffectiveness: The first is the finding that DNA topoisomerase II, with less than 7×10^3 copies per cell, was not detectable in B-CLL blood lymphocytes by immunoblotting (77). This should be compared with 36.0×10^5 copies per cell of a HeLa line. The very low enzyme level in CLL may be a reflection of the cells' quiescent state. Trapped topoisomerase II-DNA complexes are not detectable in B-CLL lymphocytes exposed to doxorubicin. Otherwise, their presence represents the initial event leading to cell death. While extremely low topoisomerase II activity seems to be associated with drug resistance in CLL, an abnormal enzyme or an increased level was also found in experimental systems studying drug resistance (78). Topoisomerase I, elevated in CLL (average of 5.3×10^5 copies/cell) and some lymphomas (e.g., diffuse histiocytic lymphoma, 16.0×10^5 copies/cell) over the level in normal lymphocytes ($2.3 \pm 1.6 \times 10^5$ copies/cell (77), may represent an alternative target for chemotherapy.

The second explanation of resistance to these drugs in CLL may be the overexpression of the multidrug resistance (mdr1) gene. This gene, investigated in CLL in several recent studies (79–84), encodes for a 170-kD phosphorylated membrane P170 glycoprotein. The P170 protein acts as an energy-dependent efflux pump for many antibiotics, including anthracyclines or epipodophyllotoxins, and participates in their intracellular binding. Holmes et al. (80) found low levels of mdr1 mRNA in lymphocytes (mostly T cells) from normal subjects, while 18/34 CLL patients (mostly B cells) had levels of mdr1 mRNA above the normal range. In three patients studied, it appeared that CLB, which is not affected by the P170 glycoprotein, also increased mdr1 expression. Perri (81) could not detect mdr1 mRNA in normal blood lymphocytes, but found the message in lymphocytes from 19 of 20 patients with CLL, regardless of disease stage or treatment. The P170 protein was present in B-lymphocytes of only 9 of 17 CLL patients. Some patients had mdr1 mRNA, but no P170 protein. This protein was not found in lymphocytes obtained from patients with Rai stage 0 disease, but it was expressed in all stage IV patients' lymphocytes. In another study, no correlation was found between the levels of mdr1 or mdr3 gene expression in lymphocytes from 17 CLL patients (82). There was no clear association between the treatment responses and mdr1 expression. A subsequent study published in an abstract form suggested that the mdr1 gene may play a role in resistance even in CLL B cells in which P170 is not detectable by standard methods (83). The treatment of CLL lymphocytes with neuraminidase, which removes sialic acid residues, quadrupled the percentage positive for the P170 protein (84). In a very recent study of 63 patients (85), 61% showed a strong reaction by immunocytochemistry for P170 in their lymphocytes, and 39% a weak reaction. It is possible that the failure to detect this protein in B lymphocytes from some CLL patients may reflect abnormal sialylation of the cells.

Many approaches have been tried to circumvent the mdr-related resistance (86). These include the use of indomethacin, calcium channel blockers, and cyclosporin. The use of high-dose verapamil in conjunction with chemotherapy has been associated with a substantial number of responses in refractory lymphoma patients whose tumors express the p-glycoprotein (87). The use of combinations of agents, such as verapamil and quinine, may even be synergistic (88). It is possible that careful selection of patients, or the use of pharmacologic agents that counteract the P170 protein's action, may eventually make the topoisomerase II-directed drugs more effective in the treatment of CLL. An alternative approach has emerged from our recent studies (89,90). Camptothecin, 9-amino-, and 10,11-methylenedioxy camptothecins overcome the mdr1-related drug resistance in in-vitro and in-vivo experiments. While clinically available anticancer agents remain ineffective, a "cure" of human colon cancer xenograft implants with the mdr1 phenotype was achieved in the nude-mouse model using 9-amino or 10,11-methylenedioxy camptothecins (91). We have also investigated the effects of camptothecin and synthetic analogs on CLL lymphocytes (92). 10,11-Methylenedioxy camptothecin is highly effective in vitro against quiescent cells such as CLL B lymphocytes.

Camptothecin itself was an active agent in preclinical testing and in early phase I trials; however, excessive toxicities, including leukopenia and cystitis, reduced enthusiasm for further clinical studies. Currently there are two derivatives of camptothecin in clinical trials, topotecan and CPT-11. Topotecan (hycamptamine, SKF 104864) is a water-soluble analog of camptothecin that is active in a variety of murine experimental systems, regardless of its route of administration. Phase I trials using a bolus or continuous infusion schedule revealed granulocytopenia to be the dose-limiting toxicity. A study using a 24-h continuous infusion is currently being completed by investigators at the M. D. Anderson Cancer Center. A phase II trial in patients with CLL who have failed fludarabine-containing regimens is planned in which the interaction of hycamptamine with human DNA topoisomerase I in patient peripheral blood leukemic cells will be analyzed and correlated with drug efficacy (M. Keating, personal communication, 1991). Ohno et al. (93) reported responses to the analog CPT-11 in a variety of histologies of lymphomas, although no cases of CLL were included in their series. An evaluation of this agent in CLL is warranted.

FUTURE DIRECTIONS

The new understanding of molecular alterations responsible for drug resistance may yield clinically useful strategies for the treatment of CLL. Several future approaches can be considered (Table 1).

Table 1 Drug Resistance in CLL and Approaches to Its Reversal

Drug(s)	Resistance mechanism(s)	Potential targets for reversal	Compounds to be developed
S-Phase inhibitors:			
Methotrexate, cytarabine, etc.	Arrest of CLL cells in G_0–G_1 phase of the cell cycle	Cycle control points; cycline-activated kinases	Modulators of cell cycle transition
Fludarabine	Loss of activating enzyme(s)	Deoxycytidine kinase	Inhibitors that bypass missing enzyme(s)
Alkylators:			
Chlorambucil	Inactivation by GSH; failure to form and/or excise alkylated nucleotides	(1) Cellular detoxicants, glutathione and protein thiols; (2) DNA repair enzymes	(1) GST inhibitors, buthionine sulfoxime (?); (2) Inhibitors of repair enzymes
Cyclophosphamide	The same as above *plus* oxidation by aldehyde dehydrogenase	Increase of hepatic microsomal activation	Aldehyde dehydrogenase inhibitors (?)
Nitrosoureas	Repair of alkylated lesions	Guanine O^6-alkyl transferase	Inhibitors of guanine O^6-alkyl transferase
DNA topoisomerase-II directed agents:			
Doxorubicin, etoposide	Low or altered DNA topoisomerase II, expressed MDR gene	(1) Topoisomerase I; (2) MDR-gene product	(1) and (2) Camptothecin analogs; (2) Ca^{2+} channel blockers, cyclosporine
Others:			
Glucocorticoids	Loss of receptors or gene-activating function	Receptors, hormone, degradation enzyme(s)	Restore receptors by gene transfer (?)
Growth factors	Loss of receptors	Lymphokine receptors	Lymphokines or IL-4

231

1. Should CLL therapy be aimed at a quiescent cell? CLL is a leukemia with a unique biological pattern of tumor cells arrested in the G_0/G_1 phase of the cell cycle. The discovery of the cyclin-cdc2 kinase system and phosphorylation/dephosphorylation reactions as regulators of the cell cycle provide a lead for studies of CLL lymphocytes. In turn, the results from these experiments may focus future drug design on agents that trigger CLL lymphocytes into mitosis, thus making them more vulnerable.
2. New antimetabolites affecting ribonucleotide/deoxyribonucleotide pathways are now available. There is a great need to further define drug action mechanisms and resistance to these novel agents at the biochemical level.
3. Further attention to the modulation of SH groups is warranted (41). Clinical studies using the combination of CLB and ethacrynic acid in CLB-refractory patients are in progress.
4. A better understanding of DNA repair in CLL cells may direct therapy at the inhibition of enzymes that catalyze these processes.
5. New therapeutic targets should be sought. Preclinical studies show an unprecedented effectiveness of camptothecin analogs, targeted at topoisomerase I. The drugs bypass the MDR1-related resistance and are effective against several human malignancies that do not respond to other drugs. Response-modulating agents, such as Ca^{2+} channel blockers or cyclosporin, may improve treatments with drugs that are otherwise ineffective against cancers with the MDR type of resistance.
6. There is a need to gain a better understanding of CLL resistance to glucocorticoids. Models of glucocorticoid-resistant cell lines are available. These should allow studies aimed at elucidating the mechanism of variable responses observed in CLL clinically.
7. CLL lymphocytes respond to some growth factors (94). If the usual impaired stimulus-transduction block could be overcome, the patients' immune response and tolerance to higher doses of chemotherapy may improve. Interleukin-4 regulates the expression of CD 23 on CLL lymphocytes (95). This lymphokine may also be inhibitory to CLL lymphocytes. It counteracts the IL-2-induced proliferation in some patients' cells (96). Human IL-4 downregulates the surface expression of CD 5-positive CLL lymphocytes (97). Research in these areas may point to new approaches in therapy.
8. A better understanding of the mechanism of action of the purine analog is essential to develop a rational approach to overcoming resistance to these active agents. For example, a potential means of reversing resistance to fludarabine is through the concurrent use of agents with the ability to act as biochemical modulators, such as cytarabine, hydroxyurea, and gallium nitrate (98–100).

REFERENCES

1. K. A. Foon, K. R. Rai, and R. P Gale, Chronic lymphocytic leukemia: New insights into biology and therapy, *Ann. Intern. Med., 113*:525 (1990).
2. M. R. Grever, J. M. Leiby, E. H. Kraut, et al., Low-dose deoxycoformycin in lymphoid malignancy, *J. Clin. Oncol., 3*:1196 (1985).
3. L. D. Piro, C. J. Carrera, E. Beutler, et al., 2-Chlorodeoxyadenosine an effective new agent for the management of chronic lymphocytic leukemia, *Blood, 72*:1069 (1988).
4. M. J. Keating, Fludarabine phosphate in the treatment of chronic lymphocytic leukemia, *Sem. Oncol., 17*:49 (1990).
5. W. Dameshek, Chronic lymphocytic leukemia: An accumulative disease of immunologically incompetent lymphocytes, *Blood, 29*:566 (1967).
6. L. S. Goodman, M. M. Wintrobe, W. Dameshek, et al., Use of methyl-bis(beta-chloro-ethylamine hydrochloride) for Hodgkin's disease, lymphosarcoma, leukemia, *J. Am. Med. Assoc., 132*:126 (1946).
7. H. E. Skipper, L. L. Bennett, and W. H. Langham, Overall tracer studies with C^{14}-labeled nitrogen mustard in normal and leukemic mice, *Cancer, 4*:1025 (1951).
8. P. Brookes and P. D. Lawley, The reaction of mono- and bifunctional alkylating agents with nucleic acids, *Biochem. J., 80*:486 (1961).
9. K. W. Kohn, N. H. Steigbigel, and C. L. Spears, Cross-linking and repair of DNA in sensitive and resistant strains of E. coli treated with nitrogen mustard, *Proc. Natl. Acad. Sci. USA, 53*:1154 (1965).
10. P. D. Lawley and P. Brookes, Cytotoxicity of alkylating agents towards sensitive and resistant strains of *Escherichia coli* in relation to extent and mode of alkylation of cellular macromolecules and repair of alkylation lesions in deoxyribonucleic acid, *Biochem. J., 109*:433 (1968).
11. S. Venitt, Interstrand cross-links in the DNA of *Escherichia coli* B/r and B_{S-1} and their removal by the resistant strain, *Biochem. Biophys. Res. Commun., 31*:355 (1968).
12. W. E. Ross, R. A. G. Ewig, and K. W. Kohn, Differences between melphalan and nitrogen mustard in the formation and removal of DNA cross-links, *Cancer Res., 38*:1502 (1978).
13. C. B. Thomas, R. Osieka, and K. W. Kohn, DNA cross-linking by in vivo treatment with 1-(2-chloroethyl)-3-(4-methylcyclohexyl)-1-nitrosourea of sensitive and resistant human colon carcinoma xenografts in nude mice, *Cancer Res., 38*:2448 (1978).
14. C. C. Erickson, M. O. Bradley, J. M. Ducore, et al., DNA cross-linking and cytotoxicity in normal and transformed human cells treated with antitumor nitrosourea, *Proc. Natl. Acad. Sci. USA, 77*:467 (1980).
15. M. Colvin, R. B. Brundrett, J. W. Cowens, et al., A chemical basis for the antitumor activity of chloroethylnitrosoureas, *Biochem. Pharmacol., 25*:695 (1976).
16. D. B. Ludlum, B. S. Kramer, J. Wang, et al., Reaction of 1,3-bis(2-chloroethyl)-1-nitrosourea with synthetic polynucleotides, *Biochemistry, 14*:5480 (1975).

17. B. B. Bank, D. Kanganis, L. F. Liebes, and R. Silber, Chlorambucil pharma-
     cokinetics and DNA binding in chronic lymphocytic leukemia lymphocytes,
     Cancer Res., 49:554 (1989).

18. D. S. Alberts, S. Y. Chang, H.-S. G. Chen, et al., Comparative pharmacoki-
     netics of chlorambucil and melphalan in man, *Recent Results Cancer Res.,
     74*:124 (1980).

19. D. S. Alberts, S. Y. Chang, H.-S. G. Chen, et al., Pharmacokinetics and
     metabolism of chlorambucil in man: A preliminary report, *Cancer Treatment
     Rev., 6*(Suppl.):9 (1979).

20. A. Begleiter and G. J. Goldenberg, Uptake and decomposition of chlorambu-
     cil by L5178Y lymphoblasts in vitro, *Biochem. Pharmacol., 32*(3):535 (1983).

21. K. R. Harrap and B. T. Hill, The selectivity of alkylating agents and drug
     resistance. III. The uptake and degradation of alkylating drugs by Yoshida
     ascites sarcoma cells in vitro, *Biochem. Pharmacol., 19*:209 (1970).

22. B. T. Hill and K. R. Harrap, The uptake and utilization of chlorambucil by
     lymphocytes from patients with chronic lymphocytic leukemia, *Br. J. Cancer,
     26*:439 (1972).

23. R. J. Rutman, E. H. L. Chun, and F. A. Lewis, Permeability differences as
     a source of resistance to alkylating agents in Ehrlich tumor cells, *Biochem.
     Biophys. Res. Commun., 32*:650 (1968).

24. G. J. Goldenberg, C. L. Vanstone, L. G. Israels, et al., Evidence for a
     transport carrier of nitrogen mustard in nitrogen mustard-sensitive and -resis-
     tant L5178Y lymphoblasts, *Cancer Res., 30*:2285 (1970).

25. M. K. Wolpert and R. W. Ruddon, A study on the mechanisms of resistance
     to nitrogen mustard (HN2) in Ehrlich ascites tumor cells: Comparison of
     uptake of HN2-^{14}C into sensitive and resistant cells, *Cancer Res., 29*:873
     (1969).

26. A. McLean, R. C. Woods, D. Catovsky, et al., Pharmacokinetics and metab-
     olism of chlorambucil in patients with malignant disease, *Cancer Treatment
     Res., 6*(Suppl.):33 (1979).

27. G. Calcutt and T. A. Connors, Tumour sulfhydryl levels and sensitivity to
     the nitrogen mustard merophan, *Biochem. Pharmacol., 12*:83a (1963).

28. M. L. Clapper and K. D. Tew, Alkylating agent resistance in drug resistance,
     in *Cancer Therapy* (R. Ozols, ed.), Kluwer Academic Publishers, Boston, p.
     125 (1989).

29. A. Meister, Glutathione metabolism and its selective modification, *J. Biol.
     Chem., 263*:17205 (1988).

30. S. L. Kelly, A. Basu, B. Teicher, M. P. Hacker, D. H. Hamer, and J.
     S. Lazo, Overexpression of metallothionein confers resistance to anticancer
     drugs, *Science, 242*:1813 (1988).

31. L. A. Cazenave, J. A. Moscow, C. E. Myers, and K. H. Cowan, Glutathione
     S-transferase and drug resistance, in *Drug Resistance in Cancer Therapy* (R.
     F. Ozols, ed.), Kluwer Academic Publishers, Boston, chap. 11, p. 171 (1989).

32. K. Suzukake, B. J. Petro, and D. T. Vistica, Reduction in glutathione content
     of L-PAM resistant L1210 cells confers drug sensitivity, *Biochem. Pharma-
     col., 31*:121 (1982).

33. L. Panasci, D. Henderson, S. J. Torres-Garcia, V. Skalski, S. Caplan, and M. Hutchinson, Transport, metabolism, and DNA interaction of melphalan in lymphocytes from patients with chronic lymphocytic leukemia, *Cancer Res., 48*:1972 (1988).

34. J. B. Johnston, L. G. Irraels, G. J. Goldenberg, et al., Glutathione S-transferase activity, sulfhydryl group and glutathione levels, and DNA cross-linking activity with chlorambucil in chronic lymphocytic leukemia, *J. Natl. Cancer Inst., 82*:779 (1990).

35. S. V. Singh, D. D. Dao, C. A. Partridge, C. Theodore, S. K. Srivastava, and Y. L. Awasthi, Different forms of human liver glutathione s-transferases arise from dimeric combinations of at least four immunologically and functionally distinct subunits, *Biochem. J., 232*:781 (1985).

36. C. B. Pickett and A. Y. H. Lu, Glutathione-S-transferases: Gene structure, regulation and biological function, *Ann. Rev. Biochem., 58*:743 (1989).

37. B. Mannervik and U. H. Danielson, Glutathione transferases-structure and catalytic activity, *CRC Crit. Rev. Biochem., 23*:283 (1985).

38. B. Ketterer, Protective role of glutathione and glutathione transferases in mutagenesis and carcinogenesis, *Mutat. Res., 202*:343 (1988).

39. C. N. Robson, A. D. Lewis, C. R. Wolf, J. D. Hayes, A. S. J. Hall, and I. D. Hickson, Reduced levels of drug-induced DNA cross-linking in nitrogen mustard-resistant Chinese hamster ovary cells expressing elevated glutathione-S-transferase activity, *Cancer Res., 47*:6022 (1987).

40. A. D. Lewis, I. D. Hickson, and C. N. Robson, Increased expression of class amplified glutathione-S-transferase encoding genes associated with resistance to nitrogen mustards, *Proc. Natl. Acad. Sci. USA, 85*:8511 (1985).

41. K. D. Tew, A. M. Bomber, and S. J. Hoffman, Ethacrynic acid and piriprost as enhancers of cytotoxicity in drug resistant and sensitive cell lines, *Cancer Res., 48*:1669 (1985).

42. R. A. Nagourney, J. C. Messenger, D. H. Kern, and L. M. Weisenthal, Enhancement of anthracycline and alkylator cytotoxicity by ethacrynic acid in primary cultures of human tissues, *Cancer Chemother. Pharmacol., 26*: 318 (1990).

43. S. McQuaid, S. McCann, P. Day, E. Lawlor, and P. Humphries, Observations on the transcriptional activity of the glutathione-S-transferase gene in human hematological malignancies and in the peripheral leukocytes of cancer patients under chemotherapy, *Br. J. Cancer, 59*:540 (1989).

44. J. A. Moscow, C. R. Fairchild, M. J. Madden, et al., Expression of anionic glutathione-S-transferase and P-glycoprotein genes in human tissues and tumors, *Cancer Res., 49*:1422 (1989).

45. J. Holmes, C. Wareing, A. Jacobs, J. D. Hayes, R. A. Padua, and C. R. Wolf, Glutathione-S-transferase pi expression in leukaemia: A comparative analysis with mdr-1 data, *Br. J. Cancer, 62*:209 (1990).

46. J. C. Schisselbauer, R. Silber, E. Papadopoulos, K. Abrams, F. P. LaCreta, and K. D. Tew, Characterization of glutathione-S-transferase expression in lymphocytes from chronic lymphocytic leukemia patients, *Cancer Res., 50*: 3562 (1990).

47. S. J. Torres, L. Cousineau, S. Caplan, et al., Correlation of resistance to nitro-gen mustards in chronic lymphocytic leukemia with enhanced removal of melphalan-induced DNA crosslinks, *Biochem. Pharmacol., 38*:3122 (1989).

48. R. Geleziunas, A. McQuillan, A. Malapetsa, M. Hutchinson, D. Kopriva, M. A. Wainberg, and J. Hiscott, Increased DNA synthesis and repair-enzyme expression in lymphocytes form patients with chronic lymphocytic leukemia resistant to nitrogen mustards, *J. Natl. Cancer Inst., 83*(8):557 (1991).

49. W. E. Ross, R. A. G. Ewig, and K. W. Kohn, Differences between melphalan and nitrogen mustard in the formation and removal of DNA crosslinks, *Cancer Res., 38*:1502 (1978).

50. L. Zwelling, S. Michaels, H. Schwartz, et al., DNA crosslinks as an indicator of sensitivity and resistance of L1210 leukemia cells to cis-diaminedichloro-platnum and L-phenylalanine mustard, *Cancer Res., 41*:640 (1981).

51. J. Hansson, R. Lewensohn, U. Ringborg, et al., Formation and removal of DNA cross-links induced by melphalan and nitrogen mustard in relation to drug-induced cytotoxicity in human melanoma cells, *Cancer Res., 47*:2631 (1987).

52. B.-J. Jiang, B. Bank, Y.-H. Hsiang, T. Shen, M. Potmesil, and R. Silber, Chlorambucil does not form DNA crosslinks in resistant Chinese hamster ovary cells, *Cancer Res., 49*:5514 (1989).

53. B. D. Cheson (ed.), Fludarabine phosphate: An effective therapy for lym-phoid malignancies, *Sem. Oncol., 17*(8):1 (1990).

54. W. Plunkett, P. Huang, and V. Gandhi, Metabolism and action of fludara-bine phosphate, *Sem. Oncol., 17*(8):3 (1990).

55. J. R. Barrueco, D. M. Jacobsen, C. H. Chang, et al., Proposed mechanism of therapeutic selectivity of 9-β-D-arabinofuranosyl-2-fluoroadenine against murine leukemia based upon lower capacities for transport and phosphoryla-tion in proliferative intestinal epithelium compared to tumor cells, *Cancer Res., 47*:700 (1987).

56. L. W. Dow, D. E. Bell, L. Poulakos, et al., Differences in metabolism and cytotoxicity between 9-β-D-arabinofuranosyladenine and 9-β-D-arabinosyl-2-fluoroadenine in human leukemic lymphoblasts, *Cancer Res., 40*:1405 (1980).

57. R. W. Brockman, Y. C. Cheng, F. M. Schabel, Jr., et al., Metabolism and chemotherapeutic activity of 9-β-D-arabinofuranosyl-2-fluoroadenine against murine leukemia L1210 and evidence for its phosphorylation by deoxycyti-dine kinase, *Cancer Res., 40*:3610 (1980).

58. S. M. El Dareer, R. F. Struck, K. F. Tillery, et al., Disposition of 9-β-D-arabinofuranosyl-2-fluoroadenine in mice, dogs, and monkeys, *Drug Metab. Dispos., 8*:660 (1980).

59. R. F. Struck, A. T. Shortnacy, M. C. Kirk, et al., Identification of metabo-lites of 9-β-D-arabinofuranosyl-2-fluoroadenine, an antitumour and antiviral agent, *Biochem. Pharmacol., 31*:1975 (1982).

60. V. I. Avramis and W. Plunkett, Metabolism of 9-β-D-arabinosyl-2-fluoroadenine 5′-monophosphate by mice bearing P388 leukemia, *Cancer Drug Del., 1*:1 (1983).

61. P. E. Noker, G. F. Duncan, S. M. El Dareer, et al., Disposition of 9-β-D-arabinofuranosyl-2-fluoroadenine 5'-phosphate in mice and dogs, *Cancer Treatment Rep., 67*:445 (1983).

62. A. D. Ho, K. Ganeshaguru, W. Knauf, G. Dietz, I. Trede, A. V. Hoffbrand, and W. Hunstein, Enzyme activities of leukemic cells and biochemical changes induced by deoxycoformycin in vitro — Lack of correlation with clinical response, *Leuk. Res., 13*:269 (1989).

63. C. J. Carrera, C. Terai, M. Lotz, J. G. Curd, L. D. Piro, E. Beutler, and D. A. Carson, Potent toxicity of 2-chlorodeoxyadenosine toward human monocytes in vitro and in vivo, *J. Clin. Invest., 86*:1480 (1990).

64. E. B. Thompson and J. M. Harmon, Glucocorticoid receptors and glucocorticoid resistance in human leukemia in vivo and in vitro, *Adv. Exp. Med. Biol., 196*:111 (1986).

65. S. K. Arya, F. Wong-Staal, and R. C. Gallo, Dexamethasone-mediated inhibition of human T-cell growth factor and gamma interferon messenger RNA, *J. Immunol., 133*:273 (1984).

66. E. B. Thompson, The structure of the human glucocorticoid receptor and its gene, *J. Steroid Biochem., 27*(1–3):105 (1987).

67. M. E. Lippman, R. H. Halterman, B. C. Leventhal, S. Perry, and E. B. Thompson, Glucocorticoid-binding proteins in human acute lymphoblastic leukemic blast cells, *J. Clin. Invest., 52*:1715 (1973).

68. A. D. Ho, W. Aunstein, and W. Schmid, Glucocorticoid receptors and sensitivity in leukemias, *Blut, 42*:183 (1981).

69. B. Terenius, B. Simonsson, and K. Nilsson, Glucocorticoid receptors in chronic lymphocytic leukaemia, in *Glucocorticoid Action and Leukemia, 7th Tenovus Workshop* (P. A. Bell and N. M. Borthwick, eds.), Alpha Omega Publishing, Cardiff, p. 155 (1978).

70. E. G. Levine, B. A. Peterson, K. A. Smith, D. D. Hurd, and C. D. Bloomfield, Glucocorticoid receptors in chronic lymphocytic leukemia, *Leuk. Res., 9*(8):993 (1985).

71. A. Klein, D. Buskila, D. Gladman, B. Bruser, and A. Malkin, Cortisol catabolism by lymphocytes of patients with SLE and RA, *J. Rheumatol., 17*:30 (1990).

72. L. F. Liu, DNA topoisomerase poisons as antitumor drugs, *Ann. Rev. Biochem., 58*:351 (1989).

73. K. M. Tewey, T. C. Rowe, L. Yang, B. D. Halligan, and L. F. Liu, Adriamycin-induced DNA damage mediated by mammalian DNA topoisomerase II, *Science, 226*:466 (1984).

74. M. E. Wall, M. C. Wani, K. H. Cooke, A. T. Palmer, L. McPhail, and G. A. Sim, The isolation and structure of camptothecin, a novel alkaloidal leukemia and tumor inhibition from *Camptotheca acuminata, J. Am. Chem. Soc., 88*:3888 (1966).

75. Y.-H. Hsiang and L. F. Liu, Identification of mammalian topoisomerase I as an intracellular target of the anticancer drug camptothecin, *Cancer Res., 48*:1722 (1988).

76. Y.-H. Hsiang, L. F. Liu, M. E. Wall, M. C. Wani, A. W. Nicholas, G.

Manikumar, S. Kirschenbaum, and M. Potmesil, DNA topoisomerase I-mediated DNA cleavage and cytotoxicity of camptothecin analogs, *Cancer Res., 49*:4385 (1989).

77. M. Potmesil, B. Bank, H. Grossberg, S. Kirschenbaum, A. Penzinger, D. Kanganis, D. Knowles, R. Silber, Y.-H. Hsiang, L. F. Liu, and F. Traganos, Resistance of human leukemic and normal lymphocytes to DNA cleavage by drugs correlates with low levels of DNA topoisomerase, *Cancer Res., 48*: 3537 (1988).

78. L. A. Zwelling, M. Hinds, D. Chan, J. Mayes, K. L. Sie, E. Parker, L. Silberman, A. Radcliffe, M. Beran, and M. Blick, Characterization of an amsacrine-resistant line of human leukemia cells. Evidence for a drug-resistant form of topoisomerase II, *J. Biol. Chem., 264*(28):16411 (1989).

79. J. L. Duechars, B. Falini, and W. M. Erber, P glycoprotein and multidrug resistance in cancer chemotherapy, *Sem. Oncol., 16*:156 (1989).

80. J. A. Holmes, A. Jacobs, G. Carter, J. A. Whittaker, D. P. Bentley, and R. A. Padua, Is the mdr 1 gene relevant in chronic lymphocytic leukemia?, *Leukemia, 4*(3):216 (1990).

81. R. T. Perri, S. W. Louie, and W. G. Espar, Relationship of the multidrug resistance (MDR) gene mdr1 in chronic lymphocytic leukemia (CLL) B cells to in vitro drug resistance/sensitivity, *Blood, 75*:308a (1989).

82. H. Herweijer, P. Sonneveld, F. Baas, and K. Nooter, Expression of mdr1 and mdr3 multidrug-resistance genes in human acute and chronic leukemias and association with stimulation of drug accumulation by cyclosporine, *J. Natl. Cancer Inst., 82*:1133 (1990).

83. R. T. Perri, S. W. Louie, and W. G. Espar, Expression of the multidrug resistance (mdr) gene mdr1 in chronic lymphocytic leukemia (CLL) B cells, *Blood, 76*:1221a (1990).

84. P. M. Cumber, A. Jacobs, T. Hoy, J. Fisher, J. A. Whittaker, T. Tsuruo, and R. A. Pauda, Expression of the multiple drug resistance gene (mdr1) and epitope masking in chronic lymphatic leukaemia, *Br. J. Haematol., 76*: 226 (1990).

85. M. Michieli, D. Raspadori, D. Damiani, A. Geromin, C. Gallizia, A. Michelutti, R. Fanin, G. Fasola, D. Russo, P. Tazzari, S. Pileri, F. Mallardi, and M. Baccarani, The expression of the multidrug resistance-associated glycoprotein in B-cell chronic lymphocytic leukaemia, *Br. J. Haematol., 77*:460 (1991).

86. T. Tsuruo, Circumvention of drug resistance with calcium channel blockers and monoclonal antibodies, in *Drug Resistance in Cancer Therapy* (R. F. Ozols, ed.), Kluwer Academic Publishers, Boston, chap. 6, p. 73 (1989).

87. T. P. Miller, T. M. Grogan, W. S. Dalton, C. M. Spier, R. J. Scheper, and S. E. Salmon, p-Glycoprotein expression in malignant lymphoma and reversal of clinical drug resistance with chemotherapy plus high-dose verapamil, *Blood, 9*:17 (1991).

88. M. Lehnert, W. S. Dalton, D. Roe, S. Emerson, and S. E. Salmon, Synergistic inhibition by verapamil and quinine of p-glycoprotein-mediated multidrug resistance in a human myeloma cell line model, *Blood, 77*:348 (1991).

89. B. C. Giovanella, J. S. Stehlin, M. E. Wall, M. C. Wani, A. W. Nicholas, L. F. Liu, R. Silber, and M. Potmesil, DNA topoisomerase I-targeted chemotherapy of human colon cancer in xenografts, *Science, 246*:1046 (1989).

90. M. Potmesil, B. C. Giovanella, L. F. Liu, M. E. Wall, R. Silber, J. S. Stehlin, Y.-H. Hsiang, and M. C. Wani, Preclinical studies of DNA topoisomerase I-targeted 9-amino and 10,11-methylenedioxy camptothecin, in *DNA Topoisomerases in Cancer* (M. Potmesil and K. W. Kohn, eds.) Oxford University Press, New York, (1991).

91. M. Potmesil, M. E. Wall, M. C. Wani, R. Silber, C. Cordon-Cardo, J. S. Stehlin, A. Kozielski, and B. C. Giovanella, DNA topoisomerase-targeted chemotherapy of human colon cancer xenografts with mdr phenotype, in *Eighty-First Annual Meeting of the American Association for Cancer Research Proceedings '31*, Washington, DC, p. 438 (1990).

92. R. Silber, M. Mani, T. Shen, and M. Potmesil, Effects of camptothecin and analogs on quiescent malignant cells, in *Eighty-Second Annual Meeting of the American Association for Cancer Research Proceedings '32*, Houston, TX, p. 337 (1991).

93. R. Ohno, K. Okada, T. Masaoka, A. Kuramoto, T. Arima, Y. Yoshida, H. Ariyashi, M. Ichimaru, Y. Sakai, M. Oguro, Y. Ito, Y. Morishima, S. Yokomaku, and K. Ota, An early phase II study of CPT-11: A new derivative of camptothecin, for the treatment of leukemia and lymphoma, *J. Clin. Oncol., 8*:1907 (1990).

94. D. W. Maher, B. L. Pike, and A. W. Boyd, The response of human B Cells to interleukin 4 is determined by their stage of activation and differentiation, *Scand. J. Immunol., 32*(6):631 (1990).

95. M. Sarfati, S. Fournier, M. Christoffersen, and G. Biron, Expression of CD23 antigen and its regulation by IL-4 in chronic lymphocytic leukemia, *Leuk. Res., 14*(1):47 (1990).

96. S. Karray, T. DeFrance, H. Merle-Béral, J. Banchereau, P. Debré, and P. Galanaud, Interleukin 4 counteracts the interleukin 2-induced proliferation of monoclonal B cells, *J. Exp. Med., 168*:85 (1988).

97. T. Defrance, B. Vanbervliet, I. Durand, and J. Banchereau, Human interleukin 4 downregulates the surface expression of CD5 on normal and leukemic B cells, *Eur. J. Immunol., 19*(2):293 (1989).

98. J. A. Streifel and S. B. Howell, Synergistic interaction between 1-b-D-arabinofuranosylcytosine, thymidine, and hydroxyurea against human B cells and leukemic blasts in vitro, *Proc. Natl. Acad. Sci. (USA), 78*:5132 (1981).

99. V. Gandhi, B. Nowak, M. J. Keating, and W. Plunkett, Modulation of arabinosylcytosine metabolism by arabinosyl-2-fluoroadenine in lymphocytes from patients with chronic lymphocytic leukemia: Implications for combination therapy, *Blood, 74*:2070 (1989).

100. J. H. Lundberg and C. R. Chitambar, Interaction of gallium nitrate with fludarabine and iron chelators: Effects on the proliferation of human leukemia HL60 cells, *Cancer Res., 50*:6466 (1990).

12

An Outline of Clinical Management of Chronic Lymphocytic Leukemia

Kanti R. Rai
*Albert Einstein College of Medicine, Bronx, New York and
Long Island Jewish Medical Center, New Hyde Park, New York*

There is a wide range of choices available to a physician today for the treatment of patients with chronic lymphocytic leukemia (CLL) (1). However, there is no universally accepted definitive treatment for this disease. I have been privileged to see a large number of CLL patients during the past several years, and this opportunity has enabled me to develop a method of approach that I find very useful in making therapeutic decisions in individual cases. In this chapter I outline my response to some of the most frequently asked questions about the clinical management of this disease.

DIAGNOSIS OF CLL

In clinical medicine, CLL is perhaps one of the easiest-made diagnoses. Until about a decade ago, a lymphocytosis in blood and bone marrow was considered sufficient to diagnose CLL, but now there is a general agreement among hematologists-oncologists that monoclonality of lymphocytes must also be demonstrated by immunophenotyping studies. The National Cancer Institute-sponsored Working Group (NCI-WG) (2), as well as the International Workshop on CLL (IWCLL) (3), have both proposed several criteria that must be met to establish the diagnosis of CLL. Listed below are these criteria and also my own efforts to reconcile a few relatively minor points of difference that were found to exist between the recommendations of these two groups.

Absolute Lymphocytosis in Blood

An absolute lymphocytosis in the peripheral blood with mature-appearing cells is required for the diagnosis of CLL. Although, in the past, an absolute lymphocyte count of $15 \times 10^9/L$ used to be considered the threshold for defining lymphocytosis, the NCI-WG (2) and the IWCLL (3) lowered this threshold to $5 \times 10^9/L$ and $10 \times 10^9/L$, respectively. NCI-WG (2) was interested in establishing objective diagnostic criteria for patients who were to be included in any future clinical research studies in CLL and, therefore, set a relatively low threshold to define lymphocytosis but added a requirement of B-cell monoclonality (described below) by immunophenotyping of lymphocytes. On the other hand, IWCLL (3) was interested in establishing a global definition (without regard for research studies) in which immunophenotyping was recommended but not mandated and, therefore, set a higher threshold to define lymphocytosis. But, from an objective point of view, if we recognize that the upper level of the range of normal absolute lymphocyte count is between 2.5 and $3.0 \times 10^9/L$, we must allow that an absolute lymphocyte count in excess of $3.0 \times 10^9/L$ is a true lymphocytosis and a diagnosis of CLL should be considered in all such cases. Although in actual practice it is rare to see a CLL case with an absolute lymphocyte count as low as $3.0 \times 10^9/L$, from a purist point of view this is the level at which a threshold defining absolute lymphocytosis should be placed.

Bone Marrow Lymphocytosis

A bone marrow aspiration examination is required for the diagnosis of CLL. The overall cellularity should be either normal or increased, and the differential count of the aspirate smear must reveal lymphocytes accounting for more than 30% of all nucleated cells.

Lymphocyte Phenotype Characteristics

Phenotyping of blood lymphocytes must reveal a majority of the population possessing features of monoclonal B cells with the following special characteristics: extremely low levels of surface membrane immunoglobulins (SmIg) with preponderance of only one light chain (either kappa or lambda) and expressing CD5, previously believed to be an antigen associated only with T cells. B cells in CLL typically also express one or more of various B-cell-associated antigens as demonstrated by CD19, CD20, CD21, or CD24 positivity.

Some Additional Comments on
Minimum Diagnostic Requirements

Sustained Nature of Blood Lymphocytosis

In the past, it was required that the blood lymphocytosis should be persistent or sustained upon repeated examinations for at least 4 weeks. This caveat was obviously introduced to avoid a misdiagnosis of CLL in cases with blood lymphocytosis that is of transient nature, as may be seen with pertussis, infectious mononucleosis, toxoplasmosis, etc. However, in none of these latter conditions is a blood lymphocytosis accompanied by a marrow lymphocytosis. Thus, I do not insist on repeated blood examinations for establishing the diagnosis of CLL because the presence of both blood and marrow lymphocytosis render the issue of sustained lymphocytosis redundant.

Is Bone Marrow Biopsy Necessary?

As described above, I consider an examination of bone marrow aspirate essential for making the initial diagnosis of CLL. Although a marrow biopsy is not necessary for diagnosing CLL, it is a good policy to include this procedure along with marrow aspiration because the results of biopsy examination provide an important prognostic tool (discussed below).

Should T-CLL Be Excluded from a Discussion of CLL?

Cases of chronic lymphocytosis with a T-cell phenotype are rare and account for less than 5% of cases of chronic lymphocytic leukemia. Based on the immunologic, biologic, and clinical differences from B-CLL, some investigators recommend that T-CLL should not be included in a discussion of CLL. There are three distinct clinical subtypes of chronic lymphocytosis with the rare T-cell phenotype: (a) adult T-cell leukemia-lymphoma (ATLL), which is associated with the human T-cell leukemia-lymphoma virus (HTLV-1); (b) Sezary syndrome, which is the leukemic manifestation of cutaneous T-cell lymphoma (CTCL); and (c) large granular lymphocytic leukemia. I agree with the view that these disorders with a T-cell phenotype are so different from B-CLL that unless specifically mentioned otherwise, a discussion of CLL should cover only the preponderant B-CLL.

DIFFERENTIAL DIAGNOSIS

Prolymphocytic leukemia, the leukemic phase of non-Hodgkin's lymphoma, and hairy cell leukemia are the three most common conditions that may sometimes present with clinical features indistinguishable from typical CLL. In most cases, morphology, cytochemistry, and bone marrow biopsy are extremely useful in arriving at the correct diagnosis. Electron microscopy has also been used, although it is expensive and frequently not readily available. If all these investigations fail to establish a diagnosis, a review of the immunophenotypic profile of the leukemic lymphocytes is of immense value. The amount of surface immunoglobulins on B cells in CLL is extremely small (faint fluorescence), whereas in all three conditions listed above, it is abundant (bright fluorescence); and CD5 positivity and rosetting with mouse erythrocytes are seen only in CLL.

STAGING AND OTHER PROGNOSTIC FACTORS

Modified Rai Staging

The two systems of clinical staging of CLL utilized most often are those proposed by Rai et al. (4) and Binet et al. (5). These systems are described elsewhere in this volume. For all clinical trials, I use the modified (6) Rai system, which consists of three risk groups as defined below:

Low-risk group: Rai stage 0
Intermediate-risk group: Rai stages I and II
High-risk group: Rai stages III and IV

Predictors of Clinical Course in Low- and Intermediate-Risk Groups

Although patients in the high-risk group uniformly tend to have active disease, those in the intermediate- and low-risk groups are known to have at least two distinct patterns of disease activity — indolent and active. Neither the Rai nor the Binet system is helpful in prospectively separating patients who are likely to have an active course from those with an indolent course. Recent studies indicate that the pattern of lymphocytic infiltration in the bone marrow biopsy specimens and the rate of increase of absolute lymphocyte count in the blood (as reflected by the lymphocyte doubling time) in patients not receiving cytotoxic therapy are predictors of clinical course of the disease. I utilize these criteria together in low- and intermediate-risk patients with CLL in the following manner:

1. Predicting an indolent course: nondiffuse (nodular or interstitial) lymphocytic infiltration in bone marrow biopsy plus prolonged (>12 months) lymphocyte doubling time
2. Predicting an active clinical course: diffuse lymphocytic infiltration in bone marrow biopsy plus short (≤ 12 months) lymphocyte doubling time

APPROACH TO THERAPY

Period of Observation

At the time of diagnosis of CLL, the disease activity is relatively indolent in about 80% of cases. It is preferable to withhold institution of cytotoxic therapy in these cases for a period that may vary from several weeks to a few years. During this period of observation, the patient is examined in the clinic and the blood counts evaluated at intervals ranging from 4 to 8 weeks. This regular follow-up also provides an opportunity to perform a bone marrow biopsy (if not done previously) and to determine the lymphocyte doubling time by charting blood lymphocyte count against time.

Indications for Therapy

Cytotoxic therapy is instituted if any of the following complications develop, which provide evidence of active disease. A minority of patients may present with some of these findings at the time of initial diagnosis of CLL, and they are started on treatment without going through an observation phase.

1. Disease-related symptoms (i.e., "B" symptoms of lymphoma — weight loss, fever without infections, night sweats, weakness, or easy fatiguability).
2. Development of anemia or thrombocytopenia resulting from bone marrow involvement.
3. Autoimmune hemolytic anemia or thrombocytopenia.
4. Progressively worsening or bulky lymphadenopathy, which poses risk to the patient from pressure on the underlying tissue, or causes pain or cosmetic discomfort.
5. Progressively increasing splenomegaly or the presence of a painfully enlarged spleen.
6. Rapidly increasing lymphocytosis (for example, blood lymphocyte count doubling in 6 months). It is not possible to set a rigid upper limit for blood lymphocyte count at which cytotoxic therapy must be instituted. However, I have seen a few cases in the past few years, of a hyperviscosity syndrome secondary to hyperlymphocytosis. Therefore, I empirically use 150×10^9/L as the threshold above which I start therapy. Nevertheless, patients may have a peripheral blood lymphocyte count of 200–300 $\times 10^9$/L and not experience symptoms related to hyperviscosity.
7. Increased susceptibility to bacterial infections.

Therapy Based on Clinical Stage

Low-Risk Group (Stage 0)

Low-risk (Stage 0) patients should not be started on cytotoxic therapy unless there is evidence of active disease (defined above). When therapy is
indicated, I recommend single-agent therapy with oral chlorambucil on an
intermittent dosage of 20 to 30 mg/m^2 in one day at intervals of 3 to 4
weeks. This therapy is stopped after a few months, as soon as the symptoms
or signs that required this intervention are resolved. If, on the other hand,
a clinical research protocol is available that is aimed at testing the value of
an investigational approach (e.g., interferon-α in low-risk CLL), I offer
that opportunity to the patient. Based on the clinical observations suggesting some benefit from interferon-α therapy in low-tumor-bearing patients
with multiple myeloma and lymphoma, it is quite justifiable to study its
role in early-stage CLL in the context of a clinical trial.

Intermediate-Risk Group (Stages I and II)

If intermediate-risk (stages I and II) patients develop evidence of active
disease (defined above), they are treated with oral chlorambucil on an intermittent dosage of 20 to 30 mg/m^2 in one day at intervals of 3 to 4 weeks.
This therapy is stopped after a few months, as soon as the symptoms
or signs that required this intervention are resolved. Cyclophosphamide is
another alkylating agent that may be as effective in CLL as chlorambucil,
and can be used in patients who cannot tolerate the latter agent. Cyclophosphamide can be given orally as well as by the intravenous route, and the
usual starting dose is 500 to 700 mg/m^2 at intervals ranging between 2 and
4 weeks.

An intergroup therapeutic protocol is currently widely available in the
United States and Canada to test whether the new drug fludarabine is
better than chlorambucil in CLL patients who have previously received no
cytotoxic or biologic therapy. I offer this protocol to all eligible patients. I
believe that fludarabine has proven to be of significant value for those
patients who have become refractory to chlorambucil or other alkylating
agent therapy. Thus, it seems appropriate now to try to determine if fludarabine, when used as the front-line therapy, will improve the natural course
of CLL, which has not changed significantly during the past three to four
decades with alkylating agents such as chlorambucil and cyclophosphamide. The intergroup protocol is a three-arm randomized study — fludarabine versus chlorambucil versus a combination of fludarabine and chlorambucil.

Intermediate-risk patients without evidence of active or progressive disease are maintained on regular observation alone without cytotoxic therapy.

High-Risk Group (Stages III and IV)

Although there are only limited data to support the use of multiple agents, I use a combination of chlorambucil and prednisone in high-risk-group (stages III and IV) patients. The dosage of chlorambucil is as described above. Prednisone is given orally at 30 to 40 mg/m^2 per day for 5 to 7 days with each cycle of chlorambucil. This therapy is continued until the maximally achievable beneficial response has become stable for about 1 to 2 months. There is no evidence for additional benefit using more intensive regimens as front-line therapy.

If a patient in the high-risk group has previously received no cytotoxic therapy, I offer the intergroup therapeutic protocol (described above).

Treatment of Autoimmune Complications of CLL

The causes of anemia and thrombocytopenia in CLL are not always clearly identifiable, but in a small minority of cases they result from autoimmune phenomena. The diagnosis of autoimmune hemolytic anemia (AIHA) is relatively easy to make because of the ready availability and reliability of the Coombs' test. However, the laboratory demonstration of autoantibodies against platelet antigens is still not a well-standardized test and, therefore, the diagnosis of immune thrombocytopenic purpura (ITP) requires a certain degree of clinical judgment. The mechanism of development of autoimmune phenomena in CLL is not clearly understood, but it is believed to be somehow related to abnormal T-cell numbers and functions in B-CLL as well as the increased number of CD5-positive B cells. The autoantibodies are polyclonal, mostly of IgG class, and bear no relation to the monoclonal immunoglobulin class present on the surface of leukemic lymphocytes.

AIHA results from the formation of warm antibodies with anti-D specificity. It should be noted that, although a positive Coombs' test is observed in nearly 20% of cases with CLL, less than half of these cases have anemia. Usually other evidence of hemolysis, such as spherocytosis, reticulocytosis, and elevations in serum lactic dehydrogenase and bilirubin, are also present. Thrombocytopenia with adequate or increased numbers of megakaryocytes in the bone marrow indicates ITP as the most likely diagnosis, and specific tests for the presence of anti-platelet antibodies, if available, should be obtained.

In most cases, AIHA and ITP respond to therapy with prednisone. The initial starting dose of prednisone may be somewhat higher (60 to 100 mg/day) than is generally used in combination with an alkylating agent in CLL, but it may be tapered after a few days when a clinical response to therapy has become manifest. When prednisone alone is not sufficient to control

AIHA or ITP, high-dose intravenous immunoglobulin (IVIG) should be added. The dose of IVIG is 0.4 g/kg and is given at 3-week intervals after an initial loading dose given daily for 5 days. Many patients also require simultaneous chemotherapy for CLL because of the presence of bulky disease or "active" disease. In a few cases when the above-noted treatments fail and the patient has a palpably enlarged spleen, splenectomy may prove beneficial. The prognosis of patients with AIHA and ITP who respond to prednisone therapy is better than that of patients whose anemia or thrombocytopenia are from causes other than autoantibodies.

Role of Splenectomy

I recommend splenectomy for patients in whom hypersplenism is believed to be the cause of anemia or thrombocytopenia, and for which chemotherapy and corticosteroids have already been tried and have failed to provide an adequate degree of control. The use of splenic irradiation has proven to be of only transient, if any, benefit. Occasionally, splenic irradiation is not even a practical option if the platelet count is already dangerously low (between 20 and 50 $\times$ 10^9/L) because, early in the course of radiation therapy, platelet counts are likely to decrease further. Splenectomy has also been occasionally beneficial when the major bulk of tumor is in the enlarged spleen and there is very little lymphadenomegaly. When splenectomy is successful in controlling CLL, the palliative effects may last for several years. Following splenectomy, the clinical course of many patients improves from active disease status of a high-risk group to indolent disease of a low- or intermediate-risk group.

Radiation Therapy

When peripheral lymph nodes are massively enlarged, are posing some risk to the patient by pressure over the underlying organs, and are painful or are cosmetically unsightly to the patient, radiation therapy may provide effective palliation. Radiation therapy is a practical option when the bulky adenopathy affects peripheral lymph nodes such as in the neck, axillae, or femoro-inguinal areas. However, for bulky intraabdominal retroperitoneal nodes, radiation therapy generally requires a large radiation field, which results in significant nausea and vomiting and other toxicities. Splenic radiation is also an effective, although transient palliative therapy for splenomegaly without significant lymphadenopathy, anemia, or thrombocytopenia. Lymphoid organs in CLL are radiosensitive and, therefore, a satisfactory response can be expected with relatively low doses of radiation. I have found a consultation with radiation oncologists always very helpful in deciding whether radiation therapy may be indicated for an individual patient.

Therapeutic Leukapheresis

There is only a limited role for therapeutic leukapheresis in CLL. However, the risk from hyperviscosity syndrome resulting from hyperleukocytosis in CLL should not be overlooked. Thus, when a patient is newly diagnosed as having CLL and the initial leukocyte count is in excess of $350 \times 10^9/L$, a therapeutic leukapheresis should be performed, to be followed immediately with chemotherapy and appropriate hydration to protect the patient from uric acid nephropathy and tumor lysis syndrome. Leukapheresis alone has an extremely transient effect in reducing blood leukocyte count and is an ineffective therapy unless the patient also receives concurrent chemotherapy.

Role of Intravenous Immunoglobulin Therapy

In properly selected patients who are believed to be at high risk to suffer from bacterial infections, intravenous immunoglobin (IVIG) therapy has been demonstrated to have a protective value (7). Patients with CLL who have previously suffered at least one major bacterial infection (such as pneumonia) and/or have a markedly decreased level of serum IgG (less than 4 g/L) should be considered for this therapy. This treatment does not provide a protective effect against viral or fungal infections. The dose of IVIG is 0.4 g/kg every 3 weeks for 1 year. There are no data available to guide us as to whether maintenance therapy, beyond 1 year, either at a lower dose or at a less frequent schedule, is beneficial.

Treatment of Pure Red Cell Aplasia in CLL

Pure red cell aplasia (PRCA) is a relatively rare cause of anemia in CLL, but when it does occur it seems to be mediated by the inhibitory effect on erythropoiesis of suppressor/cytotoxic T cells. Therapy with cyclosporine has been found to induce a reticulocyte response and eventually a significant increase in hemoglobin concentration in CLL patients with PRCA.

Newer Drugs and Second-Line Treatment Options

Fludarabine has now become widely available in the United States for all patients who have failed the initial therapy with an alkylating agent (chlorambucil or cyclophosphamide). I find it an effective agent for the control of refractory CLL. I use this drug at 25 mg/m^2/day for 5 days intravenously every month. There is some cumulative myelotoxicity after several months, but otherwise it is well tolerated. As patients with CLL are already immuno-compromised hosts and fludarabine itself is immunosuppressive, develop-ment of opportunistic infection should be kept in mind if they develop fever of unknown origin while receiving fludarabine.

2-chlorodeoxyadenosine (2-CdA) is the second most promising drug in CLL. This drug is available in the United States from the National Cancer Institute's Group C protocol mechanism for patients with hairy cell leuke-mia. NCI-sponsored clinical trials for patients with CLL will also be con-ducted. I have found it to be effective in several cases for control of refrac-tory CLL. The dose is 0.1 mg/kg/24 h for 7 days by continuous intravenous infusion every month. As with fludarabine, 2-CdA is associated with some cumulative myelotoxicity after several months of usage, and also increases the risk of opportunistic infections. The level of activity of CdA in patients who fail fludarabine is not yet known.

Deoxycoformycin (dcF) has been approved by the FDA in the United States for use in hairy cell leukemia, and it has also proven to be of some value in refractory CLL. The usual dose is 4 mg/m^2 intravenously at inter-vals of 2 to 4 weeks. This drug has some nephrotoxicity, some cumulative myelotoxicity, and a risk of opportunistic infections in patients with under-lying immunocompromised status. Whether it is active in patients who have failed fludarabine remains to be determined.

Although I have had a few successes using combination chemotherapies in patients who have become refractory to chlorambucil or cyclophospha-mide, my overall experience with COP, CHOP, M-2 protocol, etc., is not as satisfactory as has been reported by some other clinicians. However, I use one of these combinations when for some reason I cannot use fludara-bine or 2-CdA.

Experimental Therapies

The use of monoclonal antibodies (such as CAMPATH-1H) (8) is currently in experimental clinical trials at several institutions throughout the United States. Similarly, the potential role for autologous bone marrow transplan-tation in CLL is being tested by Michael Keating at the M. D. Anderson Cancer Center in Houston, Texas, and by Lee Nadler at the Dana-Farber Cancer Center in Boston, Massachusetts. When my patients appear to be eligible for one of these research studies, I refer them to the appropriate clinician leading the study.

Whenever possible, patients should be entered into clinical trials so that we may increase our understanding of the biology and immunology of CLL while improving the therapy for these patients.

ACKNOWLEDGMENTS

This work was supported by grants from Helena Rubinstein Foundation, United Leukemia Fund, Wayne Goldsmith Leukemia Research, Lauri Strauss Leukemia Fund, and Dennis Klar Memorial Fund.

REFERENCES

1. K. R. Rai, Chronic lymphocytic leukemia, in *Hematology: Basic Principles & Practice* (R. Hoffman, E. J. Benz, Jr., S. J. Shattil, B. Furie, and H. J. Cohen, eds.), Churchill Livingstone, New York, p. 990 (1991).
2. B. D. Cheson, J. M. Bennett, K. R. Rai, et al., Guidelines for clinical protocols for chronic lymphocytic leukemia (CLL). Recommendations of the NCI-Sponsored Working Group, *Am. J. Hematol., 29*:152 (1988).
3. J.-L. Binet, D. Catovsky, G. Dighiero, et al., Chronic lymphocytic leukemia: Recommendations for diagnosis, staging and response criteria, International Workshop on CLL, *Ann. Intern. Med., 110*:236 (1989).
4. K. R. Rai, A. Sawitsky, E. P. Cronkite, et al., Clinical staging of chronic lymphocytic leukemia, *Blood, 46*:219 (1975).
5. J.-L. Binet, A. Auquier, G. Dighiero, et al., A new prognostic classification of chronic lymphocytic leukemia derived from a multivariate survival analysis, *Cancer, 48*:198 (1981).
6. K. R. Rai, A critical analysis of staging in CLL, in *Chronic Lymphocytic Leukemia: Recent Progress and Future Directions*, UCLA Symposia on Molecular and Cellular Biology, New Series, Vol. 59 (R. P. Gale and K. R. Rai, eds.), Alan R. Liss, New York, p. 253 (1987).
7. Cooperative Group for the Study of Immunoglobulin in Chronic Lymphocytic Leukemia, Intravenous immunoglobulin for the prevention of infection in chronic lymphocytic leukemia. A randomized, controlled clinical trial, *N. Engl. J. Med., 319*:902 (1988).
8. M. J. S. Dyer, G. Hale, F. G. J. Hayhoe, and H. Waldmann, Effects of CAMPATH-1 antibodies in vivo in patients with lymphoid malignancies: Influence of antibody isotype, *Blood, 73*:1431 (1989).

13

Chronic Lymphocytic Leukemia: Staging and Prognostic Factors

Bruce D. Cheson
National Cancer Institute, Bethesda, Maryland

INTRODUCTION

Chronic lymphocytic leukemia (CLL) is characterized by an extremely variable clinical picture. Many patients live as long as the age-matched population without requiring treatment, and die of apparently unrelated causes, while others progress and succumb to their disease within months to a few years despite the best available therapy. Research over the past 15 years has demonstrated the biologic and immunologic heterogeneity of CLL, which is reflected in this clinical diversity. New, effective treatment approaches are currently available for CLL, making it important to precisely define and diagnose CLL, and to use the biologic characteristics of the disease as part of the basis for treatment decisions.

DIAGNOSIS

Dameshek described CLL as "a generalized self-perpetuating neoplastic proliferation of lymphoid tissue, particularly of small lymphocytes" (1); nevertheless, he also recognized that this definition would need to be revised as more was learned about the immunology of the disease. The currently accepted definition of CLL is considerably more rigorous; it requires an increase in the number of peripheral blood lymphocytes to at least 5 ×

10^9/L, sustained over at least 4 weeks. Morphologically, the majority of these cells should be small, mature-appearing lymphocytes. Immunologically, these lymphocytes are monoclonal B cells co-expressing CD5 and pan-B markers (e.g., CD19, CD20) (2). Cases characterized by increased numbers of atypical cells are generally disorders that should not be designated as CLL, but more appropriately as one of the increasing number of variants that are being recognized. Recently the French-American-British (FAB) group proposed a classification of chronic B- and T-cell leukemias using morphologic, cytochemical, and immunologic characteristics to separate CLL from other related disorders such as prolymphocytic leukemia, hairy cell leukemia and hairy cell variant, non-Hodgkin's lymphomas in a leukemic phase, splenic lymphoma with villous lymphocytes, and plasma cell leukemia (3).

STAGING SYSTEMS

It has long been recognized that certain characteristics distinguish patients with CLL into groups with differing clinical outcomes, which may require different therapeutic approaches. Nevertheless, classification schemes have evolved slowly over the years. Boggs et al. (4) reviewed 130 patients evaluated at a single institution between 1945 and 1964 and observed that certain clinical and laboratory features predicted a likelihood of dying within 5 years of diagnosis—male sex, disease-related symptoms, hepatosplenomegaly, increased lymphocytes, anemia, thrombocytopenia, and neutropenia—while the extent of lymphadenopathy or the presence of systemic symptoms did not appear to correlate with survival. Galton (5) divided 88 patients into four groups; (a) no splenomegaly or lymphadenopathy; (b) lymphadenopathy only; (c) splenomegaly only; (d) lymphadenopathy and splenomegaly. Patients in the fourth group were also more likely to have a greater number of peripheral blood lymphocytes and more frequent evidence of bone marrow failure. He also suggested that the clinical course could be predicted by the rise in peripheral blood lymphocyte count. In 1967, Dameshek (1) described the clinical course of CLL as exhibiting four stages; I, asymptomatic with lymphocytosis in the blood and bone marrow only; II, generalized lymphadenopathy with a variable degree of splenomegaly, and night sweats; III, increasing symptomatology often with large lymphoid masses, and frequent infections; IV, fever, frequent infections, autoimmune disorders, anemia, and other disease-related complications, often progressing rapidly.

In 1975, Rai and co-workers (6) published the first widely accepted, clinically relevant classification. The initially described five-stage system correlated with survival: Stage 0, lymphocytosis only (median survival > 12.5 years); stage I, with lymphadenopathy (8.5 years); stage II, with splenomegaly $+/-$ hepatomegaly (6 years); stage III, anemia (1.5 years); stage IV, thrombocytopenia (1.5 years) (Table 1). The Rai system has recently been simplified based on the observation that the original five stages segregated naturally into three groups; stage 0 (low risk), stages I and II (intermediate risk), and stages III and IV (high risk), with a median survival of > 10 years, 7 years, and 1.5 years, respectively (7) (Table 1). Binet and co-workers (8,9) developed a simpler three-stage system: stage A, < 3 node-bearing areas (> 10 years); stage B, ≥ 3 node-bearing areas (5 years); stage C, anemia and/or thrombocytopenia (2 years). The Rai classification has become the most uniformly used in the United States, whereas the Binet system is the most widely accepted in Europe; it is not clear which is more clinically relevant. The International Working Group on CLL (IWCLL) created substages of the Binet system to integrate the Rai stages: e.g., A(0), A(I), A(II), B(I), B(II), C(III), C(IV) (10). This revision has not been widely adopted.

Other staging systems that appear to correlate with survival have been proposed (11–13). Mandelli et al. (13) evaluated clinical and biological data on 1777 cases and identified four risk groups based on hemoglobin concentration, peripheral blood lymphocytosis, number of lymph node areas, and hepatomegaly: stage I, benign lymphocytosis, includes patients with hemoglobin ≥ 11 g/dL and peripheral blood lymphocytosis < 60,000/μL, < 3 lymphoid areas, without hepatomegaly (i.e., ≤ 3 cm); stage II (low risk), hemoglobin < 11 g/dL, or peripheral blood lymphocytosis $\geq 60,000/\mu$L, or > 3 involved lymphoid areas, or hepatomegaly; stage III (intermediate risk), patients with two of the four variables, and stage IV (high risk), with at least three of the four variables. The median survival for the stage I and

Table 1 Modified Rai Staging System for CLL

Rai stage	Three-stage system	Clinical features	Median survival (years)
0	Low risk	Lymphocytosis in blood and marrow only	> 10
I II	Intermediate risk	Lymphocytosis + lymphadenopathy + splenomegaly $+/-$ hepatomegaly	7
III IV	High risk	Lymphocytosis + anemia + thrombocytopenia	1.5

stage II groups had not been reached (78% and 60% alive at 84 months, respectively), but it was 59 months for stage III patients and 32 months for stage IV patients.

Jaksic and Vitale (12) suggested that the burden of CLL could be used to predict outcome. They proposed a total tumor mass (TTM) score, which is determined by calculating the sum of (a) the square root of the number of peripheral blood lymphocytes, (b) the diameter of the largest palpable lymph node, and (c) the enlargement of the spleen below the left costal margin. Patients with a high TTM at presentation had an expected median survival of 39 months compared with 101 months for those with a lower TTM. This complicated system is another that has not received wide acceptance.

PROGNOSTIC FACTORS

Clinical stage remains the strongest predictor of survival in patients with CLL (6-9,11,13-16). the substantial heterogeneity even within clinical stage has led to a search for laboratory and clinical prognostic factors to improve on currently available staging systems. A large number of factors have been reported to correlate with disease progression or survival (Table 2).

Clinical and Laboratory Prognostic Factors

Cellular Morphology

Prior to the routine availability of immunophenotyping studies, all chronic lymphoid leukemias were categorized as CLL and the morphologic variability was attributed to heterogeneity of the disease. A number of these morphologic variants appeared to be associated with a poorer prognosis, e.g., larger lymphocytes, large numbers of prolymphocytes, clefted cells, cells with a narrow rim of cytoplasm and coarse chromatin, or granular cells (17-24). However, it is not clear from these reports how many of these cases would actually be diagnosed as CLL using currently accepted definitions. Clearly, prolymphocytic leukemia is associated with a poorer prognosis than CLL (19); however, more often there is an admixture of cells observed in the peripheral blood. Melo et al. (18) designated a group of patients as CLL/PLL whose peripheral blood differential consisted of between 10% and 55% prolymphocytes. The authors' impression was that cases with fewer prolymphocytes tend to have a clinical course more similar to CLL, whereas those with larger numbers behaved more like prolymphocytic leukemia. Prospective studies are needed to better characterize the outcome of this group of patients.

Pattern of Bone Marrow Involvement

The bone marrow in CLL has traditionally been considered to be diffusely infiltrated by mature-appearing lymphocytes; however, a substantial number of patients exhibit a nondiffuse (i.e., nodular, interstitial, mixed) pattern of involvement. Rozman et al. (36) conducted a retrospective analysis of prognostic factors on 329 cases of CLL (227 without prior therapy) and found that patients with a diffuse pattern of bone marrow involvement (n = 128) had a shorter survival than those with a nondiffuse pattern (n = 201). Moreover, the pattern of bone marrow involvement appeared to be a stronger predictor of survival than hepatomegaly, hemoglobin level, lymphadenopathy, age, or thrombocytopenia. However, the bone marrow pattern did not appear to add to the predictive value of clinical stage since, while it separated patients within clinical stage, in only stage B patients was the difference significant. Pangalis et al. (37) evaluated 48 previously untreated patients, 27% of whom had a diffuse pattern, and noted that all of those with diffuse marrow involvement required therapy at presentation; however, 91% of those cases had stage C disease. In a subsequent report of 120 cases (38), these investigators noted more frequent progression from stage A and B in patients who presented with a diffuse pattern; however, they were unable to discriminate survival by pattern within stage. Their recommendation to treat all patients with diffuse disease, regardless of clinical stage, is not supportable by the available data (39). Han et al. (40) evaluated 75 cases and found the pattern of bone marrow involvement correlated with cytogenetics, lymphocyte count, tritiated thymidine incorporation, serum alkaline phosphatase, and the presence of urinary light chains. None of the 49 stage 0–II patients had received prior therapy, whereas 5 of 26 stage III–IV patients had been treated. Half (10 of 20) of those with diffuse involvement died during the period of observation, compared with 6 of 55 (11%) of those with nondiffuse disease. However, the significance of bone marrow pattern related to its correlation with clinical stage. Desablens et al. (41) evaluated 98 untreated patients and concluded that clinical stage was a better discriminant than pattern of bone marrow involvement; there was no difference in survival between diffuse and nodular patterns in stage A or B patients. Therefore, it is not clear that the pattern of bone marrow involvement contributes prognostic information beyond what is available from clinical stage.

Age and Sex

Older age has consistently been shown to confer a poorer prognosis in CLL (4,13,16,25–27). Nevertheless, the outlook for younger patients is still unsatisfactory (28–31). DeRossi et al. (29) compared the features of 133

Table 2 Prognostic Factors in Chronic Lymphocytic Leukemia

	Favorable	Unfavorable	No Effect
Clinical			
Older age		4,13,16,25–27	37,54
Male sex		13,16,26,32	4,25,27,54
Non-Caucasian		26	25
Symptoms		4,26	
Lymphadenopathy		13,26,54	4,11,16,25,27,37
Hepatomegaly		4,13,26,27,37,54	25
Splenomegaly	11	4,13,25,26,54	16,27,37,69,77
Response to therapy	16,78		
Poor performance status		26	
Hematologic			
Anemia		4,11,13,16,25–27,32,37,54,69	
Thrombocytopenia		4,11,13,16,25–27,32,54	37
Peripheral blood lymphocytosis		4,11,13,15,16,25,26,54,69	37
Percent bone marrow lymphocytes		13,25,26,54	
Diffuse bone marrow pattern		23,36–38,40,54	25,41
Morphologic variants		17–24	
Cytogenic abnormalities		64–66	
Laboratory abnormalities			
Uric acid		26,27,54	
Calcium		26	
BUN/creatinine		26	
LDH/SGOT, bilirubin, alkaline phosphatase		26	

Immunologic			
Immunophenotype	43,110	44,45,110	
surface IgM	46,47,51	45,48,49	13,54
Coombs +		13	13,14
Soluble IL-2 receptors		52,53	
Hypogammaglobulinemia		45,55,56	
Monoclonal gammopathy			13,26,54
β_2-M		57–61	45
T/NK cell number/function		62,63	
Ig gene rearrangement		67,68	14
Cellular release of TNF		72	
Kinetic			
Lymphocyte doubling time		42,50,51	
Loss of clonogenic potential		73	
Tritiated thymidine uptake		79	
Serum deoxycytidine kinase		74	
Miscellaneous			
Ribonuclease A		75	
Poly(A)-polymerase		76	

cases of CLL between the ages of 31 and 50 years (mean 46.6 years) with a group of 1777 older patients (mean age 64.2 years). An immunologic diagnosis of B-CLL was confirmed in only 26 cases. Their younger patients differed from the older group by a higher incidence of hepatosplenomegaly and lymphadenopathy, although with a lower peripheral blood lymphocyte count and a higher hemoglobin concentration and platelet count. In a univariate analysis, hemoglobin (<13 g/dL), peripheral blood lymphocytes (>40 × 10^9/L), and percent bone marrow lymphocytes (>80%) had prognostic value. In multivariate analysis, percent bone marrow lymphocytes was the strongest predictor of survival. Neither the Rai nor Binet system fit well in their younger patients (28). In a recent review by the International Working Group on CLL (IWCLL) of 454 patients under 50 years of age, 25% were Rai stage 0, 21.5% stage I, 40% stage II, 5.5% stage III, and 8% stage IV (30). The overall median survival was 12 years [expected survival for a comparable control group, 31.2 years (31)]; the probability of surviving 10 years from diagnosis was 76% for stage 0, but only 45% for stages I–II and 24% for stages III–IV. The poor outlook for younger patients, especially those with unfavorable prognostic features, provides compelling support for the development of new and more aggressive therapeutic strategies.

Most studies suggest that females with CLL survive longer with CLL than males, even matched for other known prognostic factors such as clinical stage (13,16,26,32). The reasons for this possible difference are unclear.

Lee et al. (26) performed a multivariate analysis of 325 previously untreated patients, considering clinical features (age, race, sex, performance status, lymphadenopathy, hepatosplenomegaly); hematologic values (white blood cell count, absolute lymphocyte count, absolute granulocyte count, hemoglobin, platelet count); and biochemical factors (albumin, calcium, uric acid, LDH, alkaline phosphatase, BUN, creatinine). Based on uric acid, alkaline phosphatase, lactic dehydrogenase (LDH), external lymphadenopathy, and age, patients could be separated into low-risk (0–1 poor risk features), intermediate (2–3 features), and high-risk (≥4 features) groups, with 5-year survival rates of 75%, 59%, and 14%, respectively. They felt that this system improved the predictive value of the Rai classification.

Other Prognostic Factors

Although the majority of patients with CLL eventually require therapy for their disease, it is not clear that early initiation of chemotherapy, particularly for patients with early-stage (Rai 0–I, Binet stage A) CLL, prolongs survival (33–35). The availability of newer and more effective agents for patients with advanced disease makes it potentially useful to distinguish early-stage patients who might benefit from earlier therapeutic intervention from those who are better categorized as "smoldering CLL." The French Cooperative Group on CLL (25) conducted a multivariate analysis on 309 cases with stage A disease and identified nine clinical and laboratory variables with prognostic value for either overall survival or disease progression to stage B or C disease; these included age, sex, number of nodes, presence of symptoms, hemoglobin, platelet count, lymphocyte count, splenomegaly, percent bone marrow lymphocytes, and the presence of axillary lymph nodes. The particularly favorable subset of patients, "smoldering" CLL, could be defined on the basis of four variables; hemoglobin, lymphocyte count, number of nodes, and percent bone marrow lymphocytes. However, the four variables did not provide any better distinction than prior studies using hemoglobin level and lymphocyte count alone (34). The authors suggested that biologic markers might improve on currently available clinical and laboratory features, since 10% of patients who would be considered "smoldering" by these criteria still progressed by 5 years.

Tura et al. (42) attempted to correlate lymphocyte doubling time with survival in stage 0 patients; however, although a short doubling time was associated with frequent progression to a more advanced stage, they were unable to separate patients into groups with differing survivals, since the projected median duration was 12.5 years in the group that progressed and 14 years in the group that remained stable.

The United Kingdom Medical Research Council (MRC) reported their analysis of prognostic factors for patients treated between 1978 and 1984 on the MRC CLL1 trial (16). Of 660 patients, 29% died from causes that were considered by the authors to be unrelated to CLL (including other cancers in 12%, cardiovascular disease in 16%). A large proportion of deaths in patients with stage A disease were considered unrelated to CLL, whereas the majority of deaths in patients with stage B and C disease were disease-related. This analysis is somewhat flawed in that deaths from secondary malignancies should have been considered disease-related, which would have increased the number of disease-related deaths in the early-stage patients. Clinical stage was the most important prognostic factor in their univariate analysis. Other factors that predicted a more favorable clinical outcome included younger age, female sex, as well as lower white blood cell count, hemoglobin > 10 g/dL, and response to therapy. It should be noted, however, that cases who died within 6 months of entering on study were excluded from analysis of response. The number of lymph nodes, spleen size, and platelet count were not significantly correlated with survival.

IMMUNOLOGIC FACTORS

Immunophenotype

The malignant cells in CLL exhibit a characteristic membrane phenotype with coexpression of pan-B-cell antigens such as CD19 and CD20, along with CD5 (80). CLL cells also express mouse red blood cell receptors (MRBC), but only weakly express sIg. A number of other immunophenotypic markers have been proposed to be prognostic (43–49,51). Surface IgM is characteristic of a more mature phenotype; however, it is controversial whether it confers a better prognosis (14,46–51,110). Hamblin et al. (51) evaluated 60 patients and reported that sIgM was associated with less aggressive disease. However, this may reflect the preponderance of women in this series, who generally have a more favorable prognosis with CLL than men (13,16,26). Baldini et al. (48) evaluated 76 patients and concluded that patients with $sIg\mu$ had a worse prognosis. Foa et al. (14) were also unable to support a better prognosis in association with sIgM; however, the number of patients in their series was small. Tefferi and Phyliki (45) observed that cases of CLL that expressed sIg on <20% of lymphocytes had the best prognosis. Geisler et al. (110) performed immunophenotyping on 540 newly diagnosed patients and found that high levels of IgM conferred a poor prognosis in a univariate analysis.

Cases of CLL differ in their frequency of expression of various resting and activation antigens (80). B-CLL cells express surface receptors for interleukin-2 (IL-2), and some cases also secrete soluble IL-2 receptors into the serum (52,53). Semenzato et al. (52) detected elevated levels of IL-2 receptors in the serum of 51 of 54 patients, which correlated with a number of clinical features and hematologic and immunologic data (e.g., white blood cell count, serum Ig concentration, T-cell function studies). Similarly, Kay et al. (53) noted a correlation between soluble IL-2 receptors and clinical stage.

Geisler et al. (110) noted a shorter survival for patients whose cells expressed FMC7 but who failed to express CD23. Orfao et al. (54) evaluated cells from 62 previously untreated patients with B-CLL for MRBC, HLA/DR, CD20, FMC7, CD5, CD9, but were unable to identify a relationship between immunophenotype and survival. Survival of their patients correlated with Rai stage, percent of bone marrow lymphocytes, and pattern of bone marrow involvement. Pinto et al. (81) reported that the presence of myelomonocytic antigens on CLL cells correlated with diffuse bone marrow involvement. Dadmarz and Cawley (44) studied 35 cases and found low levels of interferon-α receptors in advanced disease, while the frequency of expression of CD23 (a B-cell activation antigen) was high with more favorable disease. Faguet and Agee (82) described a common CLL antigen (cCLLa), which they suggested was a feature only of B-CLL cells, and the size of the cCLLa clone correlated with the extent of disease. This observation requires independent confirmation.

As immunophenotyping has become more routine, the immunologic diversity of CLL has become more apparent, and a number of new immunologic variants have been described (3,83–86); however, their clinical relevance remains to be determined. Wormsely et al. (83) reported that 26 of 199 consecutive cases diagnosed morphologically as CLL coexpressed CD5 and CD11c, an antigen more characteristic of hairy cells. The clinical behavior of these cases was more like CLL than hairy cell leukemia. Sun et al. (86) described another unusual "hybrid" in which hairy projections were observed in a subpopulation of peripheral blood lymphocytes that shared immunophenotypic features of CLL and hairy cell leukemia.

Immunoglobulins and Complement

Patients with CLL are at increased risk for life-threatening bacterial infections, which is related to the degree of hypogammaglobulinemia (5,55,56) and, possibly, also to defective activation of the complement system (87). Rozman et al. (55) evaluated serum concentration of immunoglobulins in 247 untreated patients and found that low IgG and IgA, but not IgM, worsened with disease progression and correlated with survival. However, this correlation held only at a cutoff level of 700 mg/dL of IgG, and did not hold up in a multivariate analysis. It did not appear that the shortened survival reflected an increased incidence of infections. Other investigators have been unable to detect a relationship between hypogammaglobulinemia and survival (13,26,54). Heath and Cheson (87) evaluated the opsonic activity of CLL serum by measuring complement activation and noted a correlation with occurrence of bacterial infections.

Beta$_2$-microglobulin

Beta$_2$-microglobulin (β_2-M) is a low-molecular-weight protein associated with the HLA complex. It is a strong prognostic factor in multiple myeloma and low-grade non-Hodgkin's lymphomas, in part by correlating with tumor mass (88,89). A number of studies suggest that it may also be prognostic in CLL (57–61). Han et al. (60) determined β_2-M levels in 65 patients (prior treatment status not noted) by radioimmunoassay and noted that increased levels (>2.3 mg/L) were associated with a median survival of 37 months, whereas the median survival had not been reached for those with a normal level. When 5 mg/L was used as a cutoff, 26 of 53 with ≤ 5 mg/L died (median survival 61 months) compared with all 12 with >5 mg/L (median survival 19 months). Di Giovanni et al. (57) found a correlation between β_2-M and Rai and Binet stage in 22 patients (five previously treated), although the values in stage A patients were the same as normal controls. The beta$_2$-M value correlated with the type of bone marrow infiltration, tumor bulk, but not with the number of peripheral blood lymphocytes. Tötterman et al. (61) demonstrated that spontaneous and TPA-induced in-vitro production of β_2-M by CLL lymphocytes correlated with disease activity.

Lymphocyte Subsets in CLL

Not only are the number and function of the malignant B cells abnormal in CLL, but abnormalities have been reported in other lymphocyte subsets as well. Tötterman et al. (62) used two-color flow cytometric analysis to evaluate natural killer (NK) and T-cell number from 23 cases of CLL and also assessed the function of these subsets. They noted a correlation between advanced Rai stage and higher numbers of activated CD4+ and CD8+ T cells and a reduced proportion of T-suppressor/effector (CD11b+) cells. Apostopoulous et al. (63) evaluated 41 newly diagnosed patients and found that the CD4/CD8 ratio and the proportion of NK cells were lower in advanced disease and were associated with hypogammaglobulinemia and more respiratory infections.

CYTOGENETICS

Recent technologic advances have permitted satisfactory cytogenetic analysis in the majority of cases of CLL. An increasing body of data supports the prognostic importance of cytogenetics in CLL, as in other forms of acute and chronic leukemias (64–66). Chromosome abnormalities occur in approximately 50% of cases of CLL. This number varies somewhat among series, based on the distribution of clinical stages; patients with early-stage disease are less likely to have a cytogenetic abnormality (20%) than those with more advanced disease (70%) (64). Nevertheless, in multivariate analyses, cytogenetics and stage are independent prognostic factors (66). The most frequently reported abnormality is trisomy 12, which occurs either alone or in combination with other defects in approximately half the cases. Other common cytogenetic abnormalities include aberrations of chromosome 13 and 8, 14q+, and t(11;14)(q13;32). Patients with a normal karyotype have a more favorable outcome than patients with single abnormalities, who live longer than those with complex karyotypic abnormalities (64,66). Han et al. (64) obtained adequate metaphases in 86 of 102 cases, and identified clonal chromosome abnormalities in half, more commonly in patients with advanced disease. Bird et al. (65) performed cytogenetic determinations on samples from 40 patients and identified clonal abnormalities in 16 of the 31 successful analyses; trisomy 12 was observed in seven and a 14q32 translocation in four. There was a significant correlation between the presence of a clonal abnormality and an increased number of bone marrow and/or peripheral blood prolymphocytes. Karyotypic evolution occurs in approximately 20% of cases, although it does not appear to correlate with disease progression (90). Patients with chromosome abnormalities may become cytogenetically normal in association with a complete remission, although it is not clear whether the disappearance of the defect influences survival (91).

Juliusson et al. (66) reported cytogenetic evaluation on 433 cases of CLL, the majority were Rai stage 0–I (258) or Binet stage A (276) disease. Analyses were successful in 391 cases, of which 218 had a clonal abnormality. Those with normal chromosomes had a median survival of >15 years, but the survival for those with a clonal abnormality was 7.7 years. Survival of the 51 cases with 13q abnormality was normal, whereas those with 14q and abnormalities of 12 had a poor survival. A high percent of cells in metaphase, reflecting proliferation, was associated with a shorter survival. Cases in which cytogenetic analyses are unsuccessful appear to have an intermediate prognosis that reflects the clinical heterogeneity of this population.

MOLECULAR BIOLOGY

The search for oncogenes in the majority of cases of B-CLL has thus far been disappointing (66,92–95). bcl-1 Is detected in fewer that 5% of cases, bcl-2 and bcl-3 in only 5–10% of cases, some of which may not be typical CLL (66,93,94,96). Approximately half the structural defects of chromosome 13 involve band 13q14, the site of the retinoblastoma anti-oncogene; however, this oncogene has been detected in only 5% of cases of CLL (66,96,98). Whether the presence of any of these oncogenes carries prognostic importance in CLL remains to be determined in a prospective analysis.

The pattern of immunoglobulin (Ig) gene rearrangements in CLL has been evaluated for prognosis. Soper et al. (67) found Ig gene rearrangements in 41 of 42 cases studied. The proportion of cells expressing the rearrangement correlated with clinical course. Rechavi et al. (68) evaluated 38 cases and concluded that there was a correlation between the loss of germline or a $C\mu$ multiband pattern and advanced disease.

CELL KINETICS AND GROWTH FACTORS

Not only has the absolute number of peripheral blood lymphocytes been reported by some investigators to correlate with survival (4,11,13,15,

16,25,26,54,69), but the rate at which the lymphocyte count increases has been suggested to have prognostic importance as well (42,70,71). Montserrat and co-workers (70) confirmed the earlier impression of Galton (5), that patients whose clinical course exhibited a progressive rise in the lymphocyte count had a poor outcome. They performed a retrospective analysis on 100 previously untreated cases and noted that cases with a lymphocyte doubling time of < 12 months had a median survival of 5 years, whereas the median was not yet reached for those with a doubling time of ≥ 12 months. A similar distinction was apparent when 6 months was used as the cutoff, but the cases were not as evenly distributed. There was a weak correlation between doubling time and stage; stages B and C as a whole had similar doubling times, and the number of patients with stage C disease was too small for a meaningful analysis. Molica and Alberti (71) conducted a similar analysis on 99 untreated patients and found the 12-month doubling time to be a significant prognostic factor even after adjustment for age, sex, lymphocyte count, anemia, and thrombocytopenia, but not after clinical stage. Similar to the observations of Montserrat et al. (70), the discriminating ability of doubling time held only for stages A and B.

The role of growth factors in the pathogenesis of CLL is unknown. Tumor necrosis factor (TNF) has been suggested to be an autocrine growth factor for CLL cells (72,98). Foa et al. (72) demonstrated that the cellular release of TNF was significantly higher in patients with Rai stages 0–I disease than those with stage II–III disease. Dadmarz et al. (73) evaluated 28 cases and noted that clinical progression was associated with a loss of clonogenic potential.

Deoxythymidine kinase, an enzyme that reflects cellular transformation from a dormant to a dividing state, has been reported to correlate with disease progression (74).

MULTIDRUG RESISTANCE

One possible explanation for the lack of effectiveness of standard chemotherapy to substantially improve the survival of patients with CLL is the presence of de-novo or acquired drug resistance (99–106). A number of investigators have evaluated CLL cells for the presence of the multidrug resistance (mdr) phenotype. Groulx et al. (102) found mdr mRNA in none of 13 previously untreated patients but in 4 of 10 previously treated patients, although their therapy had not necessarily consisted of drugs that would induce the mdr phenotype. Perri et al. (103) used RNA slot blot analysis and Northern blotting with the MDR5A probe and found mdr1 in 11 of 12 previously untreated and all 8 previously treated cases. Using the C-219 antibody, they identified the p170 glycoprotein in 8 of 17 cases, including 6 who were mdr1 positive. Clinical relevance was suggested by the fact that none of the 4 Rai stage 0 cases were positive, while all stage IV cases (denominator not given) were positive, and 4 of 8 previously untreated cases were positive.

Holmes et al. (99) reported mdr1 expression without amplification in 4 of 7 previously untreated and 14 of 27 previously treated cases. They suggested that mdr1 might increase with treatment and decrease off treatment. Herweijer et al. (100) detected mdr1 and mdr2 (referred to as mdr3) with an RNAse protection assay in all 7 cases studied. Michieli et al. (105) examined cells from 63 patients with CLL using two monoclonal antibodies—MRK, which relates to the external domains of p170, and C-219, the cytoplasmic domains. They detected a weak immunocytochemical reaction with MRK and C-219 in 61% of cases, and a strong reaction in 39%. Using flow cytometric analysis, 39% of cells with MRK, 23% with C-219.

Obviously, measures of drug resistance need to be correlated with therapeutic response. Agents that have the potential to reverse drug resistance are now available for clinical trials (e.g., ethacrynic acid and BSO for alkylator resistance; topotecan, CPT-11 as topoisomerase I inhibitors; verapamil, cyclosporine, quinine to reverse mdr).

MISCELLANEOUS

A number of other putative prognostic factors have been identified in small numbers of patients, and their importance remains to be determined. Ribonuclease H, an enzyme found in retroviruses that degrades DNA–RNA hybrids, is elevated in several forms of leukemia. Therefore, Papaphilis et al. (75) evaluated levels of the enzyme in 39 cases of CLL and found that the increased levels in 69% of cases correlated, although not strongly, with stage and disease progression. Poly(A)-polymerase is an enzyme related to mRNA stability within the cytoplasm and may be an indirect measure of protein synthesis. Pangalis et al. (76) found that the activity of this enzyme varied among CLL cases and appeared to correlate with stage and was higher in patients who required therapy.

PROBLEMS AND POTENTIAL SOLUTIONS FOR STAGING AND PROGNOSIS

The development of a meaningful classification of CLL has lagged behind our growing knowledge of the biology and immunology of this disorder. There are problems inherent to all of the currently used staging systems. Each of the currently used staging systems, and most of the additional prognostic factors, merely reflects tumor mass (e.g., size and location of lymph nodes, hepatomegaly, splenomegaly, lymphocyte count and extent of bone marrow infiltration, LDH, $beta_2$-microglobulin, circulating IL-2 receptors), or patient condition (age, performance status).

Other than the modified Rai system (7) and the Binet system (9), most classification schemes are cumbersome [e.g., IWCLL (10) and total tumor mass (12)]. The Binet system (9) does not include patients with Rai stage 0 (i.e., lymphocytosis only), whereas the Rai system (7) does not account for the occasional patient with splenomegaly but without lymphadenopathy. The systems that rely on the number of nodes (e.g., Binet, IWCLL) or the size of the largest nodes were developed prior to the availability of noninvasive radiographic techniques such as CT scans, which could identify and quantify additional node sites. Whether this information would alter the prognostic value of these systems is unknown. Most important, none of these systems provides information about the biology of the disease. Moreover, none of the systems readily permits the integration of new prognostic factors that may be responsible, in part, for the considerable heterogeneity within clinical stage.

Although a wide variety of clinical and laboratory prognostic factors have been proposed, it is difficult to determine which are worth considering when planning a therapeutic approach, either for an individual case or for clinical trials. Factors have generally been identified in small numbers of patients through retrospective analyses, without either prospective validation or independent confirmation. In addition, the factors of interest are not routinely examined in multiple series.

There is also considerable heterogeneity within patients with respect to stage, nature, and extent of prior therapy. The latter may be particularly important, since certain factors may be dependent on the type of treatment (e.g., multidrug-resistance phenotype). Most of all, the most relevant prognostic factors remain unknown, since our knowledge of the immunology and biology is still incomplete.

GUIDELINES FOR CLINICAL PROTOCOLS

Standardized protocols are essential to compare the results of clinical trials, to identify drugs or regimens worth pursuing in large-scale studies, and to permit a prospective evaluation of potentially useful prognostic factors. In 1967 (published again in 1973) (107), the Chronic Leukemia–Myeloma Task Force and in 1978 the Cancer and Leukemia Group B (108) proposed guidelines for clinical studies. Unfortunately, these did not receive universal acceptance. More recently, two independent sets of guidelines have been published (Table 3) (2,109). The National Cancer Institute (NCI)-sponsored Working Group (NCI-WG) (2) standardized eligibility, response, and toxicity criteria for use in all NCI-sponsored clinical trials to ensure patient comparability. Studies are restricted to patients with immunophenotypically characterized B-CLL with evidence of "active disease," including disease-related symptoms, progressive marrow failure, poorly responsive autoimmune anemia or thrombocytopenia, massive or progressive hepato- and/or splenomegaly, or progressive lymphocytosis. Because there is controversy as to whether the PLL/CLL (11–55% prolymphocytes) patients have a different prognosis (18), this group can be studied prospectively on a standardized protocol. Use of the modified Rai classification (7) (Table 1) is encouraged; however, others such as the Binet system can be evaluated concurrently and the clinical relevance of the two compared prospectively. The role of immunologic testing for response has not been established, but will be evaluated in a prospective fashion. A unique feature of the guidelines is that they are designed to be modified over time as additional information is gained about the disease. It is likely that investigators will adhere to these guidelines because they were developed by a committee representing the cooperative groups and cancer centers involved in the treatment of CLL, and because the NCI is the source of both financial support and drug supply for many of these trials. Most important, however, is the recognition by the investigators of a need to standardize studies so that the data are interpretable and studies are comparable.

The IWCLL (109) subsequently developed a series of recommendations that differed from that of the NCI-WG in the requisite number of circulating lymphocytes for eligibility, and the percent bone marrow lymphocytes for a complete remission (Table 3). In addition, the IWCLL uses a shift in clinical stage as the sole criterion for partial response, stable disease, or failure. In contrast, the NCI-WG guidelines provide more guidance about the initiation of treatment, eligibility criteria for clinical studies, and dose modifications for drug-related myelosuppression, and include a grading system for infectious complications, as well as other important components of clinical trials design.

CONCLUSIONS

We are currently in a period of rapid progress in our understanding of the immunology and biology of CLL. The recent development of effective treatments for this disease should provide a stimulus to apply this information to clinical trials by assisting therapeutic decision making. New response criteria are needed with a strong scientific rationale; for example, the relevance of minimal residual disease needs to be determined. Ongoing and proposed clinical trials using standardized guidelines will provide a unique opportunity to evaluate indices of tumor biology in large numbers of uni-

Table 3 Comparison of NCI Working Group and IWCLL Guidelines for CLL

	NCI	IWCLL
Diagnosis		
Lymphocytes ($\times 10^9$/L)	>5	$\geq$10 + B phenotype *or* bone marrow involved; <10 + both of above
"Atypical" cells (%) (e.g., prolymphocytes)	<55	Not stated
Duration of lymphocytosis	$\geq$2 mo.	Not stated
Bone marrow lymphocytes (%)	$\geq$30	>30
Staging	Modified Rai, correlate with Binet	IWCLL
Eligibility for trials	"Active disease" (Details in document)	A—lymphs >50 $\times$ 10^9/L; Doubling time <12 mo., diffuse marrow, B,C—all patients
Response criteria		
Complete Response		
Physical exam	Normal	Normal
Symptoms	None	None
Lymphocytes ($\times 10^9$/L)	$\leq$4	<4
Neutrophils ($\times 10^9$/L)	$\geq$1.5	>1.5
Platelets ($\times 10^9$/L)	>100	>100
Hemoglobin (g/dL)	>11 (untransfused)	Not stated
Bone marrow lymphs (%)	<30	"Normal," allowing nodules or focal infiltrates

Partial response		
Physical exam (nodes, and/or liver, spleen)	≥ 50% decrease	Downshift in stage
Plus ≥1 of:		
Neutrophils (× 10^9/L)	≥1.5	
Platelets (× 10^9/L)	>100	
Hemoglobin (g/dL)	>11 or 50% improvement	
Duration of complete or partial remission	≥2 mo.	Not stated
Progressive disease		Upshift in stage
Physical exam (nodes, liver, spleen)	≥ 50% increase or new	
Circulating lymphocytes	≥ 50% increase	
Other	Richter's syndrome	
Stable disease	All others	No change in stage

formly staged and homogeneously treated patients. Only by integrating the laboratory with the clinic can we translate this knowledge into a new and more clinically meaningful, and widely accepted, staging system.

REFERENCES

1. W. Dameshek, Chronic lymphocytic leukemia — An accumulative disease of immunologically incompetent lymphocytes, *Blood, 29*:566 (1967).
2. B. D. Cheson, J. M. Bennett, K. R. Rai, M. R. Grever, N. E. Kay, C. A. Schiffer, M. M. Oken, M. J. Keating, D. H. Boldt, S. J. Kempin, and K. A. Foon, Guidelines for clinical protocols for chronic lymphocytic leukemia: Recommendations of the National Cancer Institute-sponsored Working Group, *Am. J. Hematol., 29*:152 (1988).
3. J. M. Bennett, D. Catovsky, M-T. Daniel, G. Flandrin, D. A. G. Galton, H. R. Gralnick, and C. Sultan, Proposals for the classification of chronic (mature) B and T lymphoid leukaemias, *J. Clin. Pathol., 42*:567 (1989).
4. D. R. Boggs, S. A. Sofferman, M. M. Wintrobe, and G. E. Cartwright, Factors influencing the duration of survival of patients with chronic lymphocytic leukemia, *Am. J. Med., 40*:243 (1966).
5. D. A. G. Galton, The pathogenesis of chronic lymphocytic leukemia, *Can. Med. Assoc. J., 94*:1005 (1966).
6. K. R. Rai, A. Sawitsky, E. P. Cronkite, A. D. Chanana, R. N. Levy, and B. S. Pasternak, Clinical staging of chronic lymphocytic leukemia, *Blood, 46*:219 (1975).
7. K. R. Rai, A critical analysis of staging in CLL in *Chronic Lymphocytic Leukemia. Recent Progress and Future Direction* (R. P. Gale and K. R. Rai, eds.), Alan R. Liss, New York, p. 253 (1987).
8. J. L. Binet, M. Leporrier, G. Dighiero, D. Charron, Ph. D'Athis, G. Vaugier, H. Merle Beral, J. C. Natali, M. Raphael, B. Nizet, and J. Y. Follezou, A clinical staging system for chronic lymphocytic leukemia. Prognostic significance, *Cancer, 40*:855 (1977).
9. J. L. Binet, A. Auquier, G. Dighiero, C. Chastang, H. Piguet, J. Goasguen, G. Vaugier, G. Potron, P. Colona, F. Oberling, M. Thomas, G. Tchernia, C. Jacquillat, P. Boivin, C. Lesty, M. T. Duault, M. Monconduit, S. Belabbes, and F. Gremy, A new prognostic classification of chronic lymphocytic leukemia derived from a multivariate survival analysis, *Cancer, 48*:198 (1981).
10. J. L. Binet, D. Catovsky, P. Chandra, G. Dighiero, E. Montserrat, K. R. Rai, and A. Sawitsky, Chronic lymphocytic leukaemia: Proposals for a revised prognostic staging system, *Br. J. Haematol., 48*:365 (1981).
11. L. F. Skinnider, L. Tan, J. Schmidt, and G. Armitage, Chronic lymphocytic leukemia. A review of 745 cases and assessment of clinical staging, *Cancer, 50*:2951 (1982).
12. B. Jaksic and B. Vitale, Total tumour mass score (TIM): A new parameter in chronic lymphocytic leukaemia, *Br. J. Haematol., 49*:405 (1981).
13. F. Mandelli, G. De Rossi, P. Mancini, A. Alberti, A. Cajozzo, F. Grignani,

P. Leoni, V. Liso, M. Martelli, A. Neri, L. Resegotti, and G. Torlontano, Prognosis in chronic lymphocytic leukemia: A retrospective multicentric study from the GIMEMA group, *J. Clin. Oncol., 5*:398 (1987).

14. R. Foa, D. Catovsky, M. Brozovic, G. Marsh, T. Ooyirilangkumaran, M. Cherchi, and D. A. G. Galton, Clinical staging and immunological findings in chronic lymphocytic leukemia, *Cancer, 44*:483 (1979).

15. M. Baccarani, M. Cavo, M. Gobbi, F. Lauria, and S. Tura, Staging of chronic lymphocytic leukemia, *Blood, 59*:1191 (1982).

16. D. Catovsky, J. Fooks, and S. Richards, Prognostic factors in chronic lymphocytic leukaemia: The importance of age, sex and response to treatment in survival. A report from the MRC CLL 1 trial, *Br. J. Haematol., 72*: 141 (1989).

17. J. L. Binet, G. Vaugier, S. Dighiero, P. d'Athis, and D. Charron, Investigation of a new parameter in chronic lymphocytic leukemia: The percentage of large peripheral lymphocytes determined by the Hemalog D, *Am. J. Med., 63*:683 (1977).

18. J. V. Melo, D. Catovsky, and D. A. G. Galton, The relationship between chronic lymphocytic leukaemia and prolymphocytic leukaemia. I. Clinical and laboratory features of 300 patients and characterization of an intermediate group, *Br. J. Haematol., 63*:377 (1986).

19. J. V. Melo, D. Catovsky, W. M. Gregory, and D. A. G. Galton, The relationship between chronic lymphocytic leukaemia and prolymphocytic leukaemia. IV. Analysis of survival and prognostic features, *Br. J. Haematol., 65*:23 (1987).

20. L. C. Peterson, C. D. Bloomfield, R. D. Sundberg, K. J. Gajl-Peczalska, and R. D. Brunning, Morphology of chronic lymphocytic leukemia and its relationship to survival, *Am. J. Med., 59*:316 (1975).

21. L. C. Peterson, C. D. Bloomfield, and R. D. Brunning, Relationship of clinical staging and lymphocyte morphology to survival in chronic lymphocytic leukaemia, *Br. J. Haematol., 45*:563 (1980).

22. T. Vallespí, E. Montserrat, and M. A. Sanz, Chronic lymphocytic leukaemia: Prognostic value of lymphocyte morphological subtypes. A multivariate survival analysis in 146 patients, *Br. J. Haematol., 77*:478 (1991).

23. B. Frisch and R. Bartl, Histologic classification and staging of chronic lymphocytic leukemia, *Acta Haematol., 79*:140 (1988).

24. S. Molica and A. Alberti, Investigation of nuclear clefts as a prognostic parameter in chronic lymphocytic leukemia, *Eur. J. Haematol., 41*:62 (1988).

25. French Cooperative Group on Chronic Lymphocytic Leukaemia, Natural history of stage A chronic lymphocytic leukaemia untreated patients, *Br. J. Haematol., 76*:45 (1990).

26. J. S. Lee, D. O. Dixon, H. M. Kantarjian, M. J. Keating, and M. Talpaz, Prognosis of chronic lymphocytic leukemia: A multivariate regression analysis of 325 untreated patients, *Blood, 69*:929 (1987).

27. A. Pines, I. Ben-Bassat, M. Modan, T. Blumstein, and B. Ramot, Survival and prognostic factors in chronic lymphocytic leukemia, *Eur. J. Haematol., 38*:123 (1987).

28. G. De Rossi, F. Mandelli, A. Covelli, M. Luciani, M. Martelli, L. Resegotti, A. Alberti, A. Cajozzo, L. Deriu, R. De Biasi, G. Broccia, A. Abbadessa, F. Caronia, and P. Leone, Chronic lymphocytic leukemia (CLL) in younger adults: A retrospective study of 133 cases, *Hematol. Oncol., 7*:127 (1989).

29. G. De Rossi, Prognosis in chronic lymphocytic leukemia (CLL): Experience of the Italian cooperative group (GIMEMA), *Bone Marrow Transpl., 4*(suppl. 1):162 (1989).

30. G. A. Pangalis, J. C. Reverter, V. A. Bousiotis, and E. Montserrat, Chronic lymphocytic leukemia in younger adults: Preliminary results of a study based on 454 patients, *Leuk. and Lymph., 5*(suppl 1):175 (1991).

31. E. Montserrat, F. Gomis, T. Vallespí, A. Rios, A. Romero, J. Soler, A. Alcalá, M. Morey, C. Ferrán, J. Díaz-Mediavilla, A. Flores, S. Woessner, J. Batile, C. González-Aza, M. Rovira, J-C. Reverter, and C. Rozman, Presenting features and prognosis of chronic lymphocytic leukemia in younger adults, *Blood, 78*:1545 (1991).

32. W. Paolino, V. Infelise, A. Levis, F. Marmont, U. Vitolo, F. Paolino, M. Rossi, A. Jayme, and M. Remondino, Adenosplenomegaly and prognosis in uncomplicated and complicated chronic lymphocytic leukemia. A study of 362 cases, *Cancer, 54*:339 (1984).

33. C. Shustik, R. Mick, R. Silver, A. Sawitsky, K. Rai, and L. Shapiro, Treatment of early chronic lymphocytic leukemia: intermittent chlorambucil versus observation, *Hematol. Oncol., 6*:7 (1988).

34. French Cooperative Group on Chronic Lymphocytic Leukemia, Effects of chlorambucil and therapeutic decision in initial forms of chronic lymphocytic leukemia (stage A): Results of a randomized clinical trial on 612 patients, *Blood, 75*:1414 (1990).

35. T. Han, H. Ozer, M. Gavignan, R. Gajera, J. Minowada, M. L. Bloom, N. Samadori, A. A. Sandberg, G. A. Gomez, and E. S. Henderson, Benign monoclonal B cell lymphocytoses — A benign variant of CLL: Clinical, immunologic phenotypic, and cytogenetic studies in 20 patients, *Blood, 64*:244 (1984).

36. C. Rozman, E. Montserrat, J. M. Rodríguez-Fernández, R. Ayats, T. Vallespí, R. Parody, A. Ríos, D. Prados, M. Morey, F. Gomis, A. Alcalá, M. Gutiérrez, J. Maldonado, C. Gonzalez, M. Giralt, L. Hernández-Nieto, A. Cabrera, and J. M. Fernández-Rañada, Bone marrow histologic pattern — The best single prognostic parameter in chronic lymphocytic leukemia: A multivariate survival analysis of 329 cases, *Blood, 64*:642 (1984).

37. G. A. Pangalis, P. A. Roussou, C. Kittas, C. Mitsoulis-Mentzikoff, P. Matsouka-Alexandridis, N. Anagnostopoulos, I. Rombos, and P. Fessas, Patterns of bone marrow involvement in chronic lymphocytic leukemia and small lymphocytic (well differentiated) non-Hodgkin's lymphomas, *Cancer, 54*:702 (1984).

38. G. A. Pangalis, P. A. Roussou, C. Kittas, S. Kokkinou, and P. Fessas, B-chronic lymphocytic leukemias. Prognostic implication of bone marrow histology in 120 patients. Experience from a single hematology unit, *Cancer, 59*:767 (1987).

39. G. A. Pangalis, V. A. Boussiotis, and C. Kittas, B-chronic lymphocytic leukemia. Disease progression in 150 untreated stage A and B patients as predicted by bone marrow pattern, *Nouv. Rev. Fr. Hematol., 30*:373 (1988).

40. T. Han, M. Minowada, M. L. Bloom., N. Samadori, A. A. Sandberg, and E. S. Henderson, Bone marrow infiltration patterns and their prognostic significance in chronic lymphocytic leukemia: Correlations with clinical, immunologic, phenotypic, and cytogenetic data, *J. Clin. Oncol., 2*:562 (1984).

41. B. Desablens, J. F. Claisse, C. Piprot-Choffat, and M. F. Gontier, Prognostic value of bone marrow biopsy in chronic lymphoid leukemia, *Nouv. Rev. Fr. Hematol., 31*:179 (1989).

42. S. Tura, M. Cavo, and M. Baccarani, Stage 0 chronic lymphocytic leukemia, in *Chronic Lymphocytic Leukemia. Recent Progress and Future Direction* (R. P. Gale and K. R. Rai, eds.), Alan R. Liss, New York, p. 265 (1987).

43. F. Caligaris-Cappio, M. Gobbi, L. Bergui, D. Campana, F. Lauria, M. T. Fierro, and R. Foa, B-chronic lymphocytic leukaemia patients with stable benign disease show a distinctive membrane phenotype, *Br. J. Haematol., 56*:655 (1984).

44. R. Dadmarz and J. C. Cawley, Heterogeneity of CLL: High CD23 antigen and alpha-IFN receptor expression are features of favourable disease and of cell activation, *Br. J. Haematol., 68*:279 (1988).

45. A Tefferi and R. L. Phyliky, Role of immunophenotyping in chronic lymphocytosis: Review of the natural history of the condition in 145 adult patients, *Mayo Clin. Proc., 63*:801 (1988).

46. T. Hamblin and D. Hough, Chronic lymphatic leukaemia: Correlation of immunofluorescent characteristics and clinical features, *Br. J. Haematol., 36*:359 (1977).

47. M. B. Van Scoy-Mosher, M. Bick, V. Capostagno, R. L. Walford, and R. A. Gatti, A clinicopathologic analysis of chronic lymphocytic leukemia, *Am. J. Hematol., 10*:9 (1981).

48. L. Baldini, R. Mozzana, A. Cortelezzi, A. Neri, F. Radaelli, B. Cesana, A. T. Maiolo, and E. E. Polli, Prognostic significance of immunoglobulin phenotype in B cell chronic lymphocytic leukemia, *Blood, 65*:340 (1985).

49. E. Kimby, H. Mellstedt, B. Nilsson, M. Björkholm, G. Holm, C. Lindemalm, and B. Tribukait, Blood lymphocyte characteristics as predictors of prognosis in chronic lymphocytic leukemia of B-cell type, *Hematol. Oncol., 6*:47 (1988).

50. U. Jayaswal, S. Roath, R. D. Hyde, D. M. Chisolm, and J. L. Smith, Blood lymphocyte surface markers and clinical findings in chronic lymphoproliferative disorders, *Br. J. Haematol., 37*:207 (1977).

51. T. J. Hamblin, D. G. Oscier, J. R. Stevens, and J. L. Smith, Long survival in B-CLL correlates with surface IgMk phenotype, *Br. J. Haematol., 66*:21 (1987).

52. G. Semenzato, R. Foa, C. Agostini, R. Zambello, L. Trentin, F. Vinante, F. Benedetti, M. Chilosi, and G. Pizzolo, High serum levels of soluble interleukin 2 receptor in patients with B chronic lymphocytic leukemia, *Blood, 70*: 396 (1987).

53. N. E. Kay, J. Burton, D. Wagner, and D. L. Nelson, The malignant cells from B-chronic lymphocytic leukemia patients release TAC-soluble interleukin-2 receptors, *Blood, 72*:447 (1988).

54. A. Orfao, M. Gonzalez, J. F. San Miguel, A. Rios, M. C. Canizo, J. Hernandez, M. L. Maricato, and A. L. Borrasca, B-cell chronic lymphocytic leukemia: Prognostic values of the immunophenotype and the clinico-haematological features, *Am. J. Hematol., 31*:26 (1989).

55. C. Rozman, E. Montserrat, and N. Viñolas, Serum immunoglobulins in B-chronic lymphocytic leukemia. Natural history and prognostic significance, *Cancer, 61*:279 (1988).

56. J. E. Ultmann, W. Fish, E. Osserman, and A. Gellhorn, The clinical implications of hypogammaglobulinemia in patients with chronic lymphocytic leukemia and lymphocytic lymphosarcoma, *Ann. Intern. Med., 51*:501 (1959).

57. S. Di Giovanni, G. Valentini, P. Carducci, and P. Giallonardo, β-2-microglobulin is a reliable tumor marker in chronic lymphocytic leukemia, *Acta Haemat., 81*:181 (1989).

58. B. Simonsson, L. Wibell, and K. Nilsson, β_2-microglobulin in chronic lymphocytic leukaemia, *Scand. J. Haematol., 24*:174 (1980).

59. B. Spätl, J. A. Child, S. M. Kerruish, and E. H. Cooper, Behaviour of serum β2-microglobulin and acute phase reactant proteins in chronic lymphocytic leukaemia, *Acta Haemat., 64*:79 (1980).

60. T. Han, A. Bhargava, E. S. Henderson, E. Powell, D. Driscoll, and L. Emrich, Prognostic significance of beta-2 microglobulin (β-2m) in chronic lymphocytic leukemia (CLL) and non-Hodgkin's lymphoma (NHL), *Proc. Am. Soc. Oncol., 8*:270 (abstr. 270) (1989).

61. T. Tötterman, K. Nilsson, and B. Simonsson, Phorbol ester-induced production of beta-2-microglobulin in B-CLL cells: Relation to IgM secretory response and disease activity, *Br. J. Haematol., 62*:95 (1986).

62. T. H. Tötterman, M. Carlsson, B. Simonsson, M. Bengtsson, and K. Nilsson, T-cell activation and subset patterns are altered in B-CLL and correlate with the stage of the disease, *Blood, 74*:786 (1989).

63. A. Apostolopoulos, A. Symeonidis, and N. Zoumbos, Prognostic significance of immune function parameters in patients with chronic lymphocytic leukaemia, *Eur. J. Haematol., 44*:39 (1990).

64. T. Han, E. S. Henderson, L. J. Emrich, and A. A. Sandberg, Prognostic significance of karyotypic abnormalities in B cell chronic lymphocytic leukemia: An update, *Sem. Hematol, 24*:257 (1987).

65. M. L. Bird, Y. Ueshima, J. D. Rowley, J. M Haren, and J. W. Vardiman, Chromosome abnormalities in B cell chronic lymphocytic leukemia and their clinical correlations, *Leukemia, 3*:182 (1989).

66. G. Juliusson, D. G. Oscier, M. Fitchett, F. M. Ross, G. Stockdill, M. J. Mackie, A. C. Parker, G. L. Castoldi, A. Cuneo, S. Knuutila, E. Elonen, and G. Gahrton, Prognostic subgroups in B-cell chronic lymphocytic leukemia defined by specific chromosomal abnormalities, *N. Engl. J. Med., 323*: 720 (1990).

67. L. Soper, B. Bernhardt, A. Eisenberg, B. Cacciapaglia, L. Bennett, A. Sanda, M. Baird, R. Silver, and P. Benn, Clonal immunoglobulin gene rearrangements in chronic lymphocytic leukemia: A correlative study, *Am. J. Hematol.*, *27*:257 (1988).

68. G. Rechavi, M. Mandel, N. Katzir, F. Brok-Simoni, I. Hakim, F. Holtzman, M. Biniaminov, D. Givol, I. Ben-Bassat, and B. Ramot, Immunoglobulin heavy chain gene rearrangements in chronic lymphocytic leukaemia: Correlation with clinical stage, *Br. J. Haematol.*, *72*:524 (1989).

69. C. Rozman, E. Montserrat, E. Felíu, A. Granena, P. Marín, B. Nomdedeu, and J. L. Vives Corrons, Prognosis of chronic lymphocytic leukemia: A multivariate survival analysis of 150 cases, *Blood*, *59*:1001 (1982).

70. E. Montserrat, J. Sanchez-Bisono, N. Viñolas, and C. Rozman, Lymphocyte doubling time in chronic lymphocytic leukaemia: Analysis of its prognostic significance, *Br. J. Haematol.*, *62*:567 (1986).

71. S. Molica and A. Alberti, Prognostic value of the lymphocyte doubling time in chronic lymphocytic leukemia, *Cancer*, *60*:2712 (1987).

72. R. Foa, M. Massaia, S. Cardona, A. G. Tos, A. Bianchi, C. Attisano, A. Guarini, P. F. di Celle, and M. T. Fierro, Production of tumor necrosis factor-alpha by C-cell chronic lymphocytic leukemia cells: A possible regulatory role of TNF in the progression of the disease, *Blood,* *76*:393 (1990).

73. R. Dadmarz, S. N. Rabinowe, S. A. Cannistra, J. W. Anderson, A. S. Freeman, and L. M. Nadler, Association between clonogenic cell growth and clinical risk group in B-cell chronic lymphocytic leukemia, *Blood,* *76*:142 (1990).

74. C. R. R. Källander, B. Simonsson, H. Hagberg, and J. S. Gronowitz, Serum deoxythymidine kinase gives prognostic information in chronic lymphocytic leukemia, *Cancer,* *54*:2450 (1984).

75. A. D. Papaphilis, E. F. Kamper, C. Kattamis, and G. A. Pangalis, Activity of ribonuclease H in cells of chronic B-lymphocytic leukaemia: Correlation with clinical stage, *Br. J. Haematol.*, *70*:301 (1988).

76. G. A. Pangalis, T. Trangas, C. J. Papanastasiou, P. A. Roussou, and C. M. Tsiapalis, Poly(A)-polymerase activity in chronic lymphocytic leukemia of the B cell type, *Acta Haematol.*, *74*:31 (1985).

77. N. Patel, T. Han, E. S. Henderson, L. Emrich, U. Patel, and G. A. Gomez, Survival of patients with pure splenic form vs. combined splenomegaly and lymphadenopathy in chronic lymphocytic leukemia, *Proc. Am. Soc. Clin. Oncol.,* *6*:153 (abstr. 603) (1987).

78. J. Burghouts, E. Prüst, and H. J. J. van Lier, Response to therapy as prognostic factor in chronic lymphocytic leukemia, *Acta Haemat.,* *63*:217 (1980).

79. H. Moayeri and J. E. Sokal, In vitro leukocyte thymidine uptake and prognosis in chronic lymphocytic leukemia, *Am. J. Med.,* *66*:773 (1979).

80. A. S. Freedman and L. M. Nadler, Chronic lymphocytic leukemia: Cell surface phenotype and normal cellular counterparts, in *Chronic Lymphocytic Leukemia* (A. Polliack and D. Catovsky, eds.), Harwood Academic Pub., Chur, Switzerland, p. 47 (1988).

81. A. Pinto, V. Zagonel, A. Carbone, L. Del Vecchio, G. Marotta, U. Tirelli,

M. Roncadin, S. Monfardini, and A. Colombatti, Expression of myelomono-cytic antigens (MyAgs) on chronic lymphocytic leukemia (CLL) B cells identi-fies a subset of patients (Pts) with a "variant" CLL phenotype and different biological and clinical features, *Proc. Am. Soc. Clin. Oncol., 8*:204 (abstr. 792) (1989).

82. G. B. Faguet and J. F. Agee, Immunophenotypic diagnosis of clinical and preclinical chronic lymphatic leukemia by using monoclonal antibodies against the cCLLa, a CLL-associated antigen, *Blood, 72*:679 (1988).

83. S. B. Wormsley, S. M. Baird, N. Gadol, K. R. Rai, and R. E. Sobol, Charac-teristics of CD11c$^+$CD5$^+$ chronic B-cell leukemias and the identification of novel peripheral blood B-cell subsets with chronic lymphoid leukemia immu-nophenotypes, *Blood, 76*:123 (1990).

84. C. A. Hanson, T. E. Gribben, E. Schnitzer, J. A. Schlegelmilch, B. S. Mitchell, and L. M. Stoolman, CD11c (LEU-M5) expression characterizes a B-cell chronic lymphoproliferative disorder with features of both chronic lymphocytic leukemia and hairy cell leukemia, *Blood, 76*:2360 (1990).

85. D. Catovsky, M. Cherchi, D. Brooks, J. Bradley, and H. Zola, Heterogeneity of B-cell leukemias demonstrated by the monoclonal antibody FMC7, *Blood, 58*:406 (1981).

86. T. Sun, M. Susin, N. Shevde, and S. Teichberg, Hybrid form of hairy cell leukemia and chronic lymphocytic leukemia, *Hematol. Oncol., 8*:283 (1990).

87. M. E. Heath and B. D. Cheson, Defective complement activity in chronic lymphocytic leukemia, *Am. J. Hematol., 19*:63 (1985).

88. B. G. M. Durie, D. Stock-Novack, S. E. Salmon, P. Finley, J. Beckord, J. Crowley, and C. A. Coltman, Prognostic value of pretreatment serum β_2 microglobulin in myeloma: A Southwest Oncology Group study, *Blood, 75*: 823 (1990).

89. P. Litam, F. Swan, F. Cabanillas, S. L. Tucker, P. McLaughlin, F. B. Hagemeister, M. A. Rodriguez, and W. S. Valasquez, Prognostic value of serum β-2 microglobulin in low-grade lymphoma, *Ann. Intern. Med., 114*: 855 (1991).

90. D. Oscier, M. Fitchett, T. Herbert, and R. Lambert, Karyotypic evolution in B-cell chronic lymphocytic leukaemia, *Genes, Chrom. & Cancer, 3*:16 (1991).

91. T. Han, K. Ohtaki, N. Samadori, A. W. Block, B. Dadey, H. Ozer, and A. A. Sandberg, Cytogenetic evidence for clonal evolution in B-cell chronic lymphocytic leukemia, *Cancer. Genet. Cytogenet., 23*:321 (1986).

92. Y. Tsujimoto, Oncogenes in chronic lymphocytic leukemia, in *Chronic Lymphocytic Leukemia: Basic and Clinical Research* (B. D. Cheson, ed.), Marcel Dekker, New York (in press).

93. T. W. McKeithan, H. Ohno, and M. O. Diaz, Identification of a transcrip-tional unit adjacent to the breakpoint in the 14;19 translocation of chronic lymphocytic leukemia, *Genes, Chrom. & Cancer, 1*:247 (1990).

94. G. Rechavi, N. Katzir, F. Brok-Simoni, F. Holtzman, M. Mandel, N. Gurfin-kel, D. Givol, I. Ben-Bassat, and B. Ramot, A search for *bcl-1, bcl-2,* and *c-myc* oncogene rearrangements in chronic lymphocytic leukemia, *Leukemia, 3*:57 (1989).

95. P. J. Browett, K. Ganeshaguru, A. V. Hoffbrand, and J. D. Norton, Absence of Kirsten-*Ras* oncogene activation in B-cell chronic lymphocytic leukemia, *Leuk. Res., 12*:25 (1988).

96. S. Raghoebier, J. H. J. M. van Krieken, J. C. Kluin-Nelemans, A. Gillis, G. J. B. van Ommen, A. M. Ginsberg, M. Raffeld, and Ph. M. Kluin, Oncogene rearrangements in chronic B-cell leukemia, *Blood, 77*:1560 (1991).

97. A. M. Ginsberg, M. Raffeld, and J. Cossman, Inactivation of the retinoblastoma gene in human lymphoid neoplasms, *Blood, 77*:833 (1991).

98. F. T. Cordingly, A. V. Hoffbrand, H. E. Heslop, M. Turner, A. Bianchi, J. E. Reittie, A. Vyakarnam, A. Meager, and M. K. Brenner, Tumour necrosis factor as an autocrine tumour growth factor for chronic B-cell malignancies, *Lancet, 1*:969 (1988).

99. J. A. Holmes, A. Jacobs, G. Carter, J. A. Whittaker, D. P. Bentley, and R. A. Padua, Is the mdr 1 gene relevant in chronic lymphocytic leukemia? *Leukemia, 4*:216 (1990).

100. H. Herweijer, P. Sonneveld, F. Baas, and K. Nooter, Expression of *mdr1* and *mrd3* multidrug-resistance genes in human acute and chronic leukemias and association with stimulation of drug accumulation by cyclosporine, *J. Natl. Cancer Inst., 82*:1133 (1990).

101. R. Silber, M. Potmesil, and B. B. Bank, Studies on drug resistance in chronic lymphocytic leukemia, *Adv. Enz. Reg., 26*:267 (1989).

102. N. Groulx, J. Lemontt, C. Shustik, and P. Gros, Analysis of mdr gene expression in acute and chronic leukemias, *Blood, 72*(suppl. 1):179a (abstr. 626) (1988).

103. R. T. Perri, S. W. Louie, and W. G. Espar, Expression of the multidrug resistance (MDR) gene MDR1 in chronic lymphocytic leukemia (CLL) B cells, *Blood, 74*(supp. 1):198a (abstr. 739) (1989).

104. J. B. Johnston, L. G. Israels, G. J. Goldenberg, C. D. Anhalt, L. Verburg, M. R. A. Mowat, and A. Begleiter, Glutathione S-transferase activity, sulfhydryl group and glutathione levels, and DNA cross-linking activity with chlorambucil and chronic lymphocytic leukemia, *J. Natl. Cancer Inst., 82*:776 (1990).

105. M. Michieli, D. Raspadori, D. Damiani, A. Geromin, C. Gallizia, A. Michelutti, R. Fanin, G. Fasola, D. Russo, P. Tazzari, S. Pileri, F. Mallardi, and M. Baccarani, The expression of the multidrug resistance-associated glycoprotein in B-cell chronic lymphocytic leukaemia, *Br. J. Haematol., 77*:460 (1991).

106. P. M. Cumber, A. Jacobs, T. Hoy, J. Fisher, J. A. Whittaker, T. Tsuruo, and R. A. Padua, Expression of the multiple drug resistance gene (mdr-1) and epitope masking in chronic lymphatic leukaemia, *Br. J. Haematol., 76*:226 (1990).

107. Committee of the Chronic Leukemia-Myeloma Task Force, Proposed guidelines for protocol studies, *Cancer Chemother. Rep., 4*:141 (1973).

108. R. T. Silver, A. Sawitsky, K. Rai, J. F. Holland, and O. Glidewell, Guidelines for protocol studies in chronic lymphocytic leukemia, *Am. J. Hematol., 4*:343 (1978).

109. International Workshop on Chronic Lymphocytic Leukemia: Recommendations for diagnosis, staging, and response criteria, *Ann. Intern. Med., 110*: 236 (1989).
110. C. H. Geisler, J. K. Larsen, N. E. Hansen, M. M. Hansen, B. C. Christensen, B. Lund, T. Plesner, K. Thorling, E. Andersen, P. K. Andersen, Prognostic importance of flow cytometric immunophenotyping of 540 consecutive patients with B-cell chronic lymphocytic leukemia, *Blood, 78*:1795 (1991).

14

Chronic Lymphocytic Leukemia in Early Stage: "Smoldering" and "Active" Forms

Emilio Montserrat, Nuria Viñolas, Juan-Carlos Reverter, and Ciril Rozman
University of Barcelona Hospital Clinic, Barcelona, Spain

INTRODUCTION

Chronic lymphocytic leukemia (CLL), the most frequent form of leukemia in adults in Western countries, is a disease characterized by the progressive accumulation of neoplastic B lymphocytes, and by a heterogeneous clinical course (1). Although new agents and strategies offer promise, treatment is usually unsatisfactory and has a merely palliative effect (1–7). For years, difficulties in predicting survival made treatment decisions in individual cases difficult and hampered progress in CLL therapy.

Clinical staging systems developed by different groups are useful to establish prognosis and to plan treatment (8,9). It is recommended that, after diagnosis, patients be observed over several weeks to determine the pace of the disease and to reliably assess the stage of the disease (10), treatment being considered as indicated in patients with poor prognosis. Thus, patients with advanced clinical stages (Binet's stages B and C, Rai's stages II, III, IV) have a median survival less than 5 to 6 years and deserve treatment. In persons diagnosed at early stages of the disease (Binet's stage A, Rai's stage 0), the situation is more complex. These patients account for up to 60% of all patients with CLL and may survive for more than 10 years without major clinical problems. Some of them, however, progress and eventually die of their disease. In recent trials, on the other hand, it has been demonstrated that treatment of patients in early stage is not associated with clinical benefit, and that continuous administration of chlorambucil may even be harmful (11,12). Consequently, whether to treat these patients or not is a difficult decision. Unfortunately, none of the staging systems (8,9) used so far can identify patients in early stage who will have an indolent course and good prognosis, as compared to those who will progress rapidly. For all these reasons, the identification of patients with both a low probability of disease progression and a long survival is important: Such patients should not be treated unless progression occurs.

In the past few years, several proposals have been made to identify patients who will remain in early stage ("smoldering" CLL) as compared to those who will progress ("active" CLL) (12–14). This issue was analyzed in a meeting of the International Workshop on CLL (IWCLL) held in Egham, Surrey (U.K.) (15), and was further discussed at the Vth IWCLL held recently in Sitges, Barcelona (Spain) (16). In this chapter we will review the concept of "smoldering" CLL, its definitions, and relevance in clinical practice.

CONCEPTS

"Smoldering" CLL

It is usually considered that patients with "smoldering" CLL are those in early stage (Binet's stage A, Rai's stage 0), who are not likely to progress and have a life expectancy not different from that of sex- and age-matched controls. "Stable" CLL, "benign monoclonal B-cell lymphocytosis," and "monoclonal lymphocytosis of unknown significance" are closely related or equivalent terms (17–20).

Disease Progression

Disease progression is defined as the change of the disease to a more advanced stage (e.g., from Binet's A to B or C; from Rai's 0 to I, II, III, and IV). Although this is a practical end point when investigating the natural history of CLL, it should be noted that it defines an already progressed disease rather than disease progression.

"Active" CLL

In practice, patients with a diffuse bone marrow histologic pattern (21–26) and rapidly increasing blood lymphocyte counts (27–30) are likely to progress and should be treated regardless of their clinical stage. In addition, falling hemoglobin levels and/or platelet counts, general symptoms (fever, night sweats, weight loss), and lymphadenopathy or splenomegaly increasing in size are usually considered as criteria for initiating treatment (31).

The significance of other parameters such as lymphocyte size and morphology (32–35), phenotype of blood lymphocytes (36–39), serum B-2 microglobulin levels (40,41), activity in serum or lymphoid cells of several enzymes (e.g., lactate dehydrogenase, deoxythymidine kinase (42–45), and chromosome abnormalities (46–48) needs to be further verified, although the presence of complex cytogenetic abnormalities seems to be particularly important in terms of prognosis (48).

ANALYSIS OF DIFFERENT PROPOSALS TO SUBCLASSIFY CLL IN EARLY STAGE

The clinical heterogeneity of patients with CLL in early stage is apparent. Thus, within Binet's stage A, patients with no physical signs (A0) and patients with up to two "lymphoid" areas (either lymph nodes, spleen, or liver) involved (AI, AII) are included. As far as survival is concerned, what could be expected is that patients with high tumor mass (AI, AII) would have a poorer outcome than those with a low tumor mass (A0). In initial reports, however, the French Group on CLL claimed that survival of patients in stage A as a whole was not different from that of patients in stage 0, the advantage of stage A being that it includes approximately 60% of all CLL patients whereas Rai's stage 0 only encompasses 30% (49). In a more recent analysis, however, such differences came to light (14). Attempts to separate different prognostic groups within early-stage patients and their results are reviewed below.

International Workshop on CLL

In 1981, the IWCLL endorsed the A, B, and C Binet et al. classification and proposed the integration of this system with that of Rai et al., in the following manner: A (A0, AI, AII); B (BI, BII), and C (CIII, CIV), as it was considered that within each of the A, B, and C categories there are subsets that have a distinct biologic natural history not otherwise appreciated (50). The IWCLL also recommended the investigation of methods to predict, within each of the A, B, and C groups, subsets that develop a progressive or aggressive clinical course as compared to patients whose clinical course is benign or stable. These recommendations have recently been reemphasized by the IWCLL (51). Unfortunately, most investigators find the proposed integration cumbersome and use either Binet's or Rai's stages but not both, making the achievement of these goals difficult.

However, in the large series from the French Group, the 5-year survival rate of 127 patients in stage A0 was 89% as compared to 77% for 182 patients in stages AI–III (p = 0.005); the probability of disease progression was also different: 16% and 41%, respectively (p < 0.0001) (14). In another study based on patients followed at a single institution, an 89% survival at 8 years for patients in stage A0 as compared to 30–40% for patients in stages AI + II was found (p < 0.001) (52). In the Postgraduate School of Hematology series, the median survival of 87 patients in stage A (0) was different from that of 47 patients in stage A (I + II): 125.7 versus 91 months, although not significantly (p = NS).

Chisesi et al. (18) subclassified 92 patients in stage A as "indolent" (no general symptoms, Hb > 10 g/dL, plateles > 100×10^9/L, no disease progression for at least 24 months of observation) and "active" (patients not fulfilling all the previous criteria). Seventy patients with stage A "indolent" had a projected survival of 80% at 10 years as compared to 5.3 years for 22 stage A "active" patients (p < 0.001). Of note, A "active" disease was correlated with Rai's substages. Whereas no patients (0 of 9) in stage A0 displayed "active" disease, 2 of 29 in stage AI and 20 of 54 in stage AII had "active" disease. It can be concluded, therefore, that patients within stage A can be separated into different prognostic subsets on the basis of Rai's substages or disease "activity" criteria.

Modified Rai system

In their original 1975 paper, Rai et al. acknowledged that, on the basis of the actuarial survival curves, three different groups of patients rather than five could be distinguished: (a) low-risk (stage 0), (b) intermediate-risk (stages I, II), and (c) high-risk (stages III, IV) (8). A modification of the Rai et al. staging system in the aforementioned terms was formally published in 1987 (53), and the Working Group from the NCI recommends the use of this modified system for prospective therapeutic trials (54).

In contrast to the system of Binet et al., in this classification the prognostic importance of patients with no physical findings attributable to the disease (Rai stage 0) is emphasized. Median survival of patients in Rai stage 0 is over 10 years; most of these patients do not need therapy, and enjoy long survival.

Is Rai stage 0 equivalent to "smoldering" CLL? Han et al. (17) described 20 cases of CLL in stage 0 that did not progress for period ranging from 6.5 to 24 years ("benign monoclonal B-cell lymphocytosis"). A female sex, low level of lymphocytes in blood, normal karyotype, preserved immunity, and kappa phenotype were the most constant features of this stable CLL. However, routine clinical and laboratory data at diagnosis were not considered as useful in predicting the evolution of the disease.

Tura et al. (55), in a series of 52 patients in stage 0 observed progression to more advanced stages in 25 patients, with a cumulative risk of progression for the whole group of 34% and 53% at 4 and 6 years, respectively. Interestingly, a rapid lymphocyte doubling time was of value to predict progression. However, there was no significant difference in survival.

In the series from the Barcelona group, 28 (32%) of 87 patients in stage 0 progressed, with a cumulative risk of progression of 28% and 46% at 3 and 5 years, respectively. A lower normal Hb level was the only independent variable predicting disease progression (p = 0.015).

Recently, Oscier et al. (56) analyzed 85 stage 0 patients of whom 14 had progressive disease and 23 died. Parameters that correlated with disease progression included: initial lymphocyte count, surface immunoglobulin MD lambda phenotype, and complex cytogenetic abnormalities.

According to the results derived from these series, about one-third of patients in stage 0 progressed within 3 years after diagnosis. At present, a rapid lymphocyte doubling time and a lower normal Hb level are the most consistent predictors of disease progression in such patients. On the other hand, within stage 0, differences in survival also exist: Survival of patients in Rai stage 0 with a blood lymphocyte count less than $30 \times 10^9/L$ is not different from that of controls, whereas those with a higher lymphocyte count have shorter survival (57).

Montserrat et al.

In 1988, we proposed criteria to identify patients with CLL in early clinical stage not likely to progress and with a survival probability not different from that of sex- and age-matched controls (Table 1). Studies carried out to define "smoldering" CLL have been described elsewhere (13,58).

Among 261 patients with CLL diagnosed and followed up at the Postgraduate School of Hematology of Barcelona, 134 (51%) were in Binet stage A, and 87 (33%) were classified as in Rai stage 0. Progression and survival were correlated with the following initial variables: age, sex, symptoms, number of peripheral lymph node territories involved (left and/or right cervical, axillary, and inguinal territories, until a maximum of six

Table 1 "Smoldering" CLL (Montserrat et al.) (13)

Stage A
Nondiffuse bone marrow histology
Hemoglobin ≥ 13 g/dL
Blood lymphocytes $< 30 \times 10^9/L$
Lymphocyte doubling time > 12 months

possible involved areas), splenomegaly, hepatomegaly, Hb level, WBC, lymphocyte, neutrophil and platelet counts, LDH and uric acid levels, IgG, IgM, IgA, and percentage of lymphocytes in bone marrow aspirate, as well as lymphocyte doubling time. Variables were expressed in a categorical or, whenever possible, a continuous way. Since only 3 of 92 (3.2%) patients in whom a bone marrow biopsy was done had a diffuse bone marrow pattern, this parameter was not included in the analysis; but due to its well-known prognostic significance (21-26), it was included in the definition of "smoldering" CLL.

Thirty-three (24.6%) of 134 stage A patients progressed to more advanced stages (17 to B, and 16 to stage C), the actuarial risk of progression being 31% (95% CI: 22% to 39%) and 35% (95% CI: 22% to 44%) at 3 and 5 years, respectively (Fig. 1). In the multivariate analysis, variables associated with a more likely progression were: high number of lymph nodes involved (p < 0.001), rapid lymphocyte doubling time (p = 0.0025), and markedly increased blood lymphocyte count (p = 0.02).

When patients in Rai stage 0 were analyzed separately, 28 (32%) of 87 progressed (9 to stage I, 12 to stage II, and 7 to stage III). As mentioned before, the projected cumulative risk of disease progression was 28% (95% CI: 18% to 37%) and 46% (95% CI: 34% to 58%) at 3 and 5 years, respectively. In the multivariate analysis the only variable predictive of progression was a lower normal Hb level (in all cases, however, above 11 g/dL as per the criteria defining clinical stages) (p = 0.015).

In the survival analysis, the following independent poor prognostic variables were identified: advanced age (p = 0.011), and rapid lymphocyte

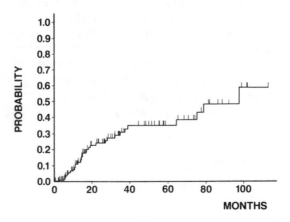

Figure 1 Cumulative proportion of patients with CLL in stage A progressing to more advanced stages.

Table 2 Characteristics of Patients in Stage A:
"Smoldering" Versus "Active"

	A "smoldering"	A "active"	p
Number	47	39	
Age (yrs)	63.3 (SD 9.8)	64.3 (SD 10.7)	NS
Sex	M 21 (45%)	M 18 (46%)	NS
	F 26 (55%)	F 21 (55%)	
Rai stages	0 38 (81%)	16 (41%)	
	I 7 (15%)	13 (33%)	<0.001
	II 1 (4%)	18 (25%)	
Lymphadenopathy	7 (15%)	21 (54%)	NS
Splenomegaly	2 (4%)	8 (20%)	0.045
Hepatomegaly	0 (0%)	4 (10%)	NS
Bone marrow histology			
Nodular	29 (61%)	27 (69%)	
Interstitial	4 (10%)	3 (7%)	NS
Mixed	14 (29%)	9 (24%)	
Doubling time >12 months	47 (100%)	16 (39%)	<0.001
Hemoglobin (g/dL)	14.7 (SD 0.9)	14.0 (SD 1.5)	0.009
Leukocytes ($\times$ 10^9/L)	22.2 (SD 6.9)	46.3 (SD 31.2)	<0.001
Lymphocytes ($\times$ 10^3/L)	17.0 (SD 6.1)	39.3 (SD 28.9)	<0.001
Platelets ($\times$ 10^3/L)	195 (SD 48)	187 (SD 59)	NS

doubling time (p = 0.0045) for stage A patients, and higher blood lymphocyte count (p = 0.005), and lower normal Hb level (p = 0.015), for stage 0.

Table 2 shows the main characteristics of 86 patients from the whole series that, according to the above definition, could be classified as in "smoldering" stage A (n = 47) in comparison to patients not fulfilling these criteria ("active" stage A) (n = 39). There were no differences in age nor sex distribution. The predominance of females among patients with early CLL has already been well documented in several series (59). Rai stage 0 accounts for the majority (38 of 47 or 81%) of patients with "smoldering" CLL.

Whereas only 6 of 47 patients with "smoldering" CLL progressed, 20 of 39 with "active" CLL did so. The cumulative risks of progression for patients with "smoldering" and "active" CLL are, respectively, 8% (95% CI: 6% to 16%) versus 57% (95% CI: 42% to 72%) at 3 years, and 13% (95% CI: 3% to 24%) versus 57% (95% CI: 42% to 72%) at 5 years (p < 0.001) (Fig. 2).

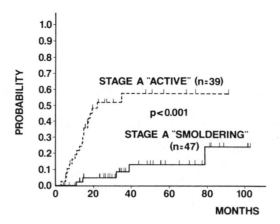

Figure 2 Disease progression in patients with "smoldering" stage A and "active" stage A.

Four of 47 patients with "smoldering" stage A died, as compared to 11 of 39 patients with "active" stage A. The projected survival at 10 years is 78% (95% CI: 56% to 99%) in the "smoldering" group as compared to 43% (95% CI: 22% to 64%) in the "active" group (p < 0.05). Median survival has not been reached in the "smoldering" CLL group and is 79

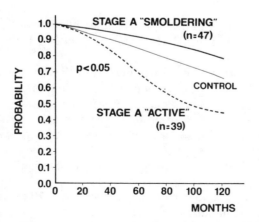

Figure 3 Survival of patients with "smoldering", "active" stage A, and control group. There is a significant difference (p < 0.05) between both "smoldering" and controls vs. "active" forms. Patients with "smoldering" CLL have a survival not different from that of a control population.

months in patients with "active" stage A (p < 0.05). Finally, survival of patients with "smoldering" CLL is not different from that of a sex- and age-matched control population (Fig. 3). Interesting enough, the "smoldering" CLL concept also applies to younger adults, in whom treatment decisions can be particularly difficult (60).

French Group on CLL

Based on their large series of patients, the French Cooperative Group on CLL carried out different studies analyzing the natural history of patients in early stage (Binet A) (12,14). In these studies the variables most strongly correlated with disease progression and survival are hemoglobin level, blood lymphocyte counts, percentage of lymphocytes in bone marrow, and number of lymphoid areas enlarged. In the statistical analysis, all these parameters behave as continuous variables. According to this analysis, two slightly different definitions of "smoldering" CLL have been proposed (Table 3).

Both definitions are able to separate among patients in stage A a "smoldering" or "stable" subgroup with a low probability of disease progression and a survival not different from matched controls. In 247 patients classified as A-1' (or "smoldering"), the 5-year rate of disease progression (to either stage B or C) is 25% as compared to 44% for 62 patients not fulfilling the proposed criteria (A-1" or "active" group), the overall survival at 5 years being 87% and 62%, respectively (p < 0.001). Similarly, in 184 patients with A-2' substage ("smoldering"), the disease progression rate at 5 years is 19% as compared to 48% for 125 patients with A-2" ("active") substage (p < 0.001), with survival also being different: 89% and 71%, respectively (p < 0.001).

Table 3 "Smoldering" CLL (French Cooperative Group on CLL) (12,14)

A-1'	Stage A
	Hemoglobin > 12 g/dL
	Blood lymphocytes $< 30 \times 10^9$/L
A-2'	Stage A
	Hemoglobin > 12 g/dL
	Blood lymphocytes $< 30 \times 10^9$/L
	Lymphocytes in bone marrow aspirate $< 80\%$
	Number of lymphoid areas[a] involved < 2

[a]Lymphoid areas considered: cervical, axillary, and inguinal lymphadenopathies (whether uni- or bilateral), spleen, and liver.

COMPARISON OF DIFFERENT PROPOSALS
TO DEFINE "SMOLDERING" CLL

The major differences between the French and the Spanish proposals to define "smoldering" CLL lay in two aspects: (a) the method of evaluating bone marrow infiltration (aspirate in the French Group proposal, biopsy in the Spanish definition), and (b) the lack of inclusion of blood lymphocyte doubling time in the French criteria, based on the fact that this parameter is not generally available at diagnosis. Concerning the evaluation of bone marrow infiltration, it should be kept in mind that bone marrow lymphocytic infiltration can be patchy and heterogeneous, thus the lymphocyte percentage may vary according to the site at which the aspirate is taken. Although overall there is a fairly good correlation between bone marrow histologic patterns and the percentage of lymphocytes in bone marrow aspirate, this correlation is not absolute. In a series of 47 patients from our group in whom bone marrow aspirate and biopsy had been done, 14 (30%) cases would have been classified differently if bone marrow aspirate rather than histology had been used to define "smoldering" CLL (unpublished results). In the larger series from the Danish Group, 86 of 296 (29%) of cases would have been misclassified as well (C. Geisler, personal communication).

Doubling time, although not available at diagnosis, is very easy to calculate by extrapolation shortly after diagnosis provided the patient is followed with no treatment for a few months and enough WBC counts are obtained (28). Doubling time is an excellent parameter for assessing the pace of the disease in daily practice, and its value in predicting disease progression and survival has been demonstrated in many studies (27–30,55,61).

Are any of the methods proposed to identify "smoldering" CLL superior to the others? A comparative analysis was carried out by both the French Cooperative Group in their large series (14) and, in a smaller number of patients followed up at a single institution, by Molica (52). These studies are summarized in Table 4. From these comparative studies, it can be concluded that all of these proposals are capable of identifying patients with a low probability of disease progression (about 15% at 5 years) and a long survival (80–90% at 5–10 years from diagnosis). It should be noted, however, that whatever the criteria used, there will be a group of patients who will progress and cannot be identified by the current criteria.

CONCLUSIONS

In the past few years, important advances have been made in the study of the natural history of early CLL. Parameters most consistently associated

Table 4 Comparison of Different Proposals to Define "Smoldering" CLL

	No. of patients	Survival (5-yr)	Progression (5-yr)
French group			
A-1'	247	87%	25%
A-1"	62	62%	54%
Molica			
A-1'	39	93%	14%
A-1"	45	53%	53%
French group			
A-2'	184	89%	19%
A-2"	125	71%	48%
Molica			
A-2'	39	93%	15%
A-2"	45	55%	52%
Montserrat et al			
"Smoldering"	47	78% (10-yr)	13%
"Active"	39	43% (10-yr)	57%
Molica			
"Smoldering"	40	85% (10-yr)	14%
"Active"	34	26% (10-yr)	53%
French group			
"Smoldering"	94	88%	20%
"Active"	68	81%	34%
Rai et al.			
0	127	89%	16%
I-III[a]	182	77%	41%
Molica			
0	41	87% (10-yr)	13%
I-II	43	28% (10-yr)	47%

[a]Patients with Hb between 10 and 11 g/dL are included. Refs: 13, 14, 52.

with disease progression are summarized in Table 5. Patients with CLL in early clinical stage (Binet stage A, Rai stage 0) with a Hb level within normal ranges (>13 g/dL), a moderate bone marrow infiltration (nondiffuse biopsy or <80% of lymphocytes in bone marrow aspirate), a low blood lymphocyte count (<30 × 10^9/L), and displaying stable blood lymphocyte counts, have a low probability of disease progression and a life expectancy not different from that of the general population ("smoldering" CLL). These patients represent up to 30% of all persons with CLL and should not be treated unless disease progression occurs.

Table 5 Parameters Associated with Disease Progression

Diffuse bone marrow infiltration
Rapid lymphocyte doubling time
High blood lymphocyte count ($>30 \times 10^9$/L)
Hemoglobin level <13 g/dL

In contrast, patients with a diffuse bone marrow infiltration, rapidly increasing high blood lymphocyte counts, or falling hemoglobin levels and/or platelet counts should be considered as having active CLL. Now that new, effective therapies are available, it is likely that these patients could gain some benefit from being treated before a change to a more advanced stage is observed, but this issue should be addressed in large randomized trials.

ACKNOWLEDGMENTS

This work was supported in part by grants from Fondo de Investigaciones de la Seguridad Social (FISS), 89/0353, and Comisión Interministerial de Ciencia y Tecnologia (CICYT), SAL 89/0963.

REFERENCES

1. K. A. Foon, K. R. Rai, and R. P. Gale, Chronic lymphocytic leukemia: New insights into biology and therapy, *Ann. Intern. Med., 113*:525–539 (1990).
2. M. J. Keating, H. M. Kantarjian, M. Talpaz, et al., Fludarabine: A new agent with major activity against chronic lymphocytic leukemia, *Blood, 74*:19–25 (1989).
3. R. O. Dillman, R. Mick, and O. R. McIntyre, Pentostatin in chronic lymphocytic leukemia: A phase II trial of cancer and leukemia group B, *J. Clin. Oncol., 7*:433–438 (1990).
4. L. D. Piro, C. J. Carrera, E. Beutler, and D. A. Carson, Chlorodeoxyadenosine: An effective new agent for the treatment of chronic lymphocytic leukemia, *Blood, 72*:1069–1073 (1988).
5. French Cooperative Group on Chronic Lymphocytic Leukaemia, Long-term results of the CHOP regimen in stage C chronic lymphocytic leukaemia, *Br. J. Haematol., 73*:334–340 (1989).
6. G. Bandini, G. Rosti, L. Albertazzi, M. Michallet, and S. Tura (International Bone Marrow Transplant Registry), Allogeneic bone marrow transplantation for chronic lymphocytic leukemia, in *New Strategies in Bone Marrow Transplantation* (R. P. Gale and R. E. Champlin, eds.), UCLA Symposium, Wiley Liss, New York, pp. 387–393 (1991).

7. C. Rozman and E. Montserrat, Chronic lymphocytic leukemia: When and how to treat, *Blut, 59*:467–474 (1990).
8. K. R. Rai, A. Sawitsky, E. P. Cronkite, et al., Clinical staging of chronic lymphocytic leukemia, *Blood, 46*:219–234 (1975).
9. J. L. Binet, A. Auquier, G. Dighiero, et al., A new prognostic classification of chronic lymphocytic leukemia derived from a multivariate survival analysis, *Cancer, 48*:198–206 (1981).
10. K. R. Rai and A. Sawitsky, Diagnosis and treatment of chronic lymphocytic leukemia, in *Neoplastic Diseases of the Blood* (P. H. Wiernik, G. P. Canellos, R. A. Kyle, and C. A. Schiffer, eds.), New York, Churchill Livingstone, New York, pp. 105–120 (1985).
11. C. Shustik, R. Mick, R. Silver, A. Sawitsky, K. R. Rai, and L. Shapiro, Treatment of early chronic lymphocytic leukemia: Intermittent chlorambucil versus observation, *Hematol. Oncol., 6*:7–12 (1988).
12. French Cooperative Group on Chronic Lymphocytic Leukemia, Effects of chlorambucil and therapeutic decision in initial forms of chronic lymphocytic leukemia (stage A): Results of a randomized trial on 612 patients, *Blood, 75*: 1414–1421 (1990).
13. E. Montserrat, N. Viñolas, J. C. Reverter, and C. Rozman, Natural history of chronic lymphocytic leukemia: On the progression and prognosis of early clinical stages, *Nouv. Rev. Fr. d'Hématol., 30*:359–361 (1988).
14. French Cooperative Group on Chronic Lymphocytic Leukemia, Natural history of stage A chronic lymphocytic leukaemia untreated patients, *Br. J. Haematol., 76*:45–57 (199=).
15. International Workshop on CLL, Prognostic features of early chronic lymphocytic leukaemia, *Lancet, ii*:968–969 (1989).
16. International Workshop on CLL, A report of Vth International Workshop, *Leukemia Res* (in press, 1992).
17. T. Han, H. Ozer, M. Gavigan, et al., Benign monoclonal B cell lymphocytosis—A benign variant of CLL: Clinical, immunologic, phenotypic, and cytogenetic studies in 20 patients, *Blood, 64*:244–252 (1984).
18. T. Chisesi, G. Capnist, and M. Vespignani, The definition of favourable stage CLL, *Haematologica, 71*:401–405 (1986).
19. H. Mellstedt, D. Pettersson, and G. Holm, Lymphocyte subpopulations in chronic lymphocytic leukemia (CLL): Relation to the activity of the disease, *Acta Med. Scand. 204*:485–491 (1978).
20. Chronic Leukemia-Myeloma Task Force, Proposed guidelines for protocol studies III. Chronic leukemia, *Cancer Chemother. Rep., 4*:159–165 (1963).
21. C. Rozman, E. Montserrat, J. M. Rodríguez-Fernández, et al., Bone marrow pattern—The best single prognostic parameter in chronic lymphocytic leukemia: A multivariate analysis of 329 cases, *Blood, 64*:642–648 (1984).
22. G. A. Pangalis, P. A. Rousso, C. Kittas, et al., B-chronic lymphocytic leukemia: Prognostic implication of bone marrow histology in 120 patients. Experience from a single hematology unit, *Cancer, 59*:767–771 (1987).
23. C. Geisler, E. Ralfkiaer, M. M. Hansen, K. Hou-Jensen, and S. Olesen Larsen, The bone marrow histological pattern has independent prognostic

value in early stage chronic lymphocytic leukemia, *Br. J. Haematol., 62*:47–54 (1986).

24. T. Han, M. Barcos, L. Emrich, et al., Bone marrow infiltration patterns and their significance in chronic lymphocytic leukemia: Correlations with clinical, immunologic, phenotypic, and cytogenetic data, *J. Clin. Oncol., 2*:562–570 (1984).

25. M. D. Lipshutz, R. Mir, K. R. Rai, and A. Sawitsky, Bone marrow biopsy and clinical staging in chronic lymphocytic leukemia, *Cancer, 46*:1422–1427 (1980).

26. M. Raphael, C. Chastang, and J. L. Binet, Is bone marrow biopsy a prognostic parameter in CLL? *Nouv. Rev. Fr. d'Hématol., 30*:377–378 (1988).

27. D. A. G. Galton, The pathogenesis of chronic lymphocytic leukemia, *Can. Med. Assoc. J., 94*:1005–1010 (1966).

28. E. Montserrat, J. Sánchez-Bisonó, N. Viñolas, et al., Lymphocyte doubling time in chronic lymphocytic leukaemia. Analysis of its prognostic significance, *Br. J. Haematol., 62*:567–575 (1986).

29. S. Molica and A. Alberti, Prognostic value of lymphocyte doubling time in chronic lymphocytic leukemia, *Cancer, 60*:2712–2716 (1987).

30. N. Viñolas, J. C. Reverter, A. Urbano-Ispizua, E. Montserrat, and C. Rozman, Lymphocyte doubling time in chronic lymphocytic leukemia: An update of its prognostic significance, *Blood Cells, 12*:457–464 (1987).

31. K. R. Rai, A. Sawitsky, K. Jagathambal, et al., Chronic lymphocytic leukemia, *Med. Clin. N. Am., 68*:697–702 (1984).

32. L. C. Peterson, C. D. Bloomfield, and R. D. Brunning, Relationship of clinical staging and lymphocyte morphology to survival in chronic lymphocytic leukaemia, *Br. J. Haematol., 45*:563–567 (1980).

33. J. V. Melo, D. Catovsky, and D. A. G. Galton, The relationship between chronic lymphocytic leukaemia and prolymphocytic leukaemia. I. Clinical and laboratory features of 300 patients and characterization of an intermediate group, *Br. J. Haematol., 63*:377–387 (1986).

34. J. M. Bennett, D. Catovsky, M. T. Daniel, et al., The French-American-British (FAB) Cooperative Group: Proposals for the classification of chronic (mature) B and T lymphoid leukemias, *J. Clin. Pathol., 42*:567–584 (1989).

35. T. Vallespí, E. Montserrat, and M. A. Sanz, Chronic lymphocytic leukaemia: Prognostic value of lymphocyte morphological subtypes. A multivariate survival analysis in 146 patients, *Br. J. Haematol., 77*:478–485 (1991).

36. R. A. Rudders and J. P. Howard, Clinical and cell surface marker characterization of the early phase of chronic lymphocytic leukemia, *Blood, 52*:25–35 (1978).

37. F. Caligaris-Cappio, M. Gobbi, L. Bergui, D. Campana, F. Lauria, M. T. Fierro, and R. Foa, B-chronic lymphocytic leukaemia patients with stable benign disease show distinctive membrane phenotype, *Br. J. Haematol., 56*:655–660 (1984).

38. L. Baldini, R. Mozzana, A. Cortelezzi, et al., Prognostic significance of immunoglobulin phenotype in B cell chronic lymphocytic leukemia, *Blood, 65*:340–344 (1985).

39. T. J. Hamblin, D. G. Oscier, J. R. Stevens, and J. L. Smith, Long survival in B-CLL correlates with surface IgMk phenotype, *Br. J. Haematol., 66*:21–26 (1987).
40. B. Simonsson, L. Wibell, and K. Nilsson, Beta-2 microglobulin in chronic lymphocytic leukemia, *Scand. J. Haemat., 24*:174–179 (1980).
41. E. Montserrat, J. P. Marques-Pereira, C. Rozman, A. M. Ballesta, J. L. Aguilar, and M. Elena, Serum beta-2 microglobulin levels in chronic lymphocytic leukaemia (letter), *Clin. Lab. Hematol., 4*:323–325 (1982).
42. J. S. Lee, D. O. Dixopn, H. M. Kantarjian, M. J. Keating, and M. Talpaz, Prognosis of chronic lymphocytic leukemia: A multivariate regression analysis of 325 untreated patients, *Blood, 69*:929–936 (1987).
43. P. H. Ellims, T. E. Gan, and M. B. van der Weyden, Thymidine kinase isoenzymes in chronic lymphocytic leukaemia, *Br. J. Haematol., 49*:479–485 (1981).
44. G. Pangalis, J. Trangas, K. Papanastasiou, P. A. Roussou, and C. M. Tsipalis, Poly (A) polymerase activity in B chronic lymphocytic leukemia, *Acta Haematol., 74*:31–35 (1985).
45. J. L. Vives-Corrons, C. Rozman, and M. A. Pujades, Combined assay of adenosine deaminase, purine nucleoside phosphorylase, and lactate dehydrogenase in the early clinical evaluation of B-chronic lymphocytic leukemia, *Am. J. Hematol., 27*:157–162 (1988).
46. T. Han, H. Ozer, N. Sadamori, et al., Prognostic importance of cytogenetic abnormalities in patients with chronic lymphocytic leukemia, *N. Engl. J. Med., 310*:288–292 (1984).
47. G. Juliusson, D. C. Oscier, M. Fitchett, et al., Prognostic subgroups in B-cell chronic lymphocytic leukemia defined by specific chromosomal abnormalities, *N. Engl. J. Med., 323*:720–724 (1990).
48. D. G. Oscier, J. Stevens, T. J. Hamblin, R. M. Pickering, R. Lambert, and M. Fitchett, Correlation of chromosome abnormalities with laboratory features and clinical course in B-cell chronic lymphocytic leukaemia, *Br. J. Haematol., 76*:352–358 (1990).
49. French Cooperative Group on CLL, Comparison of the (A, B, C) staging and the Rai's staging from a large prospective series (935 patients), *Nouv. Rev. Fr. d'Hématol., 30*:363–368 (1988).
50. International Workshop on CLL, Chronic lymphocytic leukaemia: Proposals for a revised prognostic staging system, *Br. J. Haematol., 48*:365–367 (1981).
51. International Workshop on CLL, Recommendations for diagnosis, staging, and response criteria, *Ann. Intern. Med., 110*:236–238 (1989).
52. S. Molica, On the natural history of early chronic lymphocytic leukemia, *Blood*, in press (1991).
53. K. R. Rai, A critical analysis of staging in CLL, in *Chronic Lymphocytic Leukemia: Recent Progress and Future Directions* (R. P. Gale and K. R. Rai, eds.), UCLA Symposia on Molecular and Cellular Biology, New Series, Alan R. Liss, New York, vol. 59, p. 253 (1987).
54. B. D. Cheson, J. M. Bennett, K. R. Rai, et al., Guidelines for clinical protocols for chronic lymphocytic leukemia (CLL). Recommendations of the NCI-Sponsored Working Group, *Am. J. Hematol., 29*:152–158 (1987).

55. S. Tura, M. Cavo, and M. Baccarani, Stage 0 chronic lymphocytic leukemia, in *Chronic Lymphocytic Leukemia: Recent Progress and Future Directions* (R. P. Gale and K. R. Rai, eds.), UCLA Symposia on Molecular and Cellular Biology, New Series, Alan R. Liss, New York, vol. 59, pp. 265–275 (1987).

56. D. G. Oscier, J. Stevens, T. J. Hamblin, R. M. Pickering, and M. Fitchett, Prognostic factors in stage A0 B-cell chronic lymphocytic leukaemia, *Br. J. Haematol., 76*:348–351 (1990).

57. C. Rozman and E. Montserrat, Critical factors in new therapeutic approaches in chronic lymphocytic leukemia, *Nouv. Rev. Fr. d'Hématol., 30*:453–455 (1988).

58. E. Montserrat, J. C. Reverter, N. Viñolas, M. Rovira, and C. Rozman, "Smoldering" chronic lymphocytic leukemia, *Leuk. Lymphoma* (submitted).

59. D. Catovsky, J. Fooks, and S. Richards (MRC Working Party on Leukaemia in Adults), Prognostic factors in chronic lymphocytic leukaemia: The importance of age, sex, and response to treatment in survival, *Br. J. Haematol., 72*: 141–149 (1989).

60. E. Montserrat, F. Gomis, T. Vallespí, et al., Presenting features and prognosis of chronic lymphocytic leukemia in younger adults, *Blood* in press (1991).

61. S. Molica, J. C. Reverter, A. Alberti, and E. Montserrat, Timing of diagnosis and lymphocyte accumulation patterns in chronic lymphocytic leukemia: Analysis of their clinical significance, *Eur. J. Haematol., 44*:277–281 (1990).

15

Chemotherapy of Chronic Lymphocytic Leukemia

Michael J. Keating
The University of Texas M. D. Anderson Cancer Center, Houston, Texas

INTRODUCTION

The treatment of chronic lymphocytic leukemia (CLL) is unusual in the spectrum of malignant diseases, in that the first decision to be made is whether the patient requires treatment or not. The secondary question is what treatment is appropriate for the stage of the disease. Similar approaches are taken with other chronic lymphoproliferative diseases such as the indolent lymphomas, hairy cell leukemia, and Waldenstrom's macroglobulinemia. This conservative approach is dictated by the heterogeneous outcome of CLL. While some patients with CLL are at risk of dying within the first year following diagnosis, many patients live for 20 years or more without requiring any therapeutic intervention. This variability in survival has generated a spectrum of philosophical approaches to management. Until recently, the predominant approach to the management of CLL has been "first, do no harm." Many physicians have the belief that few patients die of CLL and that palliation in terms of decreasing lymph node, liver, and spleen size, and decreasing the white cell count is all that can and should be achieved.

In the last 10 to 15 years, attempts have been made to identify which patients require treatment and the optimal timing of the initiation of treatment, while clinical trials have been conducted to identify the most effective cytoreductive programs. New treatments have provided physicians with the ability to achieve complete clinical, hematologic, and bone marrow remission in CLL. A real possibility now is that, as bone marrow remissions can be achieved, some patients would be considered eligible for autologous bone marrow transplantation, and may eventually be cured of their disease. Thus, the spectrum of approaches to CLL varies from an almost nihilistic attitude to a more "radical" approach to treatment with curative intent.

CLINICAL OUTCOME

Until very recently, the vast majority of patients with CLL who received treatment received an alkylating agent, either chlorambucil or cyclophosphamide, alone or combined with corticosteroids or vincristine. This approach has led to a monotonous treatment outcome as illustrated by Fig. 1, which shows the lack of improvement and survival of previously untreated patients referred to the M. D. Anderson Cancer Center between 1960 and 1990. These survival curves illustrate a number of points. The first is that a number of patients do die early. The second is that a number of patients still remain alive many years after diagnosis. The third is that the lack of a plateau indicates that patients are not cured of this disease, and the median survival of the total patient group is approximately 6 years.

Most therapeutic decisions are based on the information provided by the two major staging systems, those of Rai and Binet (1,2). The Rai staging system, as discussed by Cheson in this volume, is a five-stage system (1), although Rai and others feel that it is reasonable to group patients into three groups, mainly Rai 0, Rai I and II, and Rai III and IV (3). The M. D.

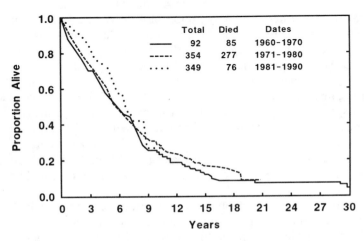

Figure 1   Survival of untreated CLL by decade – M. D. Anderson Cancer Center.

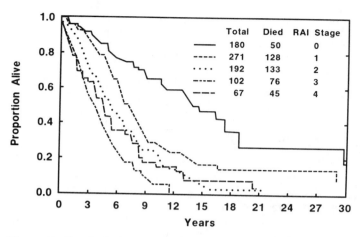

Figure 2 Survival of untreated CLL by Rai stage – M. D. Anderson Cancer Center.

Anderson data suggest that there is a distinct, significant difference between Rai stages I and II and that these should be considered separately. However, the outcome for patients with Rai stage III disease is, indeed, at least as poor as Rai stage IV (Fig. 2). The Binet staging system is a simple three-stage system, and there is obviously a clear separation into Binet stages A, B, and C when applied to the M. D. Anderson Cancer Center data (Fig. 3). The superior ability of the Rai 0 category to identify patients

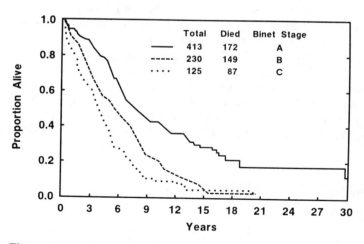

Figure 3 Survival of untreated CLL by Binet stage – M. D. Anderson Cancer Center.

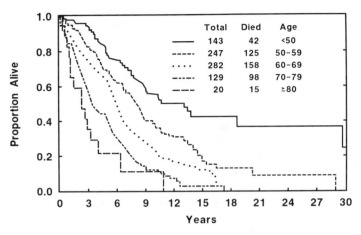

Figure 4 Survival of untreated CLL by age – M. D. Anderson Cancer Center.

who are likely to be long-term survivors when compared with the Binet A subset has led to a hybrid staging system (3), which, however, has not been widely adopted. Most clinical trials are based on one or the other of these systems, and the results should be applied specifically to the groups under investigation and not applied generally to all patients with CLL.

Although a number of other prognostic variables have been identified, the most reproducible appear to be the age of the patient, doubling time of the peripheral blood lymphocyte count, and the pattern of bone marrow involvement with CLL (4–6). In our experience, the age of the patient is a strong predictor of probability of survival, with younger patients consistently having a superior outcome to older patients (Fig. 4). While many patients with advanced age die of incidental diseases, especially cardiovascular and cerebrovascular complications, diabetes, hypertension, and second malignancies, the majority of patients who are younger appear to die of complications of their CLL. Thus, age must be taken into consideration when designing treatment programs. An expectation of survival of 5–7 years has a different impact for patients in their 70s compared to patients in their 40s or 50s.

DRUGS USED IN THE TREATMENT OF CLL

Alkylating Agents

Two alkylating agents are predominantly used in the management of chronic lymphocytic leukemia. The first is chlorambucil and the second is cyclophosphamide. Both agents are bifunctional alkylating agents and form covalent bonds with DNA, which is thought to be the mechanism of cyto-toxicity as well as of their mutagenicity and carcinogenicity. The covalent binding of the drugs to the DNA leads to a misreading of the DNA code, cross-linking of DNA, and single- and double-stranded breaks in DNA. The alkylating agents preferentially bind at sites of DNA that are actively transcribing. Alkylating agents have a greater effect on cells in the S-phase of the cell cycle than during other phases.

Chlorambucil

Chlorambucil is available in tablet form and is rapidly and almost com-pletely absorbed from the gastrointestinal (GI) tract. After a single oral dose, the peak plasma concentration occurs within 1 h. The major metabo-lite of chlorambucil is phenylacetic acid mustard, which reaches its peak level within 2–4 h of ingestion of chlorambucil. The area under the curve of the phenylacetic acid mustard derivative is approximately 50% greater than that of chlorambucil. Chlorambucil is extensively bound to plasma and tissue proteins, especially albumin in the plasma. Metabolism appears to be in the liver, with the principal metabolite being phenylacetic acid mustard, which is pharmacologically active against CLL. Chlorambucil is excreted in the urine, predominantly in the form of metabolites. One-half to two-thirds of a single oral dose is excreted in the urine within 24 h. The terminal plasma half-lives of chlorambucil and phenylacetic acid mustard are 1–1.5 and 2.5 h, respectively (7,8).

Cyclophosphamide

Cyclophosphamide is available in both parenteral and oral forms. It is 90% absorbed from the GI tract. The terminal half-life of cyclophosphamide is 5–6 h, and the terminal half-life of its active metabolite, 4-hydroxy-cyclophosphamide, is 1.5–6 h (7,8). The variability in the half-life of the 4-hydroxy-cyclophosphamide is affected by the rate of formation of the 4-hydroxy-cyclophosphamide by the liver. Thus, cyclophosphamide is ab-sorbed from the GI tract or injected intravenously, activated to 4-hydroxy-cyclophosphamide by the liver microsomes, which is then transported to the tissues, crosses the cell membrane, is converted to aldophosphamide, and spontaneously decomposes to phosphoramide mustard and acrolein. The metabolites of cyclophosphamide and 4-hydroxy-cyclophosphamide are excreted in the urine. This route of excretion leads to one of the specific toxicities of cyclophosphamide, which is hemorrhagic cystitis (8). The cysti-tis is caused by irritation from metabolites of cyclophosphamide, possibly acrolein. An effective agent to prevent this bladder toxicity is Mesna (so-dium 2-mercaptoethane sulfonate) (9). Mesna is available in parenteral and oral forms. It forms a dimer in serum but does not inactivate the active metabolite of cyclophosphamide. Upon excretion into the urine, the dimer hydrolyzes to mercaptan, which neutralizes metabolites in the urine. At the low doses of cyclophosphamide generally used to treat CLL, Mesna is usually not needed unless the patient experiences symptoms consistent with cystitis. Hydration is encouraged as well.

Toxicity of Alkylating Agents

Alkylating agents such as busulfan, cyclophosphamide, and chlorambucil have myelosuppression as their dose-limiting toxicity, with neutropenia being more marked than thrombocytopenia. If chlorambucil is administered on a chronic low-dose schedule, leukopenia often develops after 3 weeks of treatment. Myelosuppression may persist for 7–10 days after the last dose of chlorambucil. Otherwise, chlorambucil is well tolerated. Nausea, vomiting, abdominal discomfort, and diarrhea are uncommon and usually mild. Cyclophosphamide can induce cystitis (see above). Neurologic side effects are uncommon, with focal and generalized seizures having been reported. Rashes can occur. Alopecia is usually mild.

Another concern is immunosuppression, with both cellular and humoral immunity being affected. All alkylating agents appear to be carcinogenic in animals and associated with the onset of leukemia and possibly other tumors in humans. Cyclophosphamide has been reported to be associated with renal and bladder tumors in people receiving long-term treatment with cyclophosphamide.

Other alkylating agents such as ifosphamide, melphalan, and busulfan have had limited evaluation in CLL.

Prednisone

Prednisone is the most extensively studied corticosteroid in the treatment of chronic lymphocytic leukemia (10,11). Prednisone has a predominant glucocorticoid effect, although there is some mineralocorticoid activity. Other corticosteroids, such as dexamethasone and methylprednisolone, have less mineralocorticoid activity and have not been studied extensively in CLL. The main rationale for the use of prednisone in CLL is the ability of corticosteroids to produce lymphocytopenia. The other major activity is the immunosuppressive effect, which is the main reason for the use of prednisone in acquired autoimmune hemolytic anemia and immune-mediated thrombocytopenia in CLL. The use of prednisone in CLL is associated with all the general side effects of corticosteroids seen in any other disease. Prednisone is approximately five times more potent than hydrocortisone as an anti-inflammatory agent on a milligram-per-milligram basis and approximately one-tenth as potent as dexamethasone. It is approximately equivalent in potency to methylprednisolone.

As with most glucocorticoids, prednisone is rapidly absorbed when administered orally. Prednisone is widely distributed after ingestion from the bloodstream into muscles, liver, skin, intestines, and kidneys. Prednisone is metabolized in many tissues, but primarily in the liver, to biologically inactive compounds. Glucocorticoids are now seldom used alone in the management of CLL, as will be discussed later, but are used in combinations in a variety of doses and schedules.

Nucleoside Analogs

Recently, three purine analogs have been demonstrated to have major activity in the management of chronic lymphocytic leukemia. These agents, fludarabine, 2-chlorodeoxyadenosine, and pentostatin (deoxycoformycin) are illustrated in Fig. 5. While their chemical structures have similarities, pentostatin, rather than functioning as an antimetabolite of adenine, is a very potent inhibitor of adenosine deaminase.

Fludarabine

Fludarabine was developed in an attempt to identify more active derivatives of cytarabine. Arabinosyladenine was one of the first to be developed; however, it is limited in its clinical usefulness as a drug because of poor

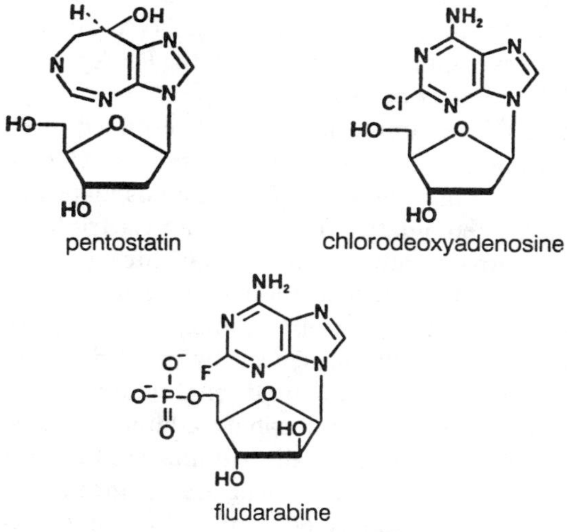

pentostatin

chlorodeoxyadenosine

fludarabine

Figure 5 Structure of nucleoside analogs useful in CLL.

solubility and rapid deamination by the enzyme adenosine deaminase to 9-β-D-arabinofuranosylhypoxanthine. Fludarabine monophosphate has a phosphate moiety to increase solubility and a fluorine atom that confers resistance to deamination by adenosine deaminase (12). Fludarabine is active in a number of mouse tumors and allows cures in L1210 leukemia. Phase I studies identified myelosuppression as the major dose-limiting toxicity of fludarabine (13). Neutropenia was more common than thrombocytopenia. Lymphocytopenia was prominent and the T lymphocyte population was more susceptible to depletion than B lymphocytes when the drug was studied in patients with solid tumors in phase I studies (14); the T lymphocyte population was decreased by 90% and the B lymphocyte population by 50%.

Following injection in humans, fludarabine monophosphate is rapidly dephosphorylated in plasma to form arabinosyl-2-fluoroadenine (F-ara-A) (15,16). F-ara-A is actively transported by a carrier-mediated process into cells and rapidly phosphorylated to its 5'-triphosphate (F-ara-ATP), which is the active metabolite of this drug responsible for its cytotoxic and therapeutic effects. The rate-limiting enzyme in the phosphorylation of F-ara-A is deoxycytidine kinase. The major action of F-ara-ATP is the inhibition of DNA synthesis. F-ara-ATP competes with deoxy-ATP for incorporation into DNA strands by DNA polymerases, and terminates DNA synthesis at the incorporation sites. In addition, F-ara-ATP is an inhibitor of ribonucleotide reductase, which consequently decreases the intracellular deoxynucleotide levels. F-ara-ATP is also incorporated in RNA, is an inhibitor of DNA repair, and decreases nicotinamide adenine dinucleotide (NAD) pools. Enzyme targets for F-ara-ATP include DNA polymerase-α, -β, -γ, and -ϵ, and DNA primase, which is an enzyme that polymerizes ribonucleotides to form the RNA primer required for the initiation of DNA replication (16).

The plasma pharmacokinetics of 2-F-ara-A have been determined in 30 patients following a rapid infusion of 2-F-ara-A monophosphate at doses of 80–260 mg/m^2 (15). Within 2 to 4 min the F-ara-A monophosphate was converted to 2-F-ara-A. F-ara-A is eliminated from plasma in a triphasic manner with an α half-life of approximately 5 min, a β half-life of 1.4 h, and a γ half-life of approximately 10.5 h. The total body clearance of F-ara-A decreases with increases in serum creatinine, indicating that these pharmacokinetic results would be markedly influenced by renal dysfunction, requiring dose reduction in patients with impaired renal function.

Studies of absorption of fludarabine monophosphate administered by mouth indicate that approximately 75% of an orally administered dose is bioavailable (17). The elimination parameters of the drug are not influenced by the route of administration. Approximately 60% of a dose of F-ara-

AMP is excreted as F-ara-A in the urine within 24 h. The major toxicity of fludarabine at this dose in humans is myelosuppression. There is a low incidence of nausea, vomiting, and almost no alopecia (18). There are minimal mucosal effects or gastrointestinal disturbances, and no evidence of direct hepatic or cardiac toxicity.

Neurotoxicity has been reported in patients treated with high doses of fludarabine. Chun and colleagues reviewed the experience of 70 patients with refractory leukemia treated with intravenous fludarabine monophosphate (19). Fourteen patients developed serious neurotoxicity. The toxicity was noted only in patients who received doses of ≥ 96 mg/m^2 per day for 5–7 days. The nervous system of three patients was submitted for postmortem examination, and the results disclosed a focal or diffuse demyelination in the brain and spinal cord. In addition, some patients have been reported to have a syndrome of fever, cough, dyspnea, and hypoxemia when receiving fludarabine for management of CLL (20). The onset of the fever varied from 3 to 28 days after receiving the doses. It usually occurred in later courses rather than the initial one or two courses. It is uncertain whether this syndrome is a toxicity of the drug or an opportunistic infection causing a diffuse interstitial pneumonitis. Tumor lysis syndrome has been observed in a small number of cases.

2-Chlorodeoxyadenosine

2-Chlorodeoxyadenosine (2-CDA), an investigational agent, is very similar in structure to F-ara-A and is an analog that is resistant to the action of adenosine deaminase. After injection 2-CDA accumulates mainly as its monophosphate in cells, and this step is catalyzed by deoxycytidine kinase; the triphosphate accumulates to a lesser extent. Synthesis and purification of 2-CDA have been carried out by workers at Scripps Clinic (21). 2-CDA has been administered as a continuous infusion, with the daily dosage of 0.05–0.4 mg/kg added to 500 cm^3 of 0.9% sodium chloride solution and given over a 24-h period. The plasma level obtained with this is < 10 mg/L (22). In one earlier study it was reported that an abrupt increase in plasma level was observed in some patients who had a tumor lysis response, presumably due to release from lysing tissue (23). The mechanism of growth inhibition of 2-CDA is probably similar to fludarabine, but it is a more potent inhibitor of ribonucleotide reductase than DNA polymerase-α (24). Through this action 2-CDA decreases deoxynucleotide pools. 2-CDA does not appear to be as potent a DNA chain terminator as fludarabine; however, it induces nucleosomal-size DNA strand breaks caused by putative endonuclease activity. 2-CDA triphosphate is a potent inhibitor of DNA polymerase-α, -β, and -γ.

Pharmacokinetics of 2-CDA.   The pharmacokinetics of 2-CDA have been studied in 12 patients with 2- and 24-h infusions of 0.14 mg/kg. If applied to a two-compartment model, the α and β half-lives were 35 min and 6.7 h, respectively. If the data were fitted to a three-compartment model, the half-lives of the α, β, and γ phases were 8 min, 1 h and 6 min, and 6.3 h, respectively. The volume at distribution was 8.9 ± 5.2 L/kg. The plasma concentration of 2-CDA during the 24-h infusion was 21.7 ± 9.8 nM. No data on excretion were presented.

Pentostatin

Pentostatin (also called 2′-deoxycoformycin or DCF) is a nucleoside analog produced by *Streptomyces antibioticus* and is a potent, irreversible inhibitor of adenosine deaminase (ADA). The major consequence of inhibition of ADA is the intracellular accumulation of adenosine and deoxyadenosine and deoxyadenosine triphosphate. Incubation of lymphocytes with DCF results in accumulation of deoxy-ATP and subsequent cytotoxicity. Deoxy-ATP is an allosteric inhibitor of ribonucleotide reductase, and this may be the mechanism of action of the drug. Deoxy-ATP also inhibits transcription and depletes nicotinamide adenine dinucleotide levels. The exact mechanism whereby DCF exerts its toxicity is uncertain. However, elevated deoxyadenosine levels inhibit S-adenosyl-homocysteine hydrolase activity. In addition, depletion of adenosine triphosphate by DCF will reduce energy levels. The triphosphate form of pentostatin is incorporated into DNA and incubation of cells with DCF causes DNA strand breaks. These activities of pentostatin have recently been reviewed (26). T cells are more susceptible than B cells to the cytotoxic and growth-inhibitory effects of pentostatin.

Inhibition of adenosine deaminase persists for more than 1 week after a single dose of pentostatin. Renal dysfunction is associated with a greater degree of ADA inhibition, presumably because of delayed excretion of pentostatin. The half-life of pentostatin is short. More than 80% of the drug is excreted unchanged in the urine. After doses of 0.25 and 2.5 mg/kg body weight, the half-lives of the α and β phases were 17 and 64 min and 18 and 104 min, respectively. Plasma decay curves are bi-exponential, with α phases of approximately 30 to 90 min; β phases are 3–9.4 h. The initial phase I studies using high doses resulted in significant toxicity, including nausea, vomiting, conjunctivitis, neurotoxicity, hepatotoxicity, and nephrotoxicity. These same studies noted significant antitumor activity in advanced leukemia and lymphoma.

WHEN TO TREAT CLL

The heterogeneity of outcome in CLL has generated a variety of opinions as to when treatment should be initiated. An additional component of the thinking involved in these decisions was the fact that conventional therapies had a low probability of achieving a complete remission, and there was no information to suggest that treatment changed the natural history of the disease. Thus, clinicians used clinical judgment as to when to initiate treatment. When the staging systems identified that anemia and/or thrombocytopenia were associated with a poor prognosis, clinicians decided to initiate treatment when these complications developed. In addition, if patients were having symptoms related to the leukemia that were interfering with their quality of life, or if there was evidence of progressive enlargement of liver, spleen, or lymph nodes, massive lymph node enlargement, or massive splenomegaly, patients were usually commenced on treatment. However, these decisions remained arbitrary.

In 1988, a National Cancer Institute-sponsored Working Group developed a series of guidelines for CLL protocols (27). A definition of "active" disease was developed that included the presence of weight loss of $\geq 10\%$ of body weight during the previous 6 months, extreme fatigue, fever $> 100.5°F$ for ≥ 2 weeks unrelated to infection, night sweats, development of anemia, thrombocytopenia, and autoimmune anemia and/or thrombocytopenia that was not responding to corticosteroid therapy. In addition, massive splenomegaly or lymphadenopathy or progressive lymphocytosis with an increase of $> 50\%$ over a 2-month period or lymphocyte doubling time of less than 6 months were indications to start treatment. Marked hypogammaglobulinemia or development of a monoclonal protein were not considered sufficient causes for initiation of treatment. These guidelines were set up to try to establish homogeneity of patients entering clinical trials in a variety of environments.

Immediate Versus Delayed Treatment

One of the few clinical trials to address the issue of timing of treatment was initiated by the French Cooperative Group on CLL (28). In 1980, a randomized clinical trial was initiated in which 612 good-prognosis patients (Binet stage A) received either no treatment (n = 309) initially or (for an indefinite period) treatment with chlorambucil at a daily dose of 0.1 mg/kg (n = 303). The "no treatment" group of patients had treatment delayed until progression was noted. Patients who progressed from stage A to stage B then received chlorambucil, and patients who evolved to stage C were treated with a cyclophosphamide–vincristine–prednisone (COP) regimen. In the chlorambucil-treated patients, those who evolved to stage B or directly to stage C received COP. Patients who had progressed to stage B and then developed stage C in the chlorambucil treatment group were then given a CHOP (COP plus adriamycin) regimen.

The major end point in this clinical trial was the survival of the patients. Although immediate chlorambucil treatment demonstrated the ability to delay progression to stage B or stage C, survival was not significantly different even after adjusting for a variety of prognostic factors. Five-year survival rates were similar for the two groups: 82% for the untreated group and 75% for the immediate chlorambucil group. After 9 months of follow-up treatment the immediate chlorambucil group had a 40% clinical and hematologic remission rate, with disappearance of adenopathy, splenomegaly, or hepatomegaly, a lymphocyte count $<4,000/\mu L$ with a hemoglobin level of $>12g\%$ and a platelet count of $>150,000/\mu L$. Another 28% of patients achieved a partial remission. The 5-year survival rate was 89% for patients who achieved clinical remission, 76% for those who achieved a partial remission, 82% for patients with stable disease, and 55% for patients with progressive disease. Survival after disease progression to stage B or stage C was significantly worse for patients with immediate chlorambucil versus those with no initial treatment.

An additional contribution of that study was to demonstrate that stage A patients with a hemoglobin level of $>12g\%$ and a lymphocyte count $<30,000/\mu L$ had a survival that was not significantly different from that of an age- and sex-matched French population. One of the issues of concern in the study was that in the "no treatment" group only 3 of the 50 deaths were associated with the development of an epithelial cancer, whereas 13 of 62 deaths in the chlorambucil treatment arm were associated with an epithelial cancer. The investigators were concerned that chlorambucil, a known mutagenic agent, may have increased the rate of development of the epithelial cancers. The recommendation from that study was that no treatment should be given to Binet stage A patients until disease progression was observed.

Catovsky has reported on the MRC–CLL trial II, in the United Kingdom (29), in which 600 patients with stage A CLL were randomized to early or delayed therapy. In that study, the effect of early treatment versus delayed therapy in stage A patients was investigated and showed no advantage for the earlier treatment. No difference in the incidence of second cancers was noted between the two groups. The conclusion from these studies is that there appears to be a subset of patients who do not have progressive disease and should not receive treatment. On the other hand, a number of patients do develop progressive disease, and the exact timing of intervention is, so far, not established. The recommendation for patients with Binet stage A and B disease and Rai stage 0–II disease is to delay treatment unless the patient has massive lymphadenopathy or hepatosplenomegaly or has symptoms of weight loss and fever related to the leukemia and not associated with infection. Most investigators would initiate treatment immediately for patients who present with Rai stage III and IV disease.

SMOLDERING LEUKEMIA

In addition to the report from the French Group of patients with a survival equivalent of an age- and sex-matched population, investigators from Spain have developed a term called "smoldering" CLL (30). They have classified Binet stage A into smoldering disease or active disease. The criteria for smoldering disease are similar to the French study, with a hemoglobin level of $\geq 12g\%$, lymphocyte count $<30,000/\mu L$, platelet count $>150,000/\mu L$. A nondiffuse pattern in the biopsy with $<80\%$ lymphocytes in the bone marrow aspirate and a prolonged doubling time of >12 months were also parameters that they found to be associated with a good life expectancy. The disease progression rate in the smoldering leukemia group is approximately 15% at 5 years, and survival is not different from controls. The Spanish investigators considered that approximately a quarter of all patients with CLL fulfilled the criteria for smoldering CLL at the time of diagnosis. One emerging feature is that an increasing number of patients are being diagnosed as having CLL coincidentally as a result of increasing use of complete blood count examinations when patients are evaluated for other conditions. Thus, more patients are likely to be diagnosed at the time that they fulfill the criteria for smoldering CLL. It is obvious from the studies that are being conducted that nothing is lost from observing these patients to establish whether they develop symptoms related to their disease or evidence of progressive disease in blood, bone marrow, or other organs, or evidence of bone marrow compromise.

The question of treating de novo patients with CLL and hypogammaglobulinemia has not been addressed. Nevertheless, relatively few patients have significant hypogammaglobulinemia at the time of initial presentation. If hypogammaglobulinemia is present, it is usually in patients with more advanced clinical stages. In addition, there is no evidence that restoring a patient to a remission status necessarily improves gamma-globulin production.

SINGLE-AGENT STUDIES IN CLL

Although many alkylating agents have been studied in CLL, including nitrogen mustard, busulfan, and triethyline-melamine, only chlorambucil and cyclophosphamide have stood the test of time and continue to be used to any large degree in the management of CLL. Most clinical studies have been conducted with chlorambucil, primarily because of the excellent tolerance of the drug, its oral route of administration, and its efficacy.

Chlorambucil

Chlorambucil has been investigated in the management of malignant lymphoproliferative diseases since the mid-1950s. The first major reports of its use in CLL were by Galton and colleagues in 1961 (11) and Ezdinli and colleagues in 1965 (31). Initially Galton used a dose of 0.03–0.3 mg/kg daily. The majority of patients received this dose on a continuous basis for 4–8 weeks. The usual dose was 4–8 mg/m^2. This study antedated the staging systems of Rai, Binet, and others. Twenty-four of 43 evaluable patients achieved "benefit" (relief of symptoms for more than 6 months) and "some benefit" (relief of symptoms for <6 months). Thus, 33 of 43 (77%) patients achieved some response. Of the 33 patients who responded initially, 23 (70%) responded to a second course, and 14 of 23 (61%) responded to a third course. Thus, approximately two-thirds of patients who had some response to the preceding course continued to respond to subsequent courses. Galton noted that the interval between courses of treatment became shorter as the disease progressed and the degree of benefit lessened. The authors documented improvement in lymph node size in approximately 60% of patients, improvement in spleen size and lymphocyte count in more than half of patients, and improvement in hemoglobin level in approximately 50% of patients. The major side effect reported was neutropenia, with thrombocytopenia being less of a problem. A number of these patients subsequently received corticosteroids in addition. The addition of the corticosteroids to the chlorambucil did not improve the response.

Ezdinli also administered chlorambucil on a continuous daily basis averaging 6–12 mg per day for 4–8 weeks (31). Fifty-one patients with CLL were treated. The overall survival was 5.2 years. Approximately three-quarters of patients had a decrease in their white cell count, one-third a decrease in lymph node enlargement, approximately one-half a decrease in splenomegaly, and 20–30% of patients experienced an improvement in their platelet count and anemia. As is customary in early-stage CLL, only five patients had subjective symptoms, and improvement occurred in one of these five patients. The authors also noted a lesser degree of lymphocyte response in patients during subsequent treatments, with only 18% of patients who received retreatment responding well. An absolute lymphocytosis usually persisted even in patients who had experienced a good response. Some patients in this study also received corticosteroids in addition to the chlorambucil without any apparent potentiation of the therapeutic response from the addition of the second agent. Five of seven patients responded to chlorambucil and prednisone when given as initial treatment, whereas only one of six had a response to the addition of corticosteroids after an unsatisfactory response to chlorambucil. Kaung treated 24 patients with a chlorambucil dose of 0.2 mg/kg per day orally on a continuous basis (32). Seventy-five percent of the patients responded to chlorambucil. Thus chlorambucil had been established as an effective treatment for controlling blood counts in the majority of patients with some improvement in hemoglobin and platelets in patients who responded.

Knospe et al. reevaluated the method of administration of chlorambucil (33). They introduced the concept of intermittent therapy, with a single dose of 0.4 mg/kg of chlorambucil every 2 weeks. Subsequent doses were increased by 0.1 mg/kg until toxicity or disease control was achieved. Six (75%) of eight previously untreated patients with indolent disease responded versus 18 of 31 (58%) of patients with inactive disease. Seven (50%) of 14 patients who had been previously treated and had not been shown to be resistant to alkylating agents responded, whereas only two (22%) of nine patients who were resistant to prolonged daily chlorambucil therapy responded. Hematologic toxicity was reported to be mild and not life-threatening. The conclusion was that biweekly oral administration was effective for CLL, with less hematologic toxicity than with daily treatment. In none of the studies of chlorambucil as a single agent was there any attempt to document bone marrow response, so a comparison of response data using modern criteria is impossible.

Cyclophosphamide

Cyclophosphamide has assumed a position as the second most widely used alkylating agent in the treatment of CLL, without any clear evidence in clinical trials of its single-agent activity. Cyclophosphamide is usually prescribed when chlorambucil is not effective or is not well tolerated by a patient. The drug is well absorbed by mouth and is, therefore, convenient for use, but induces more alopecia than chlorambucil and can be associated with hemorrhagic cystitis. Cyclophosphamide is more commonly given as part of a combination regimen.

Adrenal Corticosteroids

Galton and Ezdinli were also the investigators who contributed most to our information on corticosteroids as single agents in the management of CLL (10,11). Galton administered corticosteroids, usually prednisone or prednisolone, in a maximally tolerated daily dosage of 20–60 weeks initially, with the dose being reduced by 5 mg every 4–12 weeks until the lowest daily dose required to maintain good condition in the patient was achieved. Nearly all of the patients had been previously treated. Patients with a good initial response to therapy with chlorambucil had a response in five of nine courses administered, whereas those with a poor initial response had responses in four of nine courses and none of the nine patients who had advanced disease or who were refractory to alkylating agents achieved a response. Four patients treated for autoimmune hemolytic anemia exhibited some response. Thirty to forty percent of the courses of prednisone were associated with shrinkage of lymph nodes and, in approximately 45% of evaluable patients, splenomegaly decreased. Galton noted that the initial response to corticosteroids was an increase in the lymphocyte count for 2–10 weeks, followed by a fall. A decrease in the lymphocyte count to < 10,000/ μL was uncommon. Concern was expressed for the contribution of corticosteroids to opportunistic infections in a number of patients. Little experience was gained in this study on the use of corticosteroids in previously untreated patients.

Ezdinli also reported that one of six patients for whom prednisone was added to chlorambucil therapy responded (10). Later he reviewed the outcome of corticosteroids in 60 patients with CLL. Prednisone was administered at a dose of 40–80 mg per day. Following evidence of response, the patient was maintained on a dose of 10–30 mg per day. No complete responses were noted. A decrease in peripheral lymphadenopathy and splenomegaly was noted in two-thirds of patients. Abdominal nodes, mediastinal nodes, and pulmonary lesions responded less well. Anemia and thrombocytopenia improved in approximately 75% of patients. Improvement in anemia and thrombocytopenia was associated with a decrease in the size of the spleen. Hemoglobin and platelet count improvement were most striking when associated with significant decrease in spleen size. Approximately 6 months of treatment were required before the lymphocyte count fell below the pretreatment value. The duration of response with corticosteroids was short; the majority were shorter than 6 months in duration. The median survival was approximately 30 months. Twenty of 73 courses of prednisone were associated with major infections, and 15 of 73 courses were also associated with minor infections. Thirteen episodes of mild infection were also noted. The investigators questioned the advisability of giving high doses, since smaller initial doses of 20–30 mg per day were nearly as effective as the high doses, but with fewer anticipated complications.

Thus, corticosteroids appear to be effective in decreasing lymphadenopathy and splenomegaly and causing an improvement in hemoglobin and platelet count in a modest number of patients. No patients were able to achieve a complete remission, and, in all probability, patients resistant to alkylating agents do not respond to corticosteroids. The impact of corticosteroids on autoimmune hemolytic anemia and thrombocytopenia is probably unrelated to the cytoreductive effect in CLL. Concern persists as to the incidence of infections associated with chronic corticosteroid therapy. As with chlorambucil, no accepted optimum dose or schedule has been defined for corticosteroids as single agents.

COMBINATION THERAPY— CHLORAMBUCIL PLUS PREDNISONE

In 1973, Han reported a double-blind study in which 15 patients treated with a combination of chlorambucil and prednisone were compared with

11 patients with CLL who were treated with chlorambucil alone (34). The groups were comparable. Chlorambucil was given at a dose of 6 mg/day and prednisone as a dose of 30 mg/day. The chlorambucil dose was adjusted according to blood counts. Definition of complete remission in this study included bone marrow aspiration. Patients were evaluated after a 6-week trial period. Responding patients were maintained on chlorambucil on a daily dose of 2–4 mg/day and prednisone 15–20 mg/day. Complete remissions were observed in 3 of 15 patients (20%) in the combined group, with another 10 (67%) patients achieving a partial remission. Of the 11 chlorambucil-alone patients, one achieved a complete remission and four patients a partial response. The difference in the response rates was statistically significant. Hematologic toxicity was less frequent in the combination-therapy group. While the 2-year survival was 93% for the combination group and 54% for the chlorambucil-treated group, there was no statistically significant difference in the survival with longer follow-up. The complete remissions were sustained for up to 33 months, and the partial responses were approximately 8 months in duration. Prednisone was added for patients who did not respond to chlorambucil alone. The conclusion was that the combination was superior to chlorambucil alone.

A study comparing prednisone versus chlorambucil plus prednisone was conducted by Sawitsky et al. from the Cancer and Leukemia Group B (CALGB) (35). This study is the only one comparing the combination of chlorambucil and prednisone to prednisone alone that has been reported. In this study 96 patients with stage II to IV disease were randomized into one of three treatment schedules. Prednisone was given to all patients at a dose of 0.8 mg/kg for the first 14 days, with 50% reductions in the daily dose in the next 2 weeks and a further 50% reduction in the last 2 weeks of a total 6-week course. Subsequently, prednisone was given at a dose of 0.8 mg/kg per day for 7 days every month. In addition, patients in schedule 1 received chlorambucil once a month at a dose of 0.4–0.8 mg/kg. In schedule 2, chlorambucil was given as a continuous daily dose of 0.08 mg/kg, and patients in schedule 3 received prednisone alone. The response rate was 47% for schedule 1, 38% for schedule 2, and 11% for schedule 3 patients. In this study, as with earlier studies, responders were reported to survive longer than nonresponders. No patient in the prednisone-alone regimen achieved a complete remission. Intermittent monthly chlorambucil could be escalated to 1.5–2 mg/kg without undue marrow toxicity. In both schedule 1 and schedule 2, complete remissions were obtained. Three (8%) of 38 patients on the intermittent chlorambucil and 5 of 39 (13%) on the daily chlorambucil schedule achieved complete remission. Bone marrow criteria were used to evaluate response. The patients on chlorambucil had a shorter median time to failure of response than the prednisone-alone arm. No significant difference was noted in the survival of the three arms of the study. The conclusion of the investigators was that chlorambucil plus prednisone was superior to prednisone alone. However, there was no significant survival advantage. The major complication of treatment was reported to be episodes of infection, with one-fourth of the patients having severe infectious complications and another 30% having infections of milder degrees. Thus, the conclusion that any dosing schedule of combination therapy with chlorambucil and prednisone is superior to either agent alone is based on small numbers of patients with no survival advantage being demonstrable in either study. The chlorambucil and prednisone regimen(s) therefore, appears to be a weak "gold standard" for comparison.

High-Dose Chlorambucil Versus Intermittent Chlorambucil with Prednisone

Jaksic and collaborators, from the International Society for Chemo- and Immunotherapy (IGCS, Vienna) CLL Group, have reported a study of high-dose continuous chlorambucil versus an intermittent chlorambucil-plus-prednisone regimen. The latter was fairly similar to that used by Sawitsky et al. in the randomized comparative trial reported earlier (36). The new treatment regimen was 15 mg of chlorambucil daily until complete remission or to toxicity. Prednisone was given only when peripheral blood lymphocytes decreased below $5000/\mu L$ but significant organomegaly persisted. Regimen B was a single dose of chlorambucil, 75 mg, once every 4 weeks for 6 doses. Prednisone was given at a dose of 50 mg/day for 2 weeks, then 25 mg daily for an additional 2 weeks, then 15 mg for the last 2 weeks, then treatment was abruptly stopped. Thereafter, every 4 weeks, along with chlorambucil, 30 mg of prednisone was given daily for 1 week. Patients failing to achieve a complete remission were crossed to the alternative remission-induction regimen. Upon achieving a complete response, patients were placed on uniform maintenance therapy consisting of 15 mg of chlorambucil twice a week for at least 3 years. A marked difference in overall response was noted. Fifty-two patients were registered on regimen B with chlorambucil and prednisone and 129 on the high-dose chlorambucil regimen (a 2-to-1 randomization in favor of the high-dose chlorambucil arm). Seventy percent of the patients on the chlorambucil arm achieved a complete remission and 19% of patients a partial remission, with only 11% of patients not responding. In the combination arm, 31% of patients achieved a complete remission and 19 patients a partial remission. However, 50% of patients were classified as nonresponders. Bone marrow criteria were not used to evaluate response. There was a significant difference in survival between the two groups ($p < 0.01$), with a median survival of approximately 6 years in the chlorambucil-alone arm versus approximately

3 years for the combination-therapy arm. This difference in survival was most marked in patients with Binet stage A and Binet stage B, with no significant difference for stage C. Rather than suggesting that single-agent therapy is superior to combination therapy or that a continuous schedule is superior to an intermittent schedule of the alkylating agent, it must be recognized that the total dose of chlorambucil delivered per month was 5.6 times higher in the chlorambucil-alone arm versus the combination arm.

In this study, patients with early stage disease were also randomized to immediate-versus-delayed treatment. No significant difference in survival was found for early treatment compared with patients who were randomized to no initial treatment. An update of Jaksic's study confirms that there is still a very significant difference in response rate and survival in the high-dose chlorambucil arm (37), but that the difference is significant only for the stage A and B patients. This study emphasizes the lack of information that is available regarding the optimum dose and schedule of alkylating agents used in CLL and suggests that high-dose alkylating agents have not been explored to their full potential. The tentative approach to management of patients with CLL on the basis of their age and indolent disease may have prevented investigators from discovering the true incidence of complete responses in patients treated with alkylating agents as single agents.

SINGLE-ARM STUDIES WITH COP

Leipman and Votaw, in 1978, reported the application of the COP regimen (cyclophosphamide, vincristine, and prednisone) for CLL patients with progressive disease (38). The doses were cyclophosphamide, 400 mg/m^2, p.o., daily, days 1–5; vincristine, 1.4 mg/m^2, day 10; and prednisone, 100 mg/m^2 per day for 5 days (35). Courses were repeated at 3-week intervals. Two-thirds of the patients had Rai stage III or IV disease. After eight cycles, patients were reevaluated for extent of disease. If residual disease was present, patients were continued on COP. Some of the responding patients received COP as maintenance therapy and others received either single-drug oral chlorambucil or cyclophosphamide as maintenance therapy for a total of 2 to 5 years. Twenty-three previously untreated patients and 13 previously treated patients were studied. Nineteen patients had tissue biopsies, and eight were classified as poorly differentiated lymphocytic lymphoma. Eleven patients were documented to have well-differentiated lymphocytic lymphoma (WDLL). Nine patients had atypical peripheral lymphocyte morphology. Sixteen patients were considered to be complete responders. The response rate was 12 of 23 (52%) for previously untreated CLL and 4 of 13 (31%) for previously treated patients. Another 10 patients had good partial responses, including 6 of 23 previously untreated patients, for a total response rate of 18 of 23 (78%) for untreated patients. An additional 4 of 13 patients in the previously treated group were partial responders for a total of CR + PR rate of 8 of 13 (62%). The response rate appeared to be lower in patients whose peripheral blood had atypical lymphocytes, with 10 of 11 (91%) responding versus 12 of 19 (63%) for those with typical small lymphocytes or a mixture of small lymphocytes plus atypical lymphocytes. There was a significantly better survival of the complete responders and good partial responders than for poor partial responders and nonresponders in this study. The overall median survival of the study population was 36 months.

Oken and Kaplan reported on the use of COP in 18 patients with advanced refractory CLL (39). Eighty-nine percent of the patients had Rai stage III and IV disease. All patients had received prior alkylating agent therapy, and all but one had received chronic daily administration of an alkylating agent. Seventeen of the 18 patients were considered refractory at the time of entry on study. The dosage schedule for cyclophosphamide was 800 mg/m^2 on day 1 intravenously or 400 mg/m^2 per day orally on days 1–5. Patients received vincristine, 2 mg intravenously on day 1, and prednisone, 60–100 mg/m^2 orally on days 1–5. Cycles were repeated at 3- to 4-week intervals. Two patients achieved a clinical complete remission. No bone marrow evaluation was conducted. An additional six patients achieved a partial response, for an overall response rate of 44%. Responding patients had a median survival of 37.5 months, whereas nonresponding patients survived 5 months. In all responding patients, improvement was evident within the first month of treatment.

SINGLE-ARM STUDIES USING CHLORAMBUCIL PLUS PREDNISONE

In 1980, Michallet reported on the results of chlorambucil-plus-prednisone therapy for CLL patients (40). The chlorambucil dose was 12 mg/day combined with prednisone, 0.5 mg/kg per day for 3 to 4 days. After recovery from this course, patients received maintenance therapy of chlorambucil, 12 mg/day, and prednisone, 0.5 mg/kg per day for 10 days, each month for 5 months. One hundred and fifty-five patients were treated and approximately 64% of patients responded. Eighty-six percent of patients in Rai 0–I responded, 61% in Rai stage II, 60% in Rai stage III, and 54% in Rai stage IV disease. The definition of response was not clear in this study. The median survival of patients with Rai 0–I was 104 months and for those with Rai stage II–IV was 24 months. The survival of patients responding was 88 months from the start of treatment and was 30 months for nonresponders.

The largest single-arm study of CLL using chlorambucil and prednisone was conducted by Keller and colleagues from the Southeastern Cancer Study Group and reported in 1986 (41). One hundred and seventy-eight eligible patients were entered on the study. Seventy-eight percent were considered evaluable for response to induction therapy with a 22% hematologic complete remission rate and an overall CR-plus-PR rate of 74%. Bone marrow aspiration results were considered in the evaluation of response. Forty patients were considered nonevaluable for a variety of reasons (an unacceptably high number of nonevaluable patients). The response to treatment was 10 of 11 (91%) for Rai stage 0 disease, 27 of 31 (87%) for Rai stage I disease, 41 of 53 (77%) for Rai stage II disease, 14 of 30 (47%) for Rai stage III disease, and 10 of 13 (77%) for Rai stage IV disease. The median survival of the Rai stage IV disease patients was 41 months versus 24.5 months for the Rai stage III disease patients. The median survival of the Rai 0, I, and II groups of patients were 110+ months, 61 months, and 77 months, respectively. Only 2 of 43 (5%) patients with Rai stage III and IV disease achieved a complete response, versus 28 of 95 (29%) for Rai stages 0–II. Fifty-nine percent of the patients were classified as having active disease at the start of treatment (i.e., marrow compromise or constitutional symptoms, bulky disease, or progressive and painful enlargement of lymph nodes or spleen). The response rate was 86% for patients with indolent disease and 65% for those with active disease. There was a significant difference in survival for those considered "active" versus "indolent" patients. Again, a marked difference in survival was noted for the complete responders and partial responders versus the nonresponders, who had a median survival of approximately 14 months. The median survival of responders was 78 months. A number of patients were randomized to receive postinduction therapy with either chlorambucil and prednisone versus cyclophosphamide and cytosine arabinoside. No difference in survival was seen between the two consolidation treatments.

COMPARATIVE TRIALS IN CLL

The single-arm studies reported provided the basis for a number of comparative randomized trials in CLL. The study of Sawitzky et al. comparing prednisone alone or combined with either intermittent or continuous chlorambucil has already been described (35). The results suggested an improved freedom from progression with the combination programs when compared with the prednisone-alone arm. However, the overall survival was no different. Similarly, Han's comparative trial of chlorambucil plus prednisone versus chlorambucil alone suggested a higher response rate in the combination-therapy arm (34). However, the number of patients in that study was extremely small, and there was no survival difference between the two arms.

The comparative trial of Jaksic of high-dose single-agent chlorambucil versus intermittent chlorambucil plus prednisone has also been described, demonstrating a higher complete remission rate and improved survival for the single high-dose chlorambucil arm compared with the lower-dose combination of chlorambucil and prednisone (37). This trial is the only one that has demonstrated a survival advantage in one regimen over another using alkylating agents. Monserrat and his colleagues conducted a clinical trial of chlorambucil, 0.4 mg/kg orally as a single dose on day 6, plus prednisone, 60 mg/m^2 intravenously on day 6, vincristine 1 mg/m^2 intravenously day 6, and prednisone 60 mg/m^2 orally on days 1–5 (42). Fifty-one patients were treated with chlorambucil plus prednisone, with 4 (8%) complete remissions and 26 (51%) partial remissions. Eleven of the partial remissions were considered a good partial remission (the patient's disease improved from Binet stage C to stage A). When patients improved from stage C to stage B, they were considered to have a poor partial response. Thus, the response criteria were basically improvement in Binet stage. Complete-remission patients had no evidence of disease with a normal leukocyte count and differential count less than 3000 lymphocytes/μL, a hemoglobin level greater than 12 g/μL, and platelet count of $\geq 100,000/\mu$L with no evidence of lymphadenopathy or hepatosplenomegaly, and a bone marrow aspirate with less than 20% lymphocytes. Forty-five patients received COP treatment; only 1 of 45 (2%) patients achieved a complete remission, and 13 (29%) achieved a partial remission. Seven of the 13 PRs were "good" PRs. There was a significant difference in response to therapy in favor of the chlorambucil-plus-prednisone arm. Patients who were previously treated were included with untreated patients in the study. Of 35 patients who had received previous treatment, 5 of 18 patients responded to COP (28%). Six of 17 (35%) responded to chlorambucil plus prednisone. In the previously untreated group, 9 of 27 patients (33%) responded to COP versus 24 of 34 (71%) responding to chlorambucil plus prednisone. Thus, the chlorambucil-plus-prednisone regimen was more effective than COP in patients who had never received any prior therapy. There was no difference in the survival of the patients randomized to either group despite the higher complete response rate and partial response rate in the chlorambucil-plus-prednisone arm. The median survival was 20 months. Patients who achieved a CR or good partial response had a superior survival to those who achieved a poor partial response or who failed to respond. There was a marked difference in survival between the prior-treated group versus the no-prior-treatment group. In the previously treated group, the median survival was 13.5 months versus 32 months for the no-previous-treatment patients. Thus, there was no suggestion of any survival advantage of either treatment, but untreated patients had a high response rate to the conventional chlorambucil-plus-prednisone arm.

Monserrat and colleagues have also reported a randomized trial comparing chlorambucil plus prednisone versus cyclophosphamide, melphalan, and prednisone in the treatment of CLL stages B and C (43). Ninety-six previously untreated patients, 62 in stage B and 34 in stage C, were randomized to be treated with chlorambucil, 0.5 mg/kg orally on days 5 and 6, plus prednisone, 60 mg/m^2 orally on days 1–4, every 2 weeks, or cyclophosphamide, 160 mg/m^2 orally on days 1–4, melphalan, 6 mg/m^2 orally on days 1–4, and prednisone, 60 mg/m^2 orally on days 1–4 (CMP), every 3 weeks for 10 months. Forty-eight patients were randomized to each arm. Thirty-six (75%) of the 48 patients treated with chlorambucil plus prednisone responded with 27% complete remissions, and 26 of 48 (54%) patients treated with CMP responded, with 12.5% achieving a CR. The response rate for the chlorambucil-plus-prednisone arm was significantly higher (p = 0.054). The response rate was higher in stage B (69%, 24% CR) than in stage C (54%, 12% CR). There was no significant difference in survival between the two groups. Response to therapy was again associated with a longer survival. The investigators concluded that CMP was no better than conventional therapy.

The Eastern Cooperative Group published in 1991 the results of a comparative trial of chlorambucil, 30 mg/m^2 orally on day 1, and prednisone, 80 mg orally on days 1–5, every 2 weeks, compared with a more intensive regimen of cyclophosphamide, 300 mg/m^2 orally on days 1–5, vincristine, 1.4 mg/m^2 intravenously on day 1, and prednisone, 100 mg/m^2 orally on days 1–5, given every 3 weeks (44). Treatment was continued up to 18 months or maximum response. There were 122 eligible patients who were entered on the study. Only 2 patients were ineligible. Sixty patients received chlorambucil plus prednisone, whereas 62 received cyclophosphamide, vincristine, and prednisone. No significant difference in survival was noted, the median values being 4.8 years for the chlorambucil + prednisone (C + P) arm versus 3.9 years for the CVP patients. The CR rate was 25% versus 23% in each arm of the study. The duration of response to treatment was 2 years versus 1.9 years for C + P versus CVP. The median survival of stage III and IV patients was 4.1 years. The results were considered to be superior to those usually reported in other studies. The study confirms that, at the doses used, there was no significant difference in survival in either arm of the study. Thus, no other alkylating agent combination regimen appears at this time to be superior to a chlorambucil-plus-prednisone regimen, despite the unconfirmed results suggesting superiority of high-dose chlorambucil alone (37).

COMPARATIVE STUDIES OF FRENCH COOPERATIVE GROUP IN STAGE B AND C CLL

In addition to the clinical trial comparing immediate versus delayed treatment for Binet stage A patients (28), the French Cooperative Group has mounted two studies, one in stage B and the other in C disease (45,46). Commencing in 1980, patients with Binet stage B disease were randomized to receive an indefinite course of chlorambucil, 0.1 mg/kg per day, or 12 cycles of the COP regimen (45). The doses in the COP regimen were 300 mg/m^2 of cyclophosphamide orally on days 1–5, 1 mg/m^2 of vincristine intravenously on day 1, and 40 mg/m^2 of prednisone orally on days 1–5. Two-hundred and ninety-one patients were entered on the study. One-hundred and fifty-one were in the chlorambucil group and 140 in a COP group. The median follow-up was 53 months. One-hundred and twenty-nine patients died, 65 in the chlorambucil group and 64 in the COP group. There was no difference in survival between the two arms before and after adjusting for differences in prognostic factors and balancing the groups. Median survival was approximately 5 years. There was no difference in the rate of disease progression to stage C according to the arms of the study. There was also no difference in the incidence of death due to infection, pancytopenia, second cancers, or any other causes. Thus, COP was not shown to be superior to chlorambucil alone for stage B patients in this study.

A provocative result from a randomized comparative trial was reported in the French Cooperative Group study of Binet stage C patients (46). Patients were randomized to receive the COP regimen used in the Binet stage B study as one arm versus the same three drugs plus doxorubicin given at a dose of 25 mg/m^2 on day 1. The study was first reported in 1986 to show a significant improvement in survival for the CHOP arm compared with the COP arm, and the study was terminated at that point. This observation has now led to the French Cooperative Group moving the CHOP regimen up to Binet stage B patients. A long-term follow-up publication of this result in 1989 confirms the earlier report (47). In all, 70 stage C patients were randomized between the two treatments. Thirty-four patients received the COP regimen and 36 the CHOP regimen. The mean follow-up time was 58 months at the time of the analysis. Forty-six of the 70 patients had died, 27 in the COP group and 19 in the CHOP group. Overall survival was significantly superior for the CHOP group (P < 0.001). The 3-year survival rates were 71% for the CHOP group and 28% in the COP. The median survival time was 62 months in the CHOP group compared with 22 months in the COP group. Patients who failed to respond to COP or who had worsening of disease were subsequently treated with CHOP. CHOP was also given if patients developed stabilization or progression in less than 2 years after the initial randomization.

This study, although obviously significant, is subject to criticism by some on the basis that the median survival of the COP arm was less than 2 years (47). Recent studies of Rai stage III and IV disease or Binet stage C suggest that the median survival of Binet stage C patients treated with either chlorambucil plus prednisone or CAP is approximately 4 years (44). In addition, the number of patients in each arm of the study was small. Despite these objections, the investigators followed strict criteria for conduct of a randomized comparative trial and certainly have raised the issue as to whether anthracyclines, even at the very modest doses used in this study, are active specifically in the subset of patients who present de novo with Rai stage III and IV disease. The mechanism for anemia and thrombocytopenia in CLL patients is controversial. None of the patients in this study was Coombs positive, but some of the patients certainly could have had a response to corticosteroids if their cytopenia had been due to antibodies. However, this complication should have been randomly distributed between the two groups.

ANTHRACYCLINE COMBINATION STUDIES IN CLL

Surprisingly, there are no well-conducted clinical trials of adriamycin or any other anthracycline as single agents in CLL. The favorable survival for the French Study Group comparing CHOP with COP has prompted reevaluation of anthracyclines used in combination in CLL. Two major studies have been conducted by investigators at the M. D. Anderson Cancer Center (48,49). The first study commenced in 1974 and was a single-arm study of CAP (cyclophosphamide, 750 mg/m^2 intravenously on day 1, adriamycin, 50 mg/m^2 intravenously on day 1, and prednisone, 100 mg/day orally on days 1–5) (48). The courses were repeated at 3-week intervals until clinical complete remission, followed by maintenance with cyclophosphamide and prednisone. A total of 2 years of treatment was administered. Forty-seven patients with previously untreated CLL were treated with CAP. Forty-three percent of the patients had Rai stages III and IV and the other 57% had progressive stages 0–II. Overall, 43% of the patients obtained a CR and 23% a PR, for a total response rate of 66%. Bone marrow biopsy criteria were used to define response in addition to clinical and peripheral blood responses. At the time of final publication of this study, all patients had been followed for more than 10 years. The median survival was 5 years. No patient still remained free of disease. In keeping with the published French studies, median survival time for patients with Rai stage IV and Binet stage C disease were 93 months and 81 months, respectively.

Twelve (26%) of the patients obtained a CR on the CAP phase of the study and 36% a PR. With continued maintenance therapy with cyclophosphamide and prednisone (CP), eight of the PR patients eventually obtained a CR. Two of eight patients who had not responded to CAP responded to CP, obtaining a PR. The regimen was well tolerated, with the expected toxicities of alopecia, nausea, and vomiting. Three patients developed cardiac failure with cumulative adriamycin doses of 100 mg/m^2, 350 mg/m^2, and 450 mg/m^2. Two of the three patients had substantial risk factors for cardiac toxicity. This study was conducted at a time when the cumulative dose association of adriamycin cardiac toxicity had not been clarified. In this study, with complete follow-up, the median survival is very similar to that reported by the more conventional chlorambucil + prednisone, or COP regimens.

A subsequent study conducted at the M. D. Anderson Cancer Center evaluated a multiagent chemotherapy regimen with cyclophosphamide, adriamycin, vincristine, cytosine arabinoside, and prednisone (POACH) (49). This regimen was given to 34 previously untreated patients and 31 previously treated patients. Nineteen (56%) of the previously untreated patients responded, with 21% of patients obtaining a complete remission. The response rate for the 31 previously treated patients was 8 of 31 (26%). Two patients (7%) in the previously treated group obtained a complete remission. There was a significant difference in survival between the previously treated and the untreated patient populations. The median survival for the untreated patients was 5 years, which is almost exactly that obtained with the CAP regimen in comparable patients. The median survival for the previously treated patients was 15 months. Mortality was much higher in the previously treated patients than for the untreated patients. Pretreatment Rai stage and Binet stage were strongly predictive of death on study, but not for survival in the untreated patients. Both staging systems were predictive for survival in treated patients. The regimen was well tolerated, with the major complication being episodes of infection. While the median survival of the Binet stage C patients in this study was 27 months, only nine patients were in this category. Many of the patients on the study who died did so from complications of other diseases, which may have contributed to the lack of association of staging system with survival.

A number of other comparative trials have been initiated exploring the CHOP regimen. A Danish CLL group study was reported by Hansen to show a higher response rate for CHOP than chlorambucil plus prednisone in their study (50). Seventy-seven patients received CHOP and 80 patients received chlorambucil plus prednisone. The CHOP doses were cyclophosphamide, 750 mg/m^2 i.v. on day 1 every 4 weeks, adriamycin, 50 mg/m^2 i.v. on day 1 every 4 weeks, with both these agents being discontinued after eight courses. Vincristine, 1.5 mg, was given on day 1 every 4 weeks, and prednisolone, 40 mg/m^2, orally on days 1–5. The same prednisolone regimen was combined with chlorambucil, 10 mg/m^2, orally on days 1–5 every 4 weeks. Twenty of 68 evaluable patients obtained a clinical complete remission on the chlorambucil-plus-prednisone arm (29%). Only 3 of 20 responses were complete remissions documented by bone marrow, immunology, and CT scan. On the other hand, 43 of 64 evaluable patients responded to CHOP (67%). Thirteen of the 43 responses were confirmed to be true complete remissions. There is no survival advantage noted between the two arms on this comparative trial. These results are in apparent conflict with the French CHOP study described above (46). Kimby and colleagues, for the lymphoma group of central Sweden, reported on a comparison of chlorambucil/prednisone with CHOP in symptomatic CLL of B-cell type (51). Immunocytomas with leukemic phase were included in that study. Chlorambucil/prednisone (chlorambucil, 0.4 mg/kg per day on day 1 orally, and prednisone, 75 mg on days 1–3 every 2 weeks, with dose escalation of chlorambucil until response or toxicity) was compared with CHOP with a dose of cyclophosphamide and doxorubicin of 750 mg/m^2 and 50 mg/m^2 on day 1, respectively. The vincristine dose was 2 mg on day 1 and the prednisone dose was 50 mg/m^2 on days 1–5 every 4 weeks. The therapeutic aim was to control symptoms in the chlorambucil/prednisone arm, whereas patients who were assigned to CHOP were treated with the intent to achieve complete remission. A higher complete remission rate was noted in the CHOP group, CR + PR of 70%, compared to 50% in the chlorambucil/prednisone treatment group; however, there was no significant difference in survival between the two regimens. Toxicity was noted to be higher with the CHOP regimen. Thus, there does appear to be a suggestion of a higher complete remission rate being obtained with CHOP than was previously obtained with alkylating agents and prednisone regimens, despite a lack of impact on survival. The study of Jaksic of CHOP versus high-dose single alkylating agents will be of interest in this regard, as the higher response rates for the CHOP regimen may be due to more intensive treatment than previously reported COP or chlorambucil/prednisone regimens (37).

MULTIPLE ALKYLATING AGENT COMBINATIONS

The most prominent study reported using multiple alkylating agents is the M2 protocol of Memorial Sloan Kettering Cancer Center (52). The M2 protocol utilized vincristine, cyclophosphamide, BCNU, melphalan, and prednisone. This regimen was administered monthly to 63 evaluable patients with advanced CLL. Criteria for response in that study were clearly defined, and bone marrow biopsy had to be normal for a CR to be achieved. Eleven (17%) of the 63 evaluable patients obtained a CR. An additional 28 patients (44%) achieved a PR for an overall response rate of 61%. Seven of the CR patients had no evidence of disease when bone marrow lymphocyte subsets were analyzed using immunophenotypic methods. The CR rate for previously untreated patients was 11 of 37 (30%), versus 0 of 26 for patients who had received prior treatment. The overall response rate for untreated patients was 30 of 37 (81%), compared with 9 of 26 (35%) in the previously treated group. Unfortunately, the median survival that was reported in the study was calculated from the time of diagnosis and therefore was difficult to compare with other studies. A smaller study (MINA), based on the M2 protocol but substituting an investigational drug (Peptochemio) for BCNU, was reported from Italy (53) and was given to 20 patients with advanced CLL. Thirty-five percent of patients were reported to achieve a complete remission. Nine of 12 patients previously treated with chlorambucil and corticosteroids responded to treatment. Whether the patients were refractory to chlorambucil and corticosteroids was not stated. Five of 6 Rai stage II patients responded, 5 of 7 (71%) Rai III patients, and 4 of 7 (57%) Rai stage IV patients responded. The small number of patients in this study limits the conclusions that can be drawn regarding the usefulness of the regimen. The suggestion is that increasing the dose intensity and/or heterogeneity of the alkylating agents is associated with higher response rates than with the more conventional chlorambucil-only or chlorambucil/prednisone regimens.

NUCLEOSIDE ANALOGS

Nucleoside analogs are a major new group of drugs with activity in slow-growing lymphoid malignancies. Fludarabine monophosphate, subsequently called Fludara, has documented activity in CLL, indolent lymphoma, Waldenstrom's macroglobulinemia, and hairy cell leukemia (54). Pentostatin has marked activity in hairy cell leukemia (26), some activity in CLL (55,56), and also in indolent lymphoma and mycosis fungoides (26). 2-Chlorodeoxyadenosine has marked activity in hairy cell leukemia and substantial activity in CLL and indolent lymphoma (23). These drugs, while structurally similar, have some differences, as mentioned in the background pharmacology section. In particular, pentostatin has marked ability to inhibit adenosine deaminase, whereas this effect is not noted for the other two analogs. The common interaction in areas of purine, DNA, and RNA metabolism suggests that there is some as yet undefined common mechanism of action.

Fludarabine Monophosphate

Fludarabine was first evaluated in CLL by Grever and colleagues (57) in a Southwestern Oncology Group phase II protocol for 22 patients. All patients had received prior therapy. The characteristics of the patient population were as expected, with a median age of 63 years, a median performance status of 1. Three patients were Rai stage 0, five were stage I, six were stage II, four were stage III, and four were stage IV. Myelosuppression was noted to be the most frequent toxicity, with 13 patients having a decline in platelets and some reduction in granulocytes. One patient achieved a complete remission, 3 an excellent partial remission, and 15 patients had additional evidence of improvement. A study at the University of Texas M. D. Anderson Cancer Center, which used fludarabine to treat 68 patients with previously treated CLL, was reported in 1989 (58). Ten patients achieved a complete remission (15%) and 30 (44%) a partial response. Response rates for Rai stages 0–II, III, and IV were 64%, 58%, and 50%, respectively. Using the NCI criteria for complete remission, which allows the persistence of residual nodules in the bone marrow, the CR rate was 29%. Twenty-eight percent of patients fulfilled the NCI criteria for a partial response. The conclusion from that study was that the cytoreductive potency of fludarabine was substantial. Ten patients died during the study, seven during the first three courses of treatment. Survival was correlated with response to treatment, with those with a complete remission having a superior survival to the partial-remission patients. Median survival of the patients on the study was 16 months. In addition to stage, other factors associated with high response rates included a low white blood cell count, a limited number of lymph nodes, normal hemoglobin and platelet levels, and normal serum albumin and alkaline phosphatase levels. Factors significantly associated with survival were the serum albumin concentration, serum alkaline phosphatase level, and the platelet count. While some association of survival with Rai and Binet stage was noted, it was not significant.

The major toxicity associated with fludarabine was episodes of fever or infection. Three hundred and thirty-seven courses of treatment were evaluated for toxicity, with 25 episodes of pneumonia being noted. In addition, 28 episodes of fever of unknown origin were noted. Septicemia was uncommon, being found in only four patients, and 16 patients developed minor documented infections. Myelosuppression was the most common morbidity. Fifty-six percent of courses were associated with a nadir neutrophil count of $<500/\mu L$ and 25% with a nadir platelet count of $<50,000/\mu L$. Myelosuppression was significantly more common in patients with advanced pretreatment Rai and Binet stages. Nausea, vomiting, stomatitis, and diarrhea were noted in $<5\%$ of courses. Three patients had some symptoms suggestive of a peripheral neuropathy, but these were transient in nature.

Fludara was then used at the same dose of 30 mg/m^2 per day for 5 days intravenously every 4 weeks to treat 33 patients with previously untreated CLL (59). Patients had advanced Rai stage III or IV disease or progressive

Rai stage 0–II disease. The complete remission rate using the NCI Working Group guidelines was 75%. Fourteen of the 25 CR patients had residual lymphoid nodules in the bone marrow as their only evidence of disease. Six of the 33 patients failed to respond. Three died during the first three cycles of treatment from infection. Two patients had pneumonia, one with nocardia, and the third patient had disseminated candidiasis. All three patients were older than 75 years of age and had a pretreatment Rai stage of III–IV. Follow-up was too short to detect any association of survival advantage with the fludarabine regimen compared to the CAP and POACH regimens. The initial studies did not demonstrate any substantial difference. Since that time, an additional three patients have been treated with fludarabine as a single agent. The survival of the patients on fludarabine single-agent studies compared with CAP and POACH is illustrated in Fig. 6. The impact of fludarabine on survival of previously treated patients is difficult to establish. The survival curves of fludarabine as a single agent compared with POACH, the study immediately preceding, is illustrated in Fig. 7. Again, no significant improvement in survival has been noted.

Following the discovery of the activity of fludarabine, investigators at the M. D. Anderson Cancer Center evaluated the addition of prednisone to fludarabine for previously treated patients with CLL. One hundred and one patients were analyzed (60). Thirty-six (36%) patients obtained a complete remission, with 24 of 36 patients having persistent lymphoid nodules in the bone marrow. An additional 19% of patients obtained a PR, for a total response rate of 55%. Thus, there is no evidence of an improvement in response rate with the addition of prednisone to fludarabine. All patients

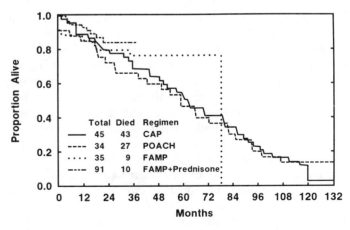

Figure 6 Survival of untreated CLL by treatment.

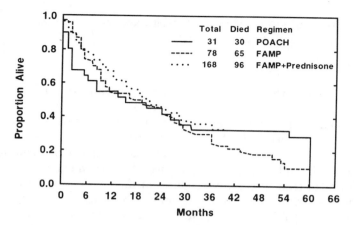

Figure 7 Survival of prior RX CLL by treatment regimen.

on the study had received prednisone previously. As with the single-agent study, the major toxicity was febrile episodes and documented infection. It is interesting that, in the more recent study with prednisone, *Pneumocytis carinii* and *Listeria* infections were noted, whereas they were not seen in the fludarabine single-agent study. Patients with Rai stage III and IV disease and those who failed to respond had a higher probability of developing infections with fludarabine.

These same investigators conducted careful immunophenotypic and molecular studies to assess the completeness of responses to fludarabine (61). No residual disease could be detected by two-color flow cytometry or surface light-chain expression in 72% of CRs, 45% of nodular CRs, but only 16% of PRs. In addition, studies of immunoglobulin gene rearrangements revealed a return to germline configuration in 83% of CRs and 20% of nodular CRs. Of note was a reversal of the CD4 : CD8, which appeared to correlate with the incidence of viral infections, but resolved postfludarabine therapy.

A group of investigators in New York has studied a different schedule of fludarabine utilizing a loading dose followed by a continuous infusion (62). Fludarabine was administered as a single bolus injection of 20 mg/m^2 intravenously on day 1, followed by a continuous infusion of 30 mg/m^2 per day for 2 days. This regimen was repeated at 4-week intervals. Forty-two patients were evaluable for response. Twenty-two obtained a partial response, with 12% having stable disease. No complete remissions were noted. Improvement in Rai stage was noted, with 6 patients achieving Rai stage 0. As with the other studies, myelosuppression was the main toxicity.

Nonhematologic toxicity was mild. Thus, fludarabine appears to be a major new agent in the management of patients with CLL.

Pentostatin (DCF)

Grever and colleagues (55) treated 25 previously treated patients with refractory CLL using 4 mg/m² of DCF every 2 weeks. Toxicity had been noted when DCF had been administered in the past at doses substantially higher than those used in this study. In this study, 1 CR and 4 PRs were noted, for an overall response rate of 20%. Seventeen of the patients had Rai stage IV disease. In addition to the 5 patients who responded, 4 had clinical improvement in their disease. No significant difference was noted in the pretreatment activity of adenosine deaminase between responding patients and patients who failed to respond. The patients entered on this study had failed standard alkylating agents, and the investigator suggested that DCF would not be cross-resistant with current agents used to treat CLL. Dillman and colleagues reported on a phase II trial of pentostatin in CLL conducted by CALGB (56). The DCF dose was 4 mg/m² i.v. weekly for 3 weeks and then every 2 weeks. Of 39 eligible patients who were evaluable, 31% were stage B and 33% had no prior treatment. Three percent of patients obtained a complete remission, 23% a partial response, 28% clinical improvement, and 38% had stable disease. Six of 13 (46%) obtained a complete or partial remission in the "no prior treatment" group, versus 4 of 26 (15%) for the prior-treated group of patients. The major toxicity noted was infection. Severe, life-threatening, or lethal bacterial infection occurred in 34% of patients. Opportunistic infections developed in 26%, including 6 patients with *Herpes simplex*, 3 with *Herpes zoster*, 2 with *Candidiasis*, and 1 with *Pneumocystis carinii*. Mostly all of these complications occurred within 6 weeks of the initiation of DCF therapy. Riddell and colleagues used a similar regimen in 16 patients, and 7 had an improvement in peripheral blood findings, but no criteria for objective responses were reported in that study (63). DCF appears to be active in refractory CLL patients. The apparently greater infectious morbidity than fludarabine makes it a less suitable agent.

2-Chlorodeoxyadenosine

2-chlorodeoxyadenosine (2-CDA) is structurally similar to fludarabine. The initial report from the Scripps clinic of 2-CDA in CLL in 1988 demonstrated that 10 (55%) of 18 patients "responded" to 2-CDA (22). The median number of courses was two, and, overall, 4 of 18 patients achieved a partial response and 6 of 18 patients achieved clinical improvement. Almost all of the patients in that study had anemia or thrombocytopenia. Patients were not maintained on therapy, and duration of remission was short (range, 2 to 15 months). Three of four patients with autoimmune hemolytic anemia demonstrated resolution of the hemolytic state. While acute toxicity was mild, the major problem was infections. One patient developed disseminated *Herpes zoster*, 2 patients had pneumonia of unknown etiology, and this was noted to be associated with *Aspergillus* infection. Twenty-eight percent of patients experienced a reduction in the platelet count during treatment. An association between failure of response and the development of progressive thrombocytopenia was noted in this study.

The Scripps investigators have subsequently enlarged their series (64). Ninety-four patients with refractory CLL have now been treated with 2-CDA. The dose given was 0.1 mg/kg per day by continuous infusion for 7 days. Patients were treated at 4-week intervals until maximum response or toxicity intervened. The median number of cycles received was two. All patients had failed prior therapy, but whether they were resistant or not was not reported. Eighty-seven patients had stage C disease. Four patients (4%) obtained a complete remission, and 41 patients (44%) a partial response. The median duration of response was 4 months. Thrombocytopenia was noted to be dose-limiting. Ten of 94 patients developed pulmonary infiltrates, four with documented infection. Six patients developed *Herpes zoster* (three dermatomal and three disseminated). In addition, three patients also developed meningitis. As with the other two agents, 2-CDA appears to be a drug with marked activity in CLL. Dose-limiting marrow toxicity and opportunistic infections are associated with the administration of the agent. The drug needs to be given by a central venous line because of the incidence of phlebitis when given by a peripheral line. Fludarabine is not associated with phlebitis or any vein irritation when given intravenously. Oral formulations of both agents are in development.

COMPARISON OF CHEMOTHERAPY WITH RADIATION

In the 1970s, Johnson reported the effects of total-body irradiation (TBI) in the management of CLL (65). Fifty of 57 (88%) patients with active CLL treated between 1964 and 1976 responded, with 22 of 57 (39%) patients achieving a complete response. It was thought that toxicity was acceptable and that a combination of TBI and chemotherapy would be possible, using a regimen of cyclophosphamide, 150 mg per day for 5 days orally and 20 mg per day orally for 5 days, and 10 Gy total body irradiation given on day 1 of each cycle. Cycles were repeated at 2-week intervals. Myelosuppression was commonly noted. Subsequently, the Eastern Cooperative Oncology Group conducted a study in which 26 evaluable patients were entered into total-body irradiation programs (66). Eleven received a course of 150 rads of total-body irradiation and 15 a lower dose of 50 rads. No complete remissions were noted, although the reported response rate was 73%. The lower dose yielded a PR rate of 47%. With the high-dose schedule, 73% of patients experienced severe thrombocytopenia and neutropenia. Twenty-six patients were also entered onto a chemotherapy arm, with patients being treated with chlorambucil plus prednisone. The overall response rate was 77%, with 6 of 26 (23%) patients achieving a complete remission and 14 of 26 a partial remission. The median duration of response was longer on the chemotherapy arm than on the total-body irradiation arm. The median survival of the two treatment populations was similar. The investigators suggested that the response rate was at least as good and probably superior for the chemotherapy arm. No difference in survival of the two studies was noted, which might be expected when such a low complete remission rate was noted. Further studies of total-body irradiation with or without chemotherapy have not been continued.

CONCLUSION

Prior to the middle 1980s, the only agents that were available for treatment of CLL were the alkylating agents and corticosteroids. Unfortunately, no studies have been conducted that demonstrate the optimum dose and schedule of any of the alkylating agents used as single agents or combined with corticosteroids. Indeed, there are very little data to support that corticosteroids add to the response rate. The gold standard of chlorambucil ± prednisone remains unchallenged by any other alkylating agent regimen. In particular, the CVP programs do not appear to be superior. Vincristine has not been demonstrated to have any significant activity in CLL, and should probably not be used in future therapeutic initiatives. Jaksic's study (36) strongly suggests that there is a strong correlation between dose intensity and response to chlorambucil, and further dose-intensification studies with alkylating agents should be considered.

Although anthracyclines, in their own right, have not been demonstrated to be active in CLL, the French studies have suggested improvement in survival in Binet stage C patients. A variety of subsequent studies comparing CHOP in various doses and schedules with COP or chlorambucil and prednisone demonstrate a higher response rate for the CHOP regimen, and they also suggest that CHOP achieves more complete remissions than were previously reported with alkylating agent regimens ± prednisone. This, however, may not be associated as much with the anthracycline as with the intensity of treatment. It is important to note, however, that in none of these studies was survival superior using CHOP. Jaksic has published preliminary data comparing high-dose chlorambucil versus CHOP and noted a higher response rate in the higher-dose alkylating agent arm (37).

Agents such as fludarabine, DCF, and 2-CDA have shown dramatic cytoreductive activity in CLL. Fludarabine is obviously the most active single agent studied to date in CLL. DCF and 2-CDA have been less extensively studied than fludarabine. Comparisons of fludarabine with CHOP are ongoing on previously treated patients in Europe, and the National Cancer Institute has initiated a comparison of chlorambucil versus fludarabine versus fludarabine + chlorambucil. The ability to achieve complete marrow remissions with nucleoside analogs raises the possibility of autologous bone marrow transplantation, and these programs are actively being explored. The encouraging preliminary results with cyclophosphamide and total-body irradiation in a small group of allogeneic transplant patients (67) suggests that bone marrow transplantation should be a useful procedure for select patients.

We are in a period of rapid development of effective therapies for CLL. Continued progress will hopefully lead to curative approaches for this disorder.

REFERENCES

1. K. R. Rai, A. Sawitsky, E. P. Cronkit, A. D. Chanana, R. N. Levy, and B. S. Pasternack, Clinical staging of chronic lymphocytic leukemia, *Blood, 46*:219 (1975).

2. J. L. Binet, D. Catovsky, P. Chandra, G. Dighiero, E. Montserrat, K. R. Rai, and A. Sawitsky, Chronic lymphocytic leukaemia: Proposals for a revised prognostic staging system, *Br. J. Haematol., 48*:365 (1981).

3. Chronic lymphocytic leukaemia: Proposals for a revised prognostic staging system, Report from the International Workshop on CLL, *Br. J. Haematol., 48*:365 (1981).

4. E. Montserrat, F. Gomis, T. Vallespi, A. Rios, A. Romero, J. Soler, A. Alcala, M. Morey, C. Ferran, J. Diaz-Mediavilla, A. Flores, S. Woessner, J. Batlle, C. Gonzalez-Aza, M. Rovira, J-C. Reverter, and C. Rozman, Presenting features and prognosis of chronic lymphocytic leukemia in younger adults, *Blood, 78*:1545 (1991).

5. E. Montserrat, J. Sanchez-Bisono, N. Vinolas, C. Rozman, Lymphocyte doubling time in chronic lymphocytic leukaemia: Analysis of its prognostic significance, *Br. J. Haematol., 62*:567 (1986).

6. C. Rozman, E. Montserrat, J. M. Rodriguez-Fernandez, R. Ayats, T. Vallespi, R. Parody, A. Rios, D. Prados, M. Morey, F. Gomis, A. Alcala, M. Gutierrez, J. Maldonado, C. Gonzalez, M. Giralt, L. Hernandez-Nieto, A. Cabrera, and J. M. Fernandez-Ranada, Bone marrow histologic pattern—The best single prognostic parameter in chronic lymphocytic leukemia: A multivariate survival analysis of 329 cases, *Blood, 64*:642 (1984).

7. D. S. Alberts, S. Y. Chang, H. S. G. Chen, B. J. Larcom, and S. E. Jones, Pharmacokinetics and metabolism of chlorambucil in man: A preliminary report, *Cancer Treatment Rep., 6*:9 (1979).

8. M. Colvin, A review of the pharmacology and clinical use of cyclophosphamide, in *Clinical Pharmacology of Antineoplastic Drugs* (H. M. Pinedo, ed.), Elsevier-North Holland, Amsterdam, p. 245 (1978).

9. N. Brock, J. Pohl, and J. Stekar, Detoxification of urotoxic oxazaphosphorines by sulfhydryl compounds, *J. Cancer Res. Clin. Oncol., 100*:311 (1981).

10. E. Z. Ezdinli, L. Stutzman, C. William Aungst, and D. Firat, Corticosteroid therapy for lymphomas and chronic lymphocytic leukemia, *Cancer, 23*:900 (1969).

11. D. A. G. Galton, E. Wiltshaw, L. Szur, and J. V. Dacie, The use of chlorambucil and steroids in the treatment of chronic lymphocytic leukaemia, *Br. J. Haematol., 7*:73 (1961).

12. S. Frederickson, Specificity of adenosine deaminase toward adenosine and 2'-deoxyadenosine analogues, *Arch. Biochem. Biophys., 113*:383 (1966).

13. M. Grever, J. Leiby, E. Kraut, E. Metz, J. Neidhart, S. Balcerzak, and L. Malspeis, A comprehensive phase I and II clinical investigation of fludarabine phosphate, *Sem. Oncol., 17*:39 (1990).

14. D. H. Boldt, D. D. Von Hoff, J. G. Kuhn, and M. Hersh, Effects on human peripheral lymphocytes of in vivo administration of 9-β-D-arabinofuranosyl-2-fluoroadenine-5'-monophosphate (NSC 312887), a new purine antimetabolite, *Cancer Res., 44*:4461 (1984).

15. L. Malspeis, M. R. Grever, A. E. Staubus, and D. Young, Pharmacokinetics of 2-F-ara-A (9-β-D-arabinofuranosyl-2- fluoroadenine) in cancer patients during the phase I clinical investigation of fludarabine phosphate, *Sem. Oncol., 17*:18 (1990).

16. W. Plunkett, P. Huang, and V. Gandhi, Metabolism and action of fludarabine phosphate, *Sem. Oncol., 17*:3 (1990).

17. A. Kemena, M. J. Keating, and W. Plunkett, Bioavailability of plasma fludarabine and fludarabine phosphate in circulating CLL cells, *Blood, 76*:288a (1990).

18. D. D. Von Hoff, Phase I clinical trials with fludarabine phosphate, *Sem. Oncol., 17*:33 (1990).

19. H. G. Chun, B. Leyland-Jones, S. M. Caryk, and D. F. Hoth, Central nervous system toxicity of fludarabine phosphate, *Cancer Treatment Rep., 70*:1225 (1986).

20. P. G. Hurst, M. P. Habib, H. Garewal, M. Bluestein, M. Paquin, and B. R. Greenberg, Pulmonary toxicity associated with fludarabine monophosphate, *Invest. New Drugs, 5*:207 (1987).

21. E. Beutler, L. D. Piro, A. Saven, A. C. Kay, R. McMillan, R. Longmire, C. J. Carrera, P. Morin, and D. A. Carson, 2-Chlorodeoxyadenosine (2-CdA): A potent chemotherapeutic and immunosuppressive nucleoside, *Leuk. Lymph., 5*:1 (1991).

22. L. D. Piro, C. J. Carrera, E. Beutler, and D. A. Carson, 2-Chlorodeoxyadenosine: An effective new agent for the treatment of chronic lymphocytic leukemia, *Blood, 72*:1069 (1988).

23. D. A. Carson, D. B. Wasson, and E. Beutler, Anti-leukemic and immunosuppressive activity of 2-chloro-2′-deoxyadenosine, *Proc. Natl. Acad. Sci. USA,* *81*:2232 (1984).
24. W. B. Parker, S. C. Shaddix, C-H. Chang, E. L. White, L. M. Rose, R. W. Brockman, A. T. Shortnacy, J. A. Montgomery, J. A. Secrist, III, and L. L. Bennett, Jr., Effects of 2-Chloro-9-(2-deoxy-2-fluoro-β-D-arabinofuranosyl) adenine on K562 cellular metabolism and the inhibition of human ribonucleotide reductase and DNA polymerases by its 5′-triphosphate, *Cancer Res., 51*: 2386 (1991).
25. J. Liliemark and G. Juliusson, On the pharmacokinetics of 2-Chloro-2′-deoxyadenosine in humans, *Cancer Res., 51*:5570 (1991).
26. P. J. O'Dwyer, B. Wagner, B. Leyland-Jones, R. E. Wittes, B. D. Cheson, and D. F. Hoth, 2′-Deoxycoformycin (Pentostatin) for lymphoid malignancies, *Ann. Intern. Med., 108*:733 (1988).
27. B. D. Cheson, J. M. Bennett, K. R. Rai, M. R. Grever, N. E. Kay, C. A. Schiffer, M. M. Oken, M. J. Keating, D. H. Boldt, S. J. Kempin, and K. A. Foon, Guidelines for clinical protocols for chronic lymphocytic leukemia: Recommendations of the National Cancer Institute-sponsored Working Group, *Am. J. Hematol., 29*:152 (1988).
28. The French Cooperative Group on Chronic Lymphocytic Leukemia, Effects of chlorambucil and therapeutic decision in initial forms of chronic lymphocytic leukemia (stage A): Results of a randomized clinical trial of 612 patients, *Blood, 75*:1414 (1990).
29. D. Catovsky, S. Richards, J. Fooks, and T. J. Hamblin, CLL trials in the United Kingdom—The Medical Research Council CLL trials 1, 2, and 3, *Leuk. Lymph., 5*:105 (1991).
30. E. Montserrat, N. Vinolas, J. C. Reverter, and C. Rozman, Natural history of chronic lymphocytic leukemia: On the progression and prognosis of early clinical stages, *Nouv. Rev. Fr. Haematol., 30*:359 (1988).
31. E. Z. Ezdinli and L. Stutzman, Chlorambucil therapy for lymphomas and chronic lymphocytic leukemia, *J. Am. Med. Assoc., 191*:444 (1965).
32. D. T. Kaung, R. M. Whittington, H. H. Spencer, and M. E. Patno, Comparison of chlorambucil and streptonigrin (NSC-45383) in the treatment of chronic lymphocytic leukemia, *Cancer, 23*:597 (1969).
33. W. H. Knospe, V. Loeb, Jr., and C. M. Huguley, Jr., Biweekly chlorambucil treatment of chronic lymphocytic leukemia, *Cancer, 33*:555 (1974).
34. T. Han, E. Z. Ezdinli, K. Shimaoka, and D. V. Desai, Chlorambucil vs. combined chlorambucil-corticosteroid therapy in chronic lymphocytic leukemia, *Cancer, 31*:502 (1973).
35. A. Sawitsky, K. R. Rai, O. Glidewell, R. T. Silver, and participating members of CALGB (Cancer and Leukemia Group B), Comparison of daily versus intermittent chlorambucil and prednisone therapy in the treatment of patients with chronic lymphocytic leukemia, *Blood, 50*:1049 (1977).
36. B. Jaksic and M. Brugiatelli, High dose continuous chlorambucil vs intermittent chlorambucil plus prednisone for treatment of B-CLL—IGCI CLL-01 trial, *Nouv. Rev. Fr. Hematol., 30*:437 (1988).

37. B. Jaksic and M. Brugiatelli, High dose chlorambucil for the treatment of B-chronic lymphocytic leukemia (CLL). Update of I.G.C.I. CLL trials, *Proc. 5th Int. Workshop on CLL — Sitges (Barcelona)*, p. 62 (1991).

38. M. Liepman and M. L. Votaw, The treatment of chronic lymphocytic leukemia with COP chemotherapy, *Cancer, 41*:1664 (1978).

39. M. M. Oken and M. E. Kaplan, Combination chemotherapy with cyclophosphamide, vincristine, and prednisone in the treatment of refractory chronic lymphocytic leukemia, *Cancer Treatment Rep., 63*:441 (1979).

40. M. Michallet, J. J. Sotto, J. J. Moulin, J. Arvieux, and D. Hollard, Management of CLL patients after chlorambucil therapy. Special value of a second Rai staging, *Eur. J. Cancer, 16*:511 (1980).

41. J. W. Keller, W. H. Knospe, M. Raney, C. M. Huguley, Jr., L. Johnson, A. A. Bartolucci, and G. A. Omura, Treatment of chronic lymphocytic leukemia using chlorambucil and prednisone with or without cycle-active consolidation chemotherapy, *Cancer, 58*:1185 (1986).

42. E. Montserrat, A. Alcala, R. Parody, A. Domingo, J. Garcia-Conde, J. Bueno, C. Ferran, M. A. Sanz, M. Giralt, D. Rubio, I. Anton, J. Estape, C. Rozman, and participating members of Pethema, Spanish Cooperative Group for Hematological Malignancies Treatment, Spanish Society of Hematology, Treatment of chronic lymphocytic leukemia in advanced stages, *Cancer, 56*: 2369 (1985).

43. E. Montserrat, A. Alcala, C. Alonso, J. Besalduch, J. M. Moraleda, J. Garcia-Conde, M. Gutierrez, F. Gomis, J. Garijo, M. C. Guzman, J. Estape, C. Rozman, and participating members of Pethema, Spanish Society of Hematology, A randomized trial comparing chlorambucil plus prednisone vs cyclophosphamide, melphalan, and prednisone in the treatment of chronic lymphocytic leukemia stages B and C, *Nouv. Rev. Fr. Hematol., 30*:429 (1988).

44. B. Raphael, J. W. Andersen, R. Silber, M. Oken, D. Moore, J. Bennett, H. Bonner, R. Hahn, W. H. Knospe, J. Mazza, and J. Glick, Comparison of chlorambucil and prednisone versus cyclophosphamide, vincristine, and prednisone as initial treatment for chronic lymphocytic leukemia: Long-term follow-up of an Eastern Cooperative Oncology Group randomized clinical trial, *J. Clin. Oncol., 9*:770 (1991).

45. The French Cooperative Group on Chronic Lymphocytic Leukemia, A randomized clinical trial of chlorambucil versus COP in stage B chronic lymphocytic leukemia, *Blood, 75*:1422 (1990).

46. French Cooperative Group on Chronic Lymphocytic Leukaemia, Effectiveness of "CHOP" regimen in advanced untreated chronic lymphocytic leukaemia, *Lancet*, 1346 (1986).

47. French Cooperative Group on Chronic Lymphocytic Leukaemia, Long-term results of the CHOP regimen in stage C chronic lymphocytic leukaemia, *Br. J. Haematol., 73*:334 (1989).

48. M. J. Keating, J. P. Hester, K. B. McCredie, M. A. Burgess, W. K. Murphy, and E. J Freireich, Long-term results of CAP therapy in chronic lymphocytic leukemia, *Leuk. Lymph., 2*:391 (1990).

49. M. J. Keating, M. Scouros, S. Murphy, H. Kantarjian, J. Hester, K. B.

McCredie, E. M. Hersh, and E. J Freireich, Multiple agent chemotherapy (POACH) in previously treated and untreated patients with chronic lymphocytic leukemia, *Leukemia, 2*:157 (1988).

50. M. M. Hansen, E. Andersen, H. Birgens, B. E. Christensen, T. G. Christensen, C. Geisler, K. Meldgaard, and D. Pedersen, CHOP versus chlorambucil + prednisolone in chronic lymphocytic leukemia, *Leuk. Lymph., 5*:97 (1991).

51. E. Kimby and H. Mellstedt, Chlorambucil/prednisone versus CHOP in symptomatic chronic lymphocytic leukemias of B-cell type. A randomized trial, *Leuk. Lymph., 5*:93 (1991).

52. S. Kempin, B. H. Lee, III, H. T. Thaler, B. Koziner, S. Hecht, T. Gee, Z. Arlin, C. Little, D. Straus, L. Reich, E. Phillips, H. Al-Mondhiry, M. Dowling, K. Mayer, and B. Clarkson, Combination chemotherapy of advanced chronic lymphocytic leukemia: The M-2 protocol (vincristine, BCNU, cyclophosphamide, melphalan and prednisone), *Blood, 60*: 1110 (1982).

53. F. Ferrara, L. D. Vecchio, G. Mele, V. Rametta, F. Ronconi, and R. Montuori, A new combination chemotherapy for advanced chronic lymphocytic leukemia (vincristine, cyclophosphamide, melphalan, peptichemio, and prednisone protocol), *Cancer, 64*:789 (1989).

54. H. M. Kantarjian, J. R. Redman, and M. J. Keating, Fludarabine phosphate therapy in other lymphoid malignancies, *Sem. Oncol., 17*:66 (1990).

55. M. R. Grever, J. M. Leiby, E. H. Kraut, H. E. Wilson, J. A. Neidhart, R. L. Wall, and S. P. Balcerzak, Low-dose deoxycoformycin in lymphoid malignancy, *J. Clin. Oncol., 3*:1196 (1985).

56. R. O. Dillman, R. Mick, and O. R. McIntyre, Pentostatin in chronic lymphocytic leukemia: A phase II trial of cancer and leukemia group B, *J. Clin. Oncol., 7*:433 (1989).

57. M. R. Grever, K. J. Kopecky, C. A. Coltman, J. C. Files, B. R. Greenberg, J. J. Hutton, R. Talley, D. D. Von Hoff, and S. P. Balcerak, Fludarabine monophosphate: A potentially useful agent in chronic lymphocytic leukemia, *Nouv. Rev. Fr. Hematol., 30*:457 (1988).

58. M. J. Keating, H. Kantarjian, M. Talpaz, J. Redman, C. Koller, B. Barlogie, W. Velasquez, W. Plunkett, E. J Freireich, and K. B. McCredie, Fludarabine: A new agent with major activity against chronic lymphocytic leukemia, *Blood, 74*:19 (1989).

59. M. J. Keating, H. Kantarjian, S. O'Brien, C. Koller, M. Talpaz, J. Schachner, C. C. Childs, E. J Freireich, and K. B. McCredie, Fludarabine: A new agent with marked cytoreductive activity in untreated chronic lymphocytic leukemia, *J. Clin. Oncol., 9*:44 (1991).

60. M. J. Keating, H. Kantarjian, S. O'Brien, J. Redman, C. Childs, and K. McCredie, Fludarabine (FLU) — Prednisone (PRED): A safe, effective combination in refractory chronic lymphocytic leukemia, *Proc. Am. Soc. Clin. Oncol.*, San Francisco, p. 201 (1989).

61. L. E. Robertson, Y. Huh, C. Hirsch-Ginsberg, H. Kantarjian, S. O'Brien, C. Koller, K. B. McCredie, and M. J. Keating, Clinical, immunophenotypic, and molecular analysis of the completeness of response in chronic lymphocytic leukemia after fludarabine, *Blood, 76*(supp. 1):314a (abstr. 1245) (1991).

62. C. A. Puccio, A. Mittelman, S. M. Lichtman, R. T. Silver, D. R. Budman, T. Ahmed, E. J. Feldman, M. Coleman, P. M. Arnold, Z. A. Arlin, and H. G. Chun, A loading dose continuous infusion schedule of fludarabine phosphate in chronic lymphocytic leukemia, *J. Clin. Oncol., 9*:1562 (1991).

63. S. Riddell, J. B. Johnston, D. Bowman, R. Glazer, and L. G. Israels, 2-Deoxycoformycin (DCF) in chronic lymphocytic leukemia (CLL) and Waldenstrom's macroglobulinemia (WM), *Proc. Am. Soc. Clin. Oncol.*, Houston, p. 167 (1985).

64. A. Saven, C. J. Carrera, D. A. Carson, E. Beutler, and L. D. Piro, 2-Chlorodeoxyadenosine treatment of refractory chronic lymphocytic leukemia, *Leuk. Lymph., 5*:133 (1991).

65. R. E. Johnson, Treatment of chronic lymphocytic leukemia by total body irradiation alone and combined with chemotherapy, *Int. J. Radiation Oncology Biol. Phys., 5*:159 (1979).

66. P. Rubin, J. M. Bennett, C. Begg, M. J. Bozdech, and R. Silber, The comparison of total body irradiation vs chlorambucil and prednisone for remission induction of active chronic lymphocytic leukemia: An ECOG study — Part I: Total body irradiation — Response and toxicity, *Int. J. Radiation Oncol. Biol. Phys., 7*:1623 (1981).

67. M. Michallet, B. Corront, L. Molina, A. Gratwohl, N. Milpied, C. Dauriac, S. Brunet, J. Soler, J. P. Jouet, H. Esperou Bourdeau, W. Arcese, F. Witz, A. Moine, and F. Zwaan, Allogeneic bone marrow transplantation in chronic lymphocytic leukemia: 17 cases. Report of the EBMT, *Leuk. Lymph., 5*:127 (1991).

16

Innovative Treatment Strategies for Chronic Lymphocytic Leukemia: Monoclonal Antibodies, Immunoconjugates, and Bone Marrow Transplantation

Susan N. Rabinowe, Michael L. Grossbard, and Lee M. Nadler
Dana-Farber Cancer Institute, Boston, Massachusetts

INTRODUCTION

Although conventional chemotherapeutic and radiotherapeutic approaches to chronic lymphocytic leukemia (CLL) often yield high response rates, virtually all patients ultimately become resistant to therapy. Moreover, these standard approaches are limited by a spectrum of nonspecific toxicities. Substantial interest exists in developing new therapeutic strategies for patients with CLL in an effort to ameliorate nonspecific toxicity, circumvent tumor cell resistance, and ultimately improve patient survival.

In contrast to chemotherapy and radiotherapy, antibodies and natural ligands bind specifically to antigens or receptors on the surface of malignant cells. Thus, antibodies and natural ligands, used either directly or conjugated to toxins or radionuclides, provide potential agents for targeted cancer therapy. Over the past decade, the advent of hybridoma technology has made available large quantities of murine monoclonal antibodies (MoAbs) (1). In addition, more recent efforts have culminated in the conjugation of a number of MoAbs to drugs, toxins, or radionuclides in an attempt to deliver cytotoxins directly to the tumor cell surface.

Simultaneous with the development of targeted therapies, progress has also been made in the use of high-dose ablative chemoradiotherapy. While these high-dose therapies are not without concomitant complications, they have the potential to overcome tumor cell resistance. Recently, extensive experience gained with autologous and allogeneic bone marrow transplantation (BMT) for hematologic malignancies has permitted the extension of this therapeutic modality to patients with CLL.

Although both targeted treatment and high-dose ablative chemoradiotherapeutic approaches are being actively investigated in non-Hodgkin's lymphomas and solid tumors (2), the ability to apply these treatment approaches to patients with CLL has been limited. The majority of patients with CLL are >60 years of age, and therefore may be ineligible for trials either secondary to the presence of co-morbid disease, or in the case of BMT, to age restrictions. Many patients are not referred for trials, since their CLL has become resistant to conventional therapy and it is felt that the toxicity of the experimental approach outweighs the potential benefit in this older population. For those asymptomatic patients with slowly progressive advanced CLL, the instinct is often to watch and wait, since these patients may feel well for a relatively long period. Each of these factors may have contributed to the fact that only small numbers of CLL patients have been treated thus far with experimental agents.

This chapter describes the conceptual basis of these new therapeutic strategies for CLL and the rationale for their clinical application. Preliminary clinical trials undertaken using unconjugated MoAbs, antibody-toxin conjugates, radioimmunoconjugates, and BMT will be discussed. Considering the limited numbers of patients studied, one must not attempt to assess the impact of these strategies but rather view them as very preliminary pilot trials.

MONOCLONAL ANTIBODIES: GENERAL CONCEPTS

MoAbs directed against antigens expressed on the surface of malignant lymphocytes can be used therapeutically in patients with CLL. In selecting an appropriate target antigen on the surface of lymphocytes, there are several important considerations (3). The specificity of the chosen target molecule and its uniformity of expression on malignant cells are both critical. The antigen should have enhanced expression on malignant cells as compared with normal cells. Indeed, the ideal situation would be one in which the targeted molecule is present exclusively on malignant cells, including the putative clonogenic tumor cell. Stem cells, which are capable of replenishing normal cells that are killed, should lack the target. By contrast, tumor cells devoid of the antigen should rarely be observed. Unfortunately, somatic cell mutation can lead to the production of antigen-negative tumor cells, thereby impairing therapeutic potential. For example, clinical trials employing antibodies directed against the unique variable region of immunoglobulin present on the surface of the malignant B cell (anti-idiotype antibodies) have had limited success due to the appearance of idiotype-negative clones of cells (4,5).

There are several potential target antigens available for the serotherapy of CLL (Table 1) (6–8). The CD5 antigen is expressed on both normal T cells and activated B cells (8–13). It is expressed in high density on virtually all CLL cells (>95%) and has been the obvious antigen to target with either MoAbs or MoAbs bound to toxins or radioisotopes. A number of B-cell antigens demonstrate B-lineage-restricted expression. The CD19 antigen is found on the surface of normal B cells and follicular dendritic cells as well as on >95% of B-CLLs, making it a suitable protein for targeted treatment strategies (8,14). Similarly, the antigen CD20 is present on normal B cells and on >95% of B-CLLs (8,15). However, CD20 lacks the capacity to internalize, thereby diminishing the capacity for a conjugated toxin to be transported into the cell cytosol to effect cytotoxicity. cClla (16–18) may be the most specific tumor antigen for B-CLL, because unlike other CLL-associated antigens, it is absent from both normal B and T lymphocytes. To date, only in-vitro studies have been performed utilizing MoAbs targeted to this antigen (19). The MoAb Lym-1 binds to a 31,000-M_r protein present on both normal B cells and 40% of B-CLLs. The MoAb Lym-2 binds to an as-yet-undefined antigen that is present on both normal B cells as well as 80% of B-CLLs. Both Lym-1 and Lym-2 (20) are therefore suitable candidate MoAbs for new treatment strategies in this disease. CD25, the IL-2 receptor, is present on normal activated T cells, activated B cells, and macrophages as well as on 50% of CLL cells and has been recently employed in new therapeutic approaches to CLL and other lymphoproliferative diseases (8,21–24). sIg is detectable on 80–90% of B-CLLs. The majority of these cells will express either sIgM or both sIgM and sIgD (Table 1) (7,8,25,26). These monoclonal surface immunoglobulins contain variable regions with antigenic determinants known as idiotypes. Idiotypes can be shared between variable regions of different immunoglobulin molecules, and panels of antibodies have been recently identified that can react with shared idiotypes present on B-CLL cells from a variety of patients (27). Finally, Dadmarz et al. (28) and others (11) have demonstrated that the clonogenic CLL cells uniformly express surface antigens including Ia, CD19, CD20, and CD5 along with the same light chain as in the original cultured CLL. Therefore, therapies directed at these antigens should have the potential for cytotoxicity against the clonogenic CLL cell.

The degree of stability of the tumor antigen within the cell membrane can be another relevant consideration. If an unconjugated MoAb is employed, the presence of a target antigen that remains fixed in the membrane may enhance antibody-mediated cytotoxicity. However, if the antibody is

Table 1 Potential Target Antigens for Serotherapy of CLL

Target antigen	Common MoAbs	Percent of CLLs positive	Normal tissue expression	References
CD5	Anti-T101 Anti-Leu1 Anti-T1 Anti-T65	>95%	T cells, activated B cells	6–13
CD19	Anti-B4 Anti-HD37 Anti-Leu12	>95%	B cells, follicular dendritic cells	6–8,14
CD20	Anti-B1 Anti-Leu16	>95%	B cells	6–8,15
cCLLa	Anti-cCLLa	>95%	None reported	16–18
Lym-1	Anti-Lym-1	40%	B cells	20
Lym-2	Anti-Lym-2	80%	B cells	20
CD25	Anti-TAC Anti-IL2R	50%	Activated T cells, activated B cells, macrophages	6–8,21–24
Surface IgM	Anti-IgM	80–90%	B cells	6–8,25–26
Surface IgD	Anti-IgD	80–90%	Resting B cells	6–8,25–26
Surface idiotype	Anti-ID	Unique for each patient or shared by several patients	None	27

used as a delivery vehicle to bring a toxin to the cell surface, it is important for the target antigen to have the capacity to internalize so that the toxin can be brought to its site of action inside the cell. Additionally, the antigen should possess only a limited capacity for shedding from the cell surface. If a significant amount of shed receptor is present in the circulation, it can compete with antigen remaining on the tumor cell surface for antibody binding. Both a minimum number of antigen receptors and a minimum number of antibody molecules binding to the cell may be necessary to achieve maximal cytotoxicity. Finally, the avidity with which the antibody binds to the receptor can be a critical determinant of the antibody's cytotoxic potential.

There are several postulated mechanisms by which MoAbs may mediate cytotoxicity: (a) through the triggering of complement-mediated cytotoxicity; (b) through antibody-dependent cell-mediated cytotoxicity; (c) via direct cytostatic or cytotoxic effects; or (d) via the delivery of drugs, toxins, or radioisotopes. When unconjugated MoAbs are used therapeutically, they rely on the potential of the antibody to effect endogenous pathways of cytotoxicity. Each of the aforementioned mechanisms has been exploited in the therapy of CLL.

Similar to the rationale underlying the therapeutic use of MoAbs has been the therapeutic application of natural ligands. These ligands, such as interleukin-2 (IL-2) and transforming growth factor alpha, are endogenous molecules that bind to a cell membrane receptor and are subsequently endocytosed (29–31). Like MoAbs, these ligands have been used therapeutically in both their native state (IL-2) or conjugated to toxins (IL-2/diphtheria toxin conjugates). However, a potential deterrent to effective cell killing is the presence of endogenous circulating ligand, which may compete with the ligand-toxin conjugate for binding to the tumor cell.

In evaluating the utility of MoAb serotherapy, one must be cognizant of several obstacles to therapy. Several of these problems have been discussed above, including those of antigen-negative tumor cells and lack of antigen specificity. Moreover, as with conventional therapeutic approaches, resistance to serotherapy can develop. For instance, antigen modulation or alteration in the ability of the antibody to mediate endogenous mechanisms of cytotoxicity can lead to reduced cell killing. Likewise, resistance can develop to a toxin or drug to which an antibody is conjugated. Finally, human antibodies can develop against the murine monoclonal, which can increase the clearance of the MoAb and limit its cytotoxicity.

We will consider the recent trials in this area from several points of interest: (a) treatment dose and infusion schedule; (b) achievement of detectable drug levels in the serum; (c) minor and major toxicities associated with treatment; and (d) human anti-mouse antibody (HAMA) and human anti-toxin antibody production. This scheme enables a clearer understanding of the results and limitations of the studies performed thus far, and more importantly, provides a perspective on future trials needed in this area.

SEROTHERAPY

CLL was one of the first diseases in which therapy with unconjugated MoAbs was attempted. Indeed, CLL could be considered to have several advantages as a prototypic disease in which to study this targeted therapy. First, CLL cells possess several tumor-associated antigens that could be targeted by MoAbs in an effort to mediate cytotoxicity. Second, the circulating malignant cells of CLL patients are readily accessible to a delivered antibody. Although bulky lymph node masses could prove to be relatively inaccessible tumor sites, this is likely to be less of a difficulty in CLL than in solid tumors. Third, patients with CLL are inherently immunosuppressed and may be less prone to the development of an immune response to a delivered murine MoAb. The development of human anti-mouse antibody (HAMA) can limit the delivery of subsequent courses of MoAb therapy both because of rapid clearance of the antibody as it is bound by the anti-mouse antibody and because of the potential occurrence of immune complex formation.

Early studies utilizing passive immunotherapy with unconjugated MoAbs affirmed both the safety of this form of therapy and the feasibility of delivering the antibody to the tumor cells. However, these preliminary trials were disappointing from the standpoint of clinical efficacy. Several trials utilized the antibody T101, an IgG2A murine MoAb that immunoprecipitates the glycoprotein antigen T65 (CD5) (Table 2). This antigen has been identified on CLL cells, benign and malignant T lymphocytes, thymocytes, and activated B cells (8–13). CD5 appeared to be a suitable target antigen in view of its high density of expression on CLL cells and possible presence on the clonogenic CLL cell (11,28). In addition, a large quantity of T101 was available for use in clinical trials. The studies demonstrated only transient decreases in the circulating leukemia cell burden, while lymph nodes, organomegaly, and bone marrow involvement remained unchanged. For the most part, toxicities were acceptable, and HAMA production was infrequent, probably secondary to the severely immunosuppressed state of these patients.

Dillman et al. (Table 2) reported several trials with T101 that examined both response rates and toxicity with various dose escalations and infusion schedules. Initially, T101 was administered to four heavily pretreated CLL patients as well as to four patients with cutaneous T-cell lymphoma (CTCL) (32). Two patients received a dose of 1–12 mg over 15 min and two received

Table 2 Serotherapeutic Trials with Unconjugated Antibodies

MoAb	Antigen	No. of pts.	Response				Antibody formation	References
			CR	PR	MR	Transient		
T101	CD5	4	—	—	—	4	0	32
T101	CD5	13	—	—	2	10	0	33
T101	CD5	6	—	—	2	4	0	34
CAMPATH	Glycoprotein	2	—	—	—	2	1 (anti-rat Ig)	35

doses of 10–100 mg as a 24-h infusion once weekly for a minimum of 1 month. Immunofluorescence studies documented antibody binding to circulating tumor cells and the subsequent elimination of these antibody-bound cells from the circulation. However, blood levels of T101 were barely detectable in these patients, secondary to binding of the antibody to the large burden of circulating tumor cells. Only the patient who received a 100-mg infusion had T101 saturation of the circulating tumor cells. In contrast, T101 levels were both detectable and maintained for longer periods of time in the patients with CTCL who had lower circulating tumor cell burdens. Two of the CLL patients who received 15-min infusions developed severe toxicity (anaphylaxis, hypotension, and dyspnea). With longer infusions, one episode of severe toxicity secondary to bronchospasm was observed. Other minor toxicities included fever, chills, malaise, and urticaria. None of the patients developed HAMA. Although all patients exhibited a transient decrease in the circulating tumor cell burden, this persisted for only a few hours to several days. Responses were likely due to clearance of antibody-bound malignant cells by the reticuloendothelial system. Antigenic modulation (the temporary loss of antigen expression from the surface of a cell in the presence of circulating antibody, with reexpression occurring upon antibody withdrawal) was documented in all patients who received 24-h infusions of T101. This occurred on cells in both the bone marrow and the circulation of one of the CLL patients, where cells were identified that expressed the CLL phenotype without expression of the T65 antigen. Interestingly, antigen reexpression was observed when cells were incubated in vitro in the absence of T101 antibody.

Foon et al. (33) (Table 2) administered T101 MoAb to 13 patients with CLL who were refractory to standard therapy. The antibody was administered twice weekly, over 2 h at escalating doses of 1, 10, 50, and 100 mg. Circulating leukemia cells (25–80%) bound T101 when exposed to doses of 50 to 100 mg of antibody. Only those patients who received the 100-mg dose of T101 exhibited measurable levels of T101 in the circulation. The majority of toxicities were mild, including fever, urticaria, and one brief episode of hypotension. However, pulmonary toxicity was observed in three patients who received 2-h infusions at the 50-mg dosage. T101 was subsequently administered over longer continuous infusions of 50 h for patients receiving 50 and 100 mg, respectively. Patients failed to produce HAMA, confirming the anticipated immunosuppression of this patient population. The majority of patients evidenced a transient decrease in circulating CLL cells, but within 1–2 days these returned to baseline. Two patients exhibited a stable 50% decrease in peripheral tumor cells for the 4 weeks of therapy. However, no reductions in lymphadenopathy or organomegaly were observed. Similarly, there were no improvements in the platelet count or hemoglobin level. In those patients who subsequently received the 50-h infusion schedule, the maximal decrement in circulating tumor cells occurred between 12 and 24 h, with a return to baseline levels by completion of the treatment. This rapid reduction and rebound was attributable to 100% modulation of the T65 antigen on both circulating and bone marrow tumor cells in response to the prolonged infusion.

Dillman et al. (34) (Table 2) reported another trial using the T101 MoAb in an additional six patients with advanced CLL as well as 10 patients with CTCL who had failed prior therapies. T101 was administered on a 24-h continuous infusion schedule at doses of 10, 50, 100, or 500 mg at 1- to 4-week intervals. Higher serum T101 levels were observed at the higher dose ranges. Receptor sites appeared to saturate rapidly, followed by a sharp rise in T101 level, which became maximal by the end of the 24-h infusion period and then rapidly declined. Minor toxicities were similar to the previous study, and severe toxicities were not observed. These CLL patients did not develop HAMA. Again, decreases in circulating lymphocytes were seen in the CLL patients, but these responses were maintained for less than 2 to 3 days in the majority of cases. Two minimal responses were observed. Although antibody saturated the circulating tumor cell population, antigenic modulation was documented in four of the six patients. Of note, antigenic modulation was documented in the bone marrow. Thus, although administration of T101 MoAb by continuous infusion appeared to both enhance binding to the bone marrow and lymph node cells as well as ameliorate side effects, it did not alter the transient nature of responses.

Another group of antibodies have also been used to treat patients with CLL. CAMPATH-1 antibodies are a family of antibodies that are exceptionally lytic when combined with human complement (Table 2) (35). These antibodies recognize a glycoprotein that is expressed on nearly all human lymphocytes. CAMPATH-1M, an IgM antibody, and CAMPATH-1G, an IgG2b antibody, have both been used clinically. In contrast to IgG2a antibodies, IgG2b antibodies not only fix human complement, but also are active in antibody-dependent cell-mediated cytotoxicity. While the T101 antibodies discussed previously were murine, these antibodies were derived from rats. One patient with B-CLL was treated with CAMPATH-1M on the first 2 days of therapy and then with CAMPATH-1G on days 3 through 12. No significant toxicities were observed, and the patient did not produce anti-rat Ig. While CAMPATH-1M infusion resulted in a rapid lowering of the white blood cell count and a decrease in serum complement levels, within 24 h after discontinuation of therapy the white blood count had returned to its baseline level. Subsequently, with CAMPATH-1G infusion, there was an equivalent reduction in the white blood cell count, but no effect on serum complement. Moreover, the increase of white blood count to baseline was less rapid after cessation of therapy, so that by day 6 no lymphocytes or prolymphocytes were detectable in the peripheral blood. A bone marrow aspirate on day 10 showed no detectable lymphoid cells. A second patient also received therapy with both CAMPATH-1M and CAMPATH-1G. In that case, the CAMPATH-1M infusion was complicated by angioedema of the lips and tongue, perhaps secondary to complement activation, and the infusion was discontinued after a small dose of antibody was delivered. The patient developed antibody directed against rat Ig. Subsequent therapy with CAMPATH-1G resulted in sustained clearance of lymphocytes from the peripheral blood, but minimal effect on bone marrow infiltration. CAMPATH-1G was also used in this trial to treat 16 other patients with lymphoid malignancies, and the side effects included fever, rigors, malaise, nausea, and vomiting. A transient rise in liver transaminases was observed in all patients up to a maximum of three times the upper limit of normal. In contrast to the trials using T101 MoAbs, the sustained reductions in tumor cells in this trial were suggestive of cell destruction rather than sequestration. Furthermore, the lack of modulation of the targeted antigen, its high density of expression, and the effective interaction of the rat MoAb with human complement are all features that should act to augment the success of this therapy.

Overall, the lack of sustained efficacy of unconjugated MoAb administration in the majority of patients with CLL could be attributed to at least two factors: antigen modulation from the cell surface membrane and insufficient binding of the antibody to the noncirculating leukemic cell compartment in lymph nodes and bone marrow. Although prolonged antibody infusions labeled CLL cells in the bone marrow and lymph nodes, antigenic modulation remained a significant problem. As stated earlier, it will be critical to select an antigen target with stability in the cell membrane in order to optimize cytotoxicity when using native MoAb serotherapy. Although the T65 antigen may meet the necessary requirement of specificity, it fails to satisfy the requirement of membrane stability. Moreover, the failure of unconjugated T101 antibody to cause significant reductions of enlarged lymph nodes and spleens, which are the bulk sites of disease, may reflect the difficulty of overcoming the presence of circulating antigen rather than the difficulty of antibody penetrating into bulky tumor masses. Nevertheless, due to the relative lack of clinical success using unconjugated MoAbs in CLL, investigators considered conjugating the antibodies to toxins and radionuclides in an effort to enhance the inherent toxicity of this form of therapy.

IMMUNOTOXIN THERAPY

Immunotoxins are conjugates between MoAbs or other natural ligands and toxins (36–38). They rely on the MoAb portion of the conjugate to deliver the toxin to the malignant cell (39). In order to develop a successful immunotoxin, three conditions must be satisfied. First, an antibody with sufficient specificity for the targeted cells must be identified, so that the damage secondary to nonspecific delivery of the toxin is minimized. Second, a potent toxin must be identified that exerts its toxicity only when it is bound to the MoAb. Third, there must be a method to stably link the antibody and toxin so that the toxin is not liberated into the circulation but rather is delivered to the targeted malignant cell.

Earlier in this review we discussed a set of characteristics that are critical in choosing an antibody and antigen for targeting malignant cells. The same qualities, including antigen specificity, membrane stability of the antigen, and absence of free circulating target, are equally essential to immunotoxin development.

In selecting an appropriate toxin, investigators were aware of several single- and multichain plant and bacterial protein toxins that are extraordinarily potent inhibitors of protein synthesis. Merely a few molecules of any of these toxins are lethal if they enter a cell. In fact, in-vitro studies have demonstrated these toxins to be 5 to 7 logs more toxic to cells than standard chemotherapeutic agents. Because of their potency, nanomolar concentrations of several of these toxins administered to a patient are likely to be lethal.

The cytotoxic mechanism of these protein toxins is best understood by considering the structure-function relationship of the various toxins. In order for native toxins to exert their cytotoxic effect, they must bind to and enter the targeted cells and the toxin must be transported to the ribosome where it inhibits protein synthesis. The single-polypeptide-chain toxins (pokeweed antiviral protein, gelonin, saporin) lack binding domains, which are essential for binding and cell entry (40). Thus, single-chain toxins are effective protein synthesis inhibitors in cell-free environments, but prove ineffective against intact cells because they are unable to translocate the cell membrane. However, when these single-chain toxins are conjugated to MoAbs, they can now specifically bind to antigens on the tumor cell surface. An optimal antibody for use in this setting is one that is readily internalized, so that the toxin can be delivered into the cytosol.

A more complex structure-function relationship is observed in the two-chain toxins. Like the single-chain toxins, these toxins, including ricin, *Pseudomonas* exotoxin, and diphtheria toxin contain a toxic moiety that inhibits protein synthesis. However, the more complex structures of these toxins provide domains that also serve the roles of binding the toxin to cells and translocating the toxin across the cell membrane to the ribosome. Immunotoxins using the toxic moiety of ricin and diphtheria toxin have been constructed and used clinically for the treatment of CLL.

Native ricin consists of two chains, referred to as the A chain and the B chain. The A chain is the toxic moiety, an enzyme that inactivates the 60S subunits of eucaryotic ribosomes and thereby disrupts protein synthesis (41). The B chain serves the roles of both binding and translocation of the toxin to the cytosol. High-affinity galactose binding sites on the B chain permit the holotoxin to bind nonspecifically to galactose-terminated oligosaccharides, which are ubiquitous on the surface of eukaryotic cells (42). In addition, the B chain functions in transporting the toxic A chain across the cell membrane into the cytosol (43).

The structure-function relationship of diphtheria toxin can be construed as conceptually similar to that of whole ricin. Diphtheria toxin is also a two-chain toxin. The A chain is the enzymatic toxic moiety, which inhibits protein synthesis by inactivating elongation factor 2 (44). As is true of ricin, the B chain of diphtheria toxin mediates cell binding and toxin translocation to the cytosol.

If either native ricin or diphtheria toxin were conjugated to a MoAb or other ligand, the resultant immunotoxin would have excessive nonspecific toxicity mediated by the intact binding chain (B chain) of the native toxin. Thus, the toxins must be altered before they are suitable for conjugation with antibodies. For example, ricin A chain alone can be used in the construction of immunotoxins (45). The toxin moiety of the immunotoxin would be supplied by ricin A chain and the binding specificity would be conferred by the antibody to which it is bound. Ricin A chain can be made available either by chemical separation from the B chain or via recombinant DNA technology. Alternatively, the nonspecific binding of the ricin B chain can be blocked either chemically or molecularly. This "blocked ricin" molecule can be conjugated to a MoAb, preserving the toxin and translocation functions of the native molecule, but ablating the binding function and replacing it with the binding of the antibody. Yet another approach is to use toxin mutants in which alterations in the amino acids comprising the toxin-binding region lead to an abolition of that function. Such diphtheria toxin mutants have been identified and conjugated to MoAbs. Again, these immunotoxins possess the binding function of the antibody and the toxic and translocation functions of the toxin. Numerous altered toxin molecules have been identified, and those described above have all been incorporated into immunotoxins used clinically against CLL. The many altered toxins have been reviewed extensively elsewhere, and will not be considered further within this chapter (38).

Single-Chain Immunotoxin Therapy

Many immunotoxins have been produced containing only ricin A chain. Unfortunately, such antibody-ricin A chain immunotoxins are cytotoxic only when conjugated to a very limited spectrum of antibodies. Because the B chain has been eliminated, not only the binding domain of the toxin but also the translocation domain is lost. Thus, any antibody to which these immunotoxins are conjugated should be internalized to assist the toxic moiety in entering the cytosol.

As noted earlier, preliminary efforts to treat patients with unconjugated T101 MoAb met with limited success. A logical extension was to conjugate that antibody to a toxin and determine whether efficacy was improved without a substantial increase in nonspecific toxicity (Table 3). Thus, the T101 MoAb was conjugated to recombinant ricin A chain (46). The binding region was replaced with T101 antibody, the translocation capability was removed with loss of the B chain, and the toxic domain was preserved in the A chain subunit (47).

Laurent et al. (48) (Table 3) described a single patient with chemotherapy-resistant Rai stage IV CLL who received 25 mg of T101-ricin A chain immunotoxin (T101-RTA) daily, over 2 h, for 3 days. T101-RTA was detectable in the serum with a plateau in concentration during the first 2 h, and a rapid decline following discontinuation of the infusion. As had been observed with unconjugated T101 antibody, complete saturation of target tumor cells was achieved for 4–6 h following the infusions. Following therapy, T65 antigen expression was reduced to 50% of its original level. The infusion was free of toxicity. The patient did not develop antibodies to either the murine monoclonal (HAMA) or to ricin A chain (HARA: human anti-ricin antibodies). A 40% reduction in the peripheral lymphocyte count was observed within 5 days and remained stable over a 2-week period. However, no improvements in hematologic parameters or in the degree of lymphadenopathy or organomegaly were seen. The patient died at day 19 due to hemorrhagic complications from thrombocytopenia.

Hertler et al. (49) (Table 3) subsequently reported a phase I trial of T101-RTA in 11 patients with T-ALL and B-CLL (4 patients). The patients with B-CLL had been previously resistant to alkylating agents and steroids. The immunotoxin was administered at a dose of 3 mg/m^2 intravenously over 1 h, twice weekly for 4 weeks. The serum half-life of T101-RTA was short, measuring only 43 min. Such rapid clearance was likely due to rapid binding of the immunotoxin to circulating malignant cells and subsequent clearance of immunotoxin-antigen complexes by the reticuloendothelial system. Intact immunotoxin was not detectable in either bone marrow or lymph node aspirates. Side effects of therapy included fever, nausea, and transient rash. Hypoalbuminemia and edema, which have been frequent accompaniments of therapy with other ricin-based immunotoxins were not evident. None of the patients developed HAMA, but one patient did develop HARA. In the setting of the rising anti-ricin A chain titer, a fall in

Table 3 Serotherapeutic Trials with Conjugated Antibodies/Ligands

MoAb/Ligand	Toxin/ radionuclide	Antigen	No. of pts.	Response				Antibody formation	References
				CR	PR	MR	Transient		
T101	Ricin A chain	CD5	1	—	—	—	1	0	48
T101	Ricin A chain	CD5	4	—	—	—	4	1 (HARA)	49
T101	Ricin A chain	CD5	5	—	—	—	4	0	47
H65	Ricin A chain	CD5	10	—	2	—	3	2 (HAMA)	51
Anti-B4	Blocked ricin	CD19	1	—	—	—	—	0	60
	Blocked ricin	CD19	5	—	1	—	3	1 (HAMA)	38
IL-2	Diphtheria	CD25	4	—	1	—	—	0	64,65
Lym-1	I131	Lym-1	5	—	—	—	5	1 (HAMA)	72, written communicatio n

serum T101-RTA levels was seen, which obviously reduced the immunotox-in's potential efficacy. All patients exhibited a 25–50% fall in white blood count, with a return to pretreatment values within 24 h. Decreases in lymph-adenopathy and organomegaly were not seen.

Hertler et al. (47) (Table 3) treated five additional CLL patients at a higher dose range (7–14 mg/m^2) with the identical infusion schedule and treatment frequency. Four of the five patients achieved complete saturation of CD5 sites by immunotoxin. Toxicities were similar to those seen at the lower dosages. Neither HAMA nor HARA was detected. Four of the five patients exhibited a 33% to 81% decrement in WBC by completion of the infusion, with a return to baseline within 24 h. No reduction in lymphade-nopathy or organomegaly was seen. In-vitro studies confirmed that T101-RTA was not cytotoxic to leukemic cells from these patients. Leukemic cells obtained from an additional 14 patients were insensitive as well. How-ever, with the addition of the enhancers monensin or monensin linked to human serum albumin, cytotoxicity was observed. Monensin raises intraly-sosomal pH, thereby potentially protecting the immunotoxin from proteo-lytic inactivation (50). The relatively low CD5 surface antigen density on the patients' leukemic cells was also believed to contribute to the limited T101-RTA cytotoxicity.

Another immunotoxin tested against CLL employs a different MoAb directed against the T65 antigen. H65-RTA is an immunotoxin comprised of a murine IgG$_1$ MoAb that recognizes CD5 (T65) and ricin A chain. LeMaistre et al. (51) (Table 3) performed a phase I study in which this agent was administered intravenously to 10 patients with CLL over 1 h daily for 14 days at doses of 0.2 0.33, 0.4, or 0.5 mg/kg. Patients were retreated at 28-day intervals. All patients had Rai stage II or III disease that was resistant to conventional therapy. At doses equal to or less than the maximum tolerated dose (MTD), only mild side effects were noted, including arthralgias, dyspnea, fever, malaise, nausea, rash, and fluid re-tention. The MTD was determined to be 0.33 mg/kg, due to the develop-ment of rhabdomyolysis. Of particular interest, the two patients who achieved a partial response to therapy were treated above the MTD, and developed rhabdomyolysis with concomitant renal insufficiency. These re-sponses were maintained for 3 and 8 months, respectively.

The lack of substantial efficacy for T101-RTA immunotoxins can be attributed to several factors. First, after intravenous administration, immu-notoxin bioavailability is shortened due to a rapid clearance from the circu-lation (52). As noted above, rapid clearance can occur if the immunotoxin binds to circulating malignant cells and the resultant complexes are taken up by the reticuloendothelial system. Moreover, carbohydrate residues in the ricin A chain component are recognized and taken up by reticuloendothelial and parenchymal cells of the liver. To circumvent this problem, investigators have developed immunotoxins with deglycosylated ricin A chain with resultant reduced hepatic clearance (53).

Second, in-vitro data have documented weak cytotoxicity against tumor cells, even when saturating doses of immunotoxin are administered. This may be due, in part, to degradation of the immunotoxin by lysosomal proteases (54). In vitro, this destruction can be reduced by the addition of ammonium chloride, chloroquine, amantidine, or monensin to the incubation media. All of these agents operate by increasing intralysosomal pH and protect the immunotoxin from proteolytic inactivation (54).

Third, tumor cells residing in the bone marrow may not be exposed to the immunotoxin due to its rapid clearance from the circulation. These cells may subsequently be released from the marrow, leading to a renewed appearance of tumor cells in the circulation (55). Greater efficacy may therefore be possible with administration of higher doses of immunotoxin for prolonged durations.

Fourth, it is apparent from in-vitro studies that many antibody-ricin A chain conjugates demonstrate less cytotoxicity than conjugates constructed between the same antibody and whole ricin. Indeed, only a few ricin A chain immunotoxins have been demonstrated to kill 3 logs of cells at concentrations that can feasibly be achieved in a patient's circulation. Again, this may be reflective of the limited ability of the MoAbs chosen thus far for clinical testing to internalize. Unless the antibody undergoes sufficient internalization, ricin A chain cannot be efficiently translocated to the cytosol.

Thus, early studies with ricin A-chain immunotoxins in CLL indicated that therapeutic efficacy could be optimized by enhancing resistance to inactivation and improving pharmacokinetic characteristics of the immunotoxin. A deglycosylated ricin A-chain immunotoxin that meets these requirements has been developed. cCLLa is a 69-kD glycoprotein that is expressed by all B-CLL cells and is common to both prolymphocytic leukemias and hairy cell leukemias of B-cell derivation. Unlike other antigens expressed on CLL cells, it is absent from normal B and T lymphocytes (16–18,56). These characteristics, in addition to its high density of expression on CLL cells, high affinity for specific MoAbs, and modulating capacity, make it a potentially effective target of immunotoxin therapy. Faguet et al. (19) evaluated the in-vitro cytotoxicity of an immunotoxin consisting of an IgG$_{2a}$ anti-cCLLa MoAb (CLL2m) and deglycosylated ricin A chain against the malignant lymphocytes from two patients with CLL. Eighty-one percent and 95% cell kill were achieved, respectively. In comparison, normal B cells were unaffected by in-vitro exposure to the immunotoxin. The potential efficacy of this agent in CLL has yet to be confirmed by clinical trials.

Two-Chain Immunotoxin Therapy

An alternative approach to construction of ricin-based immunotoxins is the production of a toxin containing both the A and B chains, but in which the nonspecific galactose-binding sites of ricin have been blocked. Anti-B4-blocked ricin (Anti-B4-bR) is a recently developed immunoconjugate that links the anti-B4 MoAb to the toxin-blocked ricin. Anti-B4 provides the tumor cell binding domain, the B chain contributes its toxin translocation function without its binding function, and ricin A chain remains the toxic moiety.

This conjugate exhibits only a slight decrease in cytotoxicity in comparison to intact ricin, yet possesses toxicity that significantly exceeds that of ricin A-chain immunotoxins. Hence, the ability of the B chain to assist in A-chain transport across the cell membrane remains intact. The murine IgG$_1$ anti-B4 (CD19) MoAb recognizes a B-cell lineage-restricted glycoprotein of 95 kD (14,57). B4 antigen is expressed throughout normal B-cell development on nearly all peripheral blood B cells and B cells of lymphoid organs. It is expressed on 95% of B-cell malignancies (58,59).

At the Dana-Farber Cancer Institute we have recently completed two phase I trials utilizing Anti-B4-bR in patients with B4-positive leukemias or lymphomas refractory to or relapsed from prior therapy (Table 3) (38,60). In the first phase I trial, the agent was administered as a daily bolus infusion over 1 h for 5 days. A total of 25 patients were treated, and one patient had the diagnosis of CLL. Therapeutic blood levels of the immunotoxin were maintained for only 3 to 4 h following the infusion. The dose-limiting toxicity was defined by transient elevations in hepatic transaminases. The MTD was 50 μg/kg per day for 5 consecutive days. In addition, side effects included low-grade fevers, transient thrombocytopenia, and hypoalbuminemia without edema. Nine patients produced HAMA and HARA. The single patient with CLL who was treated on this protocol had progressive disease after one course of therapy and failed to develop HAMA or HARA.

Because preclinical data suggested that increased doses of Anti-B4-bR could be administered with reduced nonspecific toxicity if delivered by prolonged continuous infusion, a second phase I trial utilized a 7-day continuous infusion schedule (Table 3). Patients received doses ranging from 10 μg/kg per day to 70 μg/kg per day for 7 days. A total of 43 patients with relapsed and refractory B-cell malignancies were treated, five of whom had the diagnosis of CLL. The majority of patients who received the agent at the MTD achieved sustained therapeutic blood levels until the discontinuation of the infusion. All patients developed transient rises of hepatic transaminase persisting for 7–14 days. This level of hepatic injury ultimately defined the MTD of 50 μg/kg per day for 7 days by continuous infusion. Thus, a higher dose of Anti-B4-bR could be delivered when the drug was administered by prolonged continuous infusion. Eleven patients developed peripheral edema, and 23 patients developed transient hypoalbuminemia as defined by a 20% or greater decrease in serum albumin. Thirty patients experienced fevers of 101° or greater. Again, modest reductions in platelet counts occurred, with two patients requiring platelet transfusions. Twenty-five patients produced HAMA or HARA after a single course of therapy and therefore were not re-treated. Approximately 50% of those patients with low- and intermediate-grade NHL or CLL responded to therapy (2 complete responses, 5 partial responses, 12 transient responses).

Of the five patients with CLL, one had Rai stage IV disease, one had Rai stage II disease, and three had bulky Rai stage I disease, with one patient having severe concomitant autoimmune hemolytic anemia. All patients had been heavily pretreated, having received a minimum of three prior chemotherapy regimens, while one patient had received six prior regimens. Two of the patients had failed prior fludarabine therapy. The doses administered to these patients were 10, 30, 40, 50, and 60 μg/kg per day by 7-day continuous infusion, respectively. Of the five patients treated, one had a partial response, three had transient responses (documented regression of adenopathy, but maintained for less than 4 weeks), and one patient did not respond. One of the patients produced HAMA. A phase II study has recently begun to assess the efficacy of therapy with Anti-B4-bR in patients with previously untreated CLL or patients who have received no more than one prior chemotherapy regimen for their disease. The dose to be administered is 50 μg/kg per day, the MTD determined in the continuous-infusion phase I study.

With the availability of recombinant DNA technology, a fusion protein has been produced in which the receptor-binding domain of diphtheria toxin has been replaced with the DNA sequences for human interleukin-2 (IL-2) (31). This immunotoxin preserves the toxin domain of diphtheria toxin. However, the B chain of diphtheria toxin, which provides the non-specific binding capability to cells (although the actual receptor is unknown), is deleted and replaced by the binding function of IL-2. The fusion toxin ($DAB_{486}IL$-2) has been expressed in and isolated from recombinant *Escherichia coli* and retains the toxin and translocation capability of diphtheria toxin in conjunction with the binding ability of IL-2. This agent can bind to and kill cells that express the high-affinity receptor for IL-2 (61). The high affinity IL-2 receptor contains two glycoprotein subunits: p55, a low-affinity subunit; and p75, an intermediate-affinity subunit (62). A number of hematologic malignancies express the high-affinity IL-2 receptor, including B-CLL and lymphomas (8,63). Although the receptor may be expressed on activated T or B lymphocytes and macrophages, it is not present on normal tissues (21,23,24).

LeMaistre et al. (Table 3) (C. F. LeMaistre, written communication, 1991) (64) performed a phase I study in which escalating-dose $DAB_{486}IL-2$ was administered to 18 patients, four of whom had CLL (three B-CLL, one T-CLL). IL-2 receptor expression was identified prior to therapy in all patients by immunostaining with an antibody directed against the p55 subunit of the IL-2 receptor. However, the p55 subunit is only part of the high-affinity IL-2 receptor complex, and more definitive techniques to detect the high-affinity receptor were not undertaken. The patients had all received prior therapy with conventional agents. The immunotoxin was administered intravenously, over 1–5 min daily. Elevated levels of soluble IL-2 receptors were identified in all patients, but the clearance of $DAB_{486}IL-2$ was not affected (22). The half-life of this agent in the circulation was approximately 5 min. Of note, in-vitro studies indicated that a 30-min exposure time was necessary to achieve adequate tumor cell kill. Due to elevations of hepatic transaminases, a dose of 0.1 mg/kg per day was documented to be the MTD. Mild side effects included nausea, fever, and rash. Three patients developed chest tightness when treated at the highest dose, but when the infusion time was extended to 20 min, this symptom did not recur. Prior to therapy, four patients had evidence of antidiphtheria toxin, and two patients had evidence of anti-$DAB_{486}IL-2$ antibodies. Although these patients exhibited an amnestic response during treatment, the presence of antidiphtheria toxin antibodies did not influence immunotoxin clearance or inhibit efficacy. A total of nine patients had evidence of antibody to both diphtheria toxin and $DAB_{486}IL-2$ by the end of the trial. Anti-IL-2 antibodies were detected prior to and following therapy in two of the 18 patients, without adverse sequelae. Four patients responded to therapy, including a patient with follicular large cell lymphoma who achieved a complete remission that is maintained at 18 months. Future trials using longer infusion schedules may improve the therapeutic index.

One of the above four CLL patients achieved a partial remission (by the CLL Working Group Criteria) (65,66) of 5 months' duration. The patient had Rai stage III CLL that had been previously treated with interferon-γ, combination chemotherapy, and fludarabine. Fifty-five percent of the leukemia cells expressed low-affinity IL-2 receptor, and the high-affinity receptor was identifiable through the use of Scatchard analysis. The patient initially received 3 daily intravenous boluses at a dose of 0.05 mg/kg per day, followed 1 week later by 7 daily intravenous boluses. The second cycle (0.1 mg/kg per day) had to be delayed until day 45 secondary to illness from a community acquired pneumonia. In addition, the patient received a maintenance course of 0.1 mg/kg per day for a 7-day period every 28 days, beginning on day 80 and day 113. Intravenous gamma-globulin (also containing antidiphtheria toxin antibodies) was administered between the first and second doses of the second maintenance course as prophylaxis against further pulmonary infections. Effective serum concentrations were achieved for more than 1 h. The only side effect observed was an asymptomatic, transient elevation of hepatic transaminases. The patient did not develop antibodies to diphtheria toxin or the fusion protein. The initial response was evidenced by a fall in the peripheral tumor cell count from $54,280/\mu L$ to less than $11,000/\mu L$, reduction in marrow involvement (64–29%) and greater than a 50% reduction in lymphadenopathy. These parameters continued to improve with each successive course of therapy, even in the face of gamma-globulin administration. A reduction in splenomegaly was also observed. In addition, although this patient had known elevations of soluble IL-2 receptor in the serum prior to therapy (9355 U/μL), the presence of shed receptor did not appear to diminish the response (level fell to 4500 U/μL). Therefore, even with a large population of circulating leukemia cells, $DAB_{486}IL-2$ was able to bind to and effect cytotoxicity against bulky tumors.

An understanding of the toxicity spectrum of this fusion protein has been broadened by considering the toxicities seen in 47 patients with IL-2 receptor bearing malignancies who are presently evaluable for treatment response (J. C. Nichols, Seragen, Inc., written communication, 1991). The primary toxicities observed at the MTD have been transient elevations of hepatic transaminases (30%), hypoalbuminemia (10%), hypersensitivity-like syndromes including fever, chest tightness, rash (20%), and occasionally transient elevations of serum creatinine or thrombocytopenia. Since all patients have been previously immunized against diphtheria toxin, one concern had been that the presence of antibodies to diphtheria toxin could then inhibit therapeutic efficacy or lead to serum sickness. Approximately 30% of patients had evidence of antibodies to diphtheria toxin and DAB_{486}-IL-2 prior to administration, while 60% of patients produced them after one or more treatment cycles. Nevertheless, the development of these antibodies apparently has not led to either toxicity or inhibition of therapeutic benefit.

These preliminary reports of immunotoxin therapy in patients with CLL demonstrate that immunotoxins can be safely administered to patients with a tolerable toxicity profile. Although immune responses to the delivered toxin and antibody have occurred frequently, they do not appear to be the limiting factor in enhanced response rates. Preliminary results from studies with both Anti-B4-bR and $DAB_{486}IL-2$ suggest that clinical efficacy may be enhanced and toxicity may be reduced by administering these agents by prolonged continuous infusion.

RADIOIMMUNOCONJUGATE THERAPY

Radiotherapy can frequently provide effective reduction of symptomatic adenopathy in patients with CLL. Both local as well as total nodal and total body irradiation have been delivered, with often gratifying results (67–69). The radionuclide^{32}P was administered in the 1950s to CLL patients, with evidence of efficacy (70,71). Recently, clinical trials have been undertaken to examine the potential efficacy of radioisotopes conjugated to MoAbs in the therapy of lymphoma and CLL. The murine IgG$_{2a}$ MoAb Lym-1 recognizes and binds to an antigen that is present on the majority of B-cell leukemias and lymphomas (20), but does not appear to bind to normal tissues. The antigen to which Lym-1 binds is neither shed nor modulated. The aforementioned characteristics of the antigen, in conjunction with the known stability of Lym-1 after conjugation with radioisotopes, made Lym-1 a suitable MoAb for radioimmunoconjugate therapy. There are several issues that need to be kept in mind when trying to assess the efficacy and overall utility of this form of therapy for CLL patients. In CLL, unlike solid tumors, the radioimmunoconjugate will bind to both circulating and marrow tumor cells and therefore both normal hematopoietic and tumor tissues will be vulnerable to its cytotoxic effects. Consequently, there is great potential for hematologic toxicity. In addition, if responses are seen, it remains difficult to discern if these responses are secondary to the conjugate that is meant to "target" the tumor cell versus the cytotoxicity of the radioisotope alone.

DeNardo et al. (G. L. DeNardo, written communication, 1991) (72) (Table 3) have administered ^{131}I conjugated Lym-1 to five patients with Rai stage III or IV CLL that was refractory to chemotherapy. The peripheral blood lymphocytes from all patients were shown to react with LYM-1. Due to the observation that LYM-1 binds nonspecifically to receptor sites in the liver, 5 mg or greater of cold antibody was given prior to the radioimmunoconjugate. The radioimmunoconjugate was administered 5 min later, with dose ranges varying from 20 to 65 mCi ^{131}I conjugated to 1–8 mg of antibody. Treatments were repeated at 2- to 6-week intervals until significant toxicity occurred, the antibody failed to localize at sites of tumor, HAMA was produced, or patients deteriorated clinically. Patients were also monitored with whole-body planar imaging. Significant decrements in peripheral white blood count were observed, with counts returning to pretreatment levels after a several-month period. All patients were noted to have significant reductions in adenopathy, both by physical examination and on CT scanning. In the majority of patients, decreases in lymphadenopathy were noted within the first week of therapy. Severe, persistent thrombocytopenia developed in three patients who received radionuclide doses of >300 mCi, requiring intermittent platelet support. One patient developed HAMA. No other significant toxicities developed.

These preliminary results suggest the potential utility of radioimmuno-conjugates as a therapeutic modality in CLL. However, as mentioned above, it remains unclear if the observed responses could have been second-ary to ^{131}I administration alone. Ultimately, a comparison with ^{131}I alone would be necessary to truly assess efficacy. In addition, hematologic toxic-ity remains a major problem. This mode of therapy may be of greatest benefit to those patients who have achieved a minimal disease state in the bone marrow with other treatment modalities, with subsequent administra-tion of the radioimmunoconjugate to eradicate the remainder of the tumor cell burden without fear of severe hematologic toxicity. Alternatively, pe-ripheral blood stem cells and/or hematopoietic growth factors could be administered in an effort to rescue the patient from hematologic side ef-fects.

BONE MARROW TRANSPLANTATION

The use of MoAbs bound to immunotoxins or radioisotopes is likely to have a future place in the therapeutic armamentarium for CLL. Further trials remain necessary to optimize proper dosage and schedule of adminis-tration as well as to maximize efficacy and minimize toxicity. However, at present, none of the modalities discussed offers the potential for cure in this disease.

Over the past decade, high-dose ablative therapy rescued with autolo-gous or allogeneic bone marrow has become a standard treatment modality for many patients with lymphoma or leukemia (2,73–75). Lymphoma has become the most common malignancy for which an autologous BMT is performed. Similarly, thousands of patients with leukemia have undergone allogeneic BMT in an effort to cure their disease. In contrast, fewer than 30 patients with CLL have undergone BMT worldwide (76–78). Several factors limit the use of BMT as a standard approach to the management of this disease. The majority of patients with CLL are above the age of 60, making them ineligible for this approach. Indeed, only 43% of patients with CLL have been reported to be less than or equal to the age of 60 (79). BMT continues to be excluded as a treatment option in this group for several reasons, including: (a) the relatively long-term median survival of patients with this disease; (b) the presence of co-morbid disease; and (c) concerns regarding potential morbidity and mortality secondary to trans-plant-related toxicity. However, prognostic factors such as Rai (80) or Binet stage (81), lymphocyte doubling time (82,83), chromosomal abnormalities

(84), and pattern of marrow involvement on bone marrow biopsy (85) can help distinguish those patients who are most likely to have rapidly progressive disease and/or suffer an earlier demise. These poor-prognosis patients, if younger than age 60, may be candidates for BMT. Over the past several years, investigators have begun to assess the curative potential of BMT for this disease. Thus, it is essential that those patients who undergo BMT are carefully assessed for remission status following transplant, utilizing not only routine physical examination, X-ray, CT, and bone marrow evaluations, but also the techniques of flow cytometric analysis and immunoglobulin gene rearrangements. Clearly, the concept of cure cannot be considered in this disease without very long-term assessment (5–10 years).

The largest series has been recently reported by Michallet et al. (78), who undertook a clinical trial utilizing allogeneic BMT in a cohort of 17 patients with CLL. The majority of patients were male, with an overall mean age of 40. Fifteen of the patients were immunologically classified as B-CLL, and 15 were previously resistant to chemotherapy, including chlorambucil, COP, and CHOP. In addition, four of the patients had undergone splenectomy, while two had received prior total nodal irradiation. Twelve patients had Rai stage III or IV disease, two had Rai stage II disease, and three had Rai stage 0 or I disease. Only the Rai stage 0 patient and one Rai stage III patient had not received prior therapy. The median interval between the time of the diagnosis and BMT was 44 months, with a range of 5 to 96 months. The preparative regimen consisted of cyclophosphamide (11 patients), cyclophosphamide and etoposide (4 patients), cyclophosphamide and chlorambucil (1 patient), or cyclophosphamide and melphalan (1 patient) in addition to total body irradiation (TBI) at a dose of 800–1400 cGy. All patients were rescued with bone marrow from HLA-matched sibling donors. Prophylaxis for graft-versus-host disease (GVHD) varied, and included long-term methotrexate (MTX) (1 patient), cyclosporine and short-term MTX (11 patients), cyclosporine alone (2 patients), and cyclosporine and physical T-cell depletion (3 patients).

Fifteen of the 17 patients evidenced stable engraftment. One patient died at day 15 (prior to engraftment), and another had documented graft failure at day 34. The median time to achieve an ANC of $500/mm^3$ was 25 (with a range of day 12–38), while the median time to reach a platelet count of $50/mm^3$ was day 70 (range 30–395). Peripheral blood lymphocytosis persisted until 13 to 28 days after marrow infusion. Except for one patient, all patients demonstrated resolution of lymphadenopathy and organomegaly within 3 to 20 days following bone marrow infusion. All of the 15 evaluable patients developed acute GVHD (grade I, 5; grade II, 5; grade III, 3; grade IV, 2). The two patients with grade IV GVHD died. Five patients developed chronic GVHD.

Fifteen of 16 evaluable patients achieved a complete remission post-BMT. At a median follow-up of 25.6 months (4–48), nine patients remain in continuous complete remission and in good health. Unfortunately, six of these patients died after BMT, including two from relapse of their disease, one from graft failure by day 34, one from intracerebral hemorrhage at day 31, and two from acute GVHD by days 71 and 82, respectively. Of the two relapses, one occurred 7 months following marrow infusion, and the patient died 1 month later. The second relapse occurred 54 months following marrow infusion, and the patient died at 60 months following a second BMT. Nevertheless, the many durable remissions obtained in this population, which included many poor-prognosis patients, is encouraging. However, the procedure was not free of toxicity, particularly an extremely high incidence of GVHD.

Complete chimerism was detected in eight patients either by red blood cell markers (3), sex markers (2) or restriction fragment length polymorphism (RFLP) (3). Two patients who continued in complete remission at 19 and 48 months, respectively, did not show evidence for immunoglobulin gene rearrangements.

Since August 1989, the Dana-Farber Cancer Institute has been conducting a pilot study utilizing high-dose chemoradiotherapy and autologous or allogeneic BM support in patients with Rai stage II, III, or IV B-CLL who were >18 and <60 years of age. Documentation of B-CLL was provided by flow cytometric analysis. All patients were required to achieve a minimal disease state prior to admission for BMT. A minimal disease state was defined as (a) tumor masses <2 cm in greatest diameter as assessed by physical examination, X-ray or CT scanning; (b) BM involvement of 20% or less of the intertrabecular space as assessed by standard bilateral BM biopsies; (c) no CNS involvement; (d) no splenomegaly (as defined by CT scanning). Patients underwent anti-T12 (CD6) antibody-depleted allogeneic BMT (75) if an HLA-identical sibling donor could be identified. All other patients underwent an autologous marrow harvest followed by marrow purging with anti-B1, J5, and B5 MoAbs plus complement (2). The BMT preparative regimen for all patients has been cyclophosphamide (60 mg/kg × 2) and fractionated TBI (total of 1400 cGy).

To date, a total of thirteen patients (ten male, three female) have undergone BMT for CLL. The median age was 40 (range 27–54). All patients had documentation of Rai stage II, III, or IV disease prior to embarking on outpatient therapy to achieve a minimal disease state. Three of the patients had a known family history of CLL, and three patients had trisomy 12 upon cytogenetic analysis. Four patients required splenectomy prior to BMT and were found to have residual CLL in the specimen. Six of the patients underwent autologous BMT, and seven of the patients underwent allogeneic BMT. At the time of BMT, six of the thirteen patients had only <5% involvement of the intertrabecular space by bilateral bone marrow biopsies, while five patients had 5–10% involvement and two patients had complete remission biopsies.

Following bone marrow infusion, all patients showed evidence of engraftment. Within 1 month of marrow infusion, eleven of the twelve evaluable patients had no evidence of CLL by bilateral bone marrow biopsies, aspirates, peripheral blood and bone marrow phenotyping. The patients with trisomy 12 pre-transplant had normal cytogenetics 1 month and 1 year post-transplant. One patient who underwent autologous BMT died at day 60, secondary to severe interstitial pneumonitis. Eleven of the twelve evaluable patients are in complete remission by physical examination, abdominal/pelvic CT, CXR, bilateral bone marrow biopsies, peripheral blood and bone marrow phenotyping at a median of 8 months respectively. Three patients studied for evidence of immunoglobulin gene rearrangements were found to be negative. One of the seven patients who underwent allogeneic BMT developed acute and chronic GVHD of the skin and gastrointestinal tract but remains alive 18 months post-marrow infusion. The other six patients who underwent allogeneic bone marrow transplant did not develop GVHD and remain alive and well at a maximum of 8 months following marrow infusion.

CONCLUSIONS

Standard chemotherapeutic agents in conventional doses remain limited in their ability to have a substantial impact on the survival of the majority of patients with CLL. Factors including common mechanisms of tumor cell resistance, the relatively limited cytotoxic potency of standard therapeutic agents, and the significant nonspecific toxicity of chemoradiotherapy have led to the preliminary evaluation of new modalities of therapy in this disease.

Although the therapies discussed in this chapter have completed only preliminary clinical testing, several conclusions can already be made. First, these therapies can be safely administered to patients, with a tolerable side-effect profile. Indeed, even patients who have had end-organ damage from prior therapies have been able to tolerate the administration of MoAbs, immunotoxins, and radioimmunoconjugates. Second, responses have been observed in patients who were refractory to prior conventional therapies, suggesting that these new modalities may complement rather than replace standard approaches to therapy in patients with CLL. Third, high-dose ablative therapy appears able to induce sustained clinical and cytogenetic remissions in patients with CLL.

Much remains to be learned regarding the application of these new modalities of therapy. The schedule of immunotoxin administration may be critical in evaluating its efficacy, and studies continue to explore the utility of prolonged continuous infusion of these agents. The low serum levels of immunotoxin that have been achieved in patients suggest that these agents might be even more efficacious in a minimal disease state, where therapeutic blood levels could be more easily achieved. BMT may have enhanced efficacy if it can be performed earlier in the patient's disease course, before resistance to chemotherapy develops.

In the past 5 years, immunotoxins, radioimmunoconjugates, and BMT have been introduced to the clinical arena for use in patients with CLL. A remarkable amount of information concerning the use of these agents has already been accumulated. The next decade should witness their broader application in patients with CLL.

ACKNOWLEDGMENT

This work was supported by National Institute of Health CA 34183.

REFERENCES

1. G. Kohler and C. Milstein, Continuous cultures of fused cells secreting antibody of predefined specificity, *Nature, 256*:495–497 (1972).
2. A. S. Freedman, T. Takvorian, K. C. Anderson, et al., Autologous bone marrow transplantation in B-cell non-Hodgkin's lymphoma: Very low treatment-related morality in 100 patients in sensitive relapse, *J. Clin. Oncol., 8*: 784–791 (1990).
3. A. Houghton and D. Scheinberg, Monoclonal antibodies in the treatment of hematopoietic malignancies, *Sem. Hematol., 25*:23–29 (1988).
4. T. Meeker, J. Lowder, M. L. Cleary, et al., Emergence of idiotype variants during treatment of B cell lymphomas with anti-idiotype antibodies, *N. Engl. J. Med. 312*:1658–1665 (1985).
5. S. L. Brown, R. A. Miller, S. J. Horning, et al., Treatment of B-cell lymphomas with anti-idiotype antibodies alone and in combination with alpha interferon, *Blood, 73*:651–661 (1989).
6. A. S. Freedman and L. M. Nadler, B cell development in chronic lymphocytic leukemia. *Sem. Hematol., 24*:230–239 (1987).
7. A. S. Freedman and L. M. Nadler, The relationship of chronic lymphocytic leukemia to normal activated B cells, *Leuk. Lymph., 1*:293–300 (1990).
8. A. S. Freedman, A. W. Boyd, F. Bieber, et al., Normal cellular counterparts of B cell chronic lymphocytic leukemia, *Blood, 70*:418–427 (1987).
9. L. Boumsell, A. Bernard, E. R. Reinherz, et al., Surface antigens on malignant Sezary and T-CLL cells correspond to those of mature T cells, *Blood, 57*:526–530 (1981).
10. M. Kamoun, M. F. Kadin, P. J. Martin, J. Nettleton, and J. A. Hansen, A

novel human T cell antigen preferentially expressed on mature T cells and also on (B type) chronic lymphatic leukemic cells, *J. Immunol., 127*:987–996 (1981).

11. R. T. Perri, I. Royston, T. LeBien, and N. E. Kay, Chronic lymphocytic leukemia progenitor cells carry the antigens T65, BA-1, and Ia, *Blood, 61*: 871–875 (1983).

12. A. S. Freedman, G. Freeman, J. Whitman, et al., Expression and regulation of CD5 on in vitro activated human B cells. *Eur. J. Immunol., 19*:849–855 (1989).

13. A. S. Freedman, G. Freeman, J. Whitman, J. Segil, J. Daley, and L. M. Nadler, Studies on in vitro activated CD5 + B cells, *Blood, 73*:202–208 (1989).

14. L. M. Nadler, K. C. Anderson, G. Marti, et al., B4, a human B cell associated antigen expressed on normal, mitogen activated, and malignant B lymphocytes, *J. Immunol., 131*:244–250 (1983).

15. L. M. Nadler, P. Stashenko, J. Ritz, R. Hardy, J. M. Pesando, and S. F. Schlossman, A unique cell surface antigen identifying lymphoid malignancies of B cell origin, *J. Clin. Invest., 67*:134–140 (1981).

16. G. B. Faguet and J. F. Agee, Monoclonal antibodies against the chronic lymphatic leukemia antigen cCLLa: Characterization and reactivity, *Blood, 70*:437–443 (1987).

17. G. B. Faguet and J. F. Agee, Immunophenotypic diagnosis of clinical and preclinical chronic lymphatic leukemia by using monoclonal antibodies against the cCLLa, a CLL-associated antigen, *Blood, 72*:679–684 (1988).

18. G. B. Faguet and J. F. Agee, Modulation, shedding and serum titers of the chronic lymphatic leukemia associated antigen: Characterization and clinical correlations, *Blood, 74*:2493–2500 (1989).

19. G. B. Faguet and J. F. Agee, A deglycosylated ricin A-chain based immunotoxin directed against the common chronic lymphocytic leukemia antigen (cCLLa): In vitro specificity and cytotoxic activity. *Blood, 76*(suppl. 7):268 (1990).

20. A. L. Epstein, R. J. Marder, J. N. Winter, et al., Two new monoclonal antibodies Lym-1 and Lym-2, reactive with human B-lymphocytes and derived tumors, with immunodiagnostic and immunotherapeutic potential, *Cancer Res., 47*:830–840 (1987).

21. A. W. Boyd, D. C. Fisher, D. Fox, S. F., Schlossman, and L. M. Nadler, Structural and functional characterization of Il-2 receptors on activated B cells, *J. Immunol., 134*:2387–2392 (1985).

22. G. Semenzato, R. Foa, C. Agostini, et al., High serum levels of soluble interleukin-2 receptor in patients with B chronic lymphocytic leukemia, *Blood, 70*: 396–400 (1987).

23. J. W. Lowenthal, R. H., Zubler, H., Nabholz, and H. R. MacDonald, Similarities between interleukin-2 receptor and a number of activated B and T lymphocytes, *Nature, 315*:669–672 (1985).

24. W. Holter, C. K. Goldman, L. Casabo, D. L. Nelson, W. C. Greene, and T. A. Waldmann, Expression of functional IL-2 receptors by lipopolysaccharide and interferon stimulated human monocytes, *J. Immunol., 138*:2917–2922 (1987).

25.   J. L. Preud'homme and M. Seligmann, Surface bound immunoglobulins as a cell marker in human lymphoproliferative diseases, *Blood, 40*:777–791 (1972).

26.   J. L. Preud'homme, J. C. Brouet, J. P. Clauvel, and M. Seligmann, Surface IgD immunoproliferative disorders, *Scand. J. Immunol., 3*:853–859 (1974).

27.   E. M. Swisher, D. L. Shawler, H. A. Collins, et al., Expression of shared idiotypes in chronic lymphocytic leukemia and small lymphocytic lymphoma, *Blood, 77*:1977–1982 (1991).

28.   R. Dadmarz, S. N. Rabinowe, S. A. Cannistra, J. W. Andersen, A. S. Freedman, and L. M. Nadler, Association between clonogenic cell growth and clinical risk group in B-cell chronic lymphocytic leukemia, *Blood, 76*:142–149 (1990).

29.   C. B. Siegall, D. J. FitzGerald, and I. Pastan, Selective killing of tumor cells using EGF or TGF alpha-*Pseudomonas* exotoxin chimeric molecules, *Sem. Cancer Biol., 1*:345–350 (1990).

30.   H. Loberboum-Galski, D. J. FitzGerald, V. Chaudhary, S. Adhya, and I. Pastan, Cytotoxic activity of an interleukin 2 *Pseudomonas* exotoxin chimeric protein produced in *E. coli, Proc. Natl. Acad. Sci. USA, 85*:1922–1926 (1988).

31.   D. P. Williams, P. Parker, P. Bacha, et al., Diphtheria toxin receptor binding domain substitution with interleukin-2: Genetic construction and properties of a diphtheria toxin-related interleukin-2 fusion protein, *Protein Eng., 1*:493–498 (1987).

32.   R. O. Dillman, D. L. Shawler, J. B. Dillman, and I. Royston, Therapy of chronic lymphocytic leukemia and cutaneous T-cell lymphoma with T101 monoclonal antibody, *J. Clin. Oncol., 2*:881–891 (1984).

33.   K. A. Foon, R. W. Schroff, P. A. Bunn, et al., Effects of monoclonal antibody therapy in patients with chronic lymphocytic leukemia, *Blood, 64*:1085–1093 (1984).

34.   R. O. Dillman, J. Beauregard, D. L. Shawler, et al., Continuous infusion of T101 monoclonal antibody in chronic lymphocytic leukemia and cutaneous T-cell lymphoma, *J. Biol. Resp. Modif., 5*:394–410 (1986).

35.   M. J. S. Dyer, G. Hale, F. G. J. Hayhoe, and H. Waldman, Effects of CAMPATH-1 antibodies in vivo in patients with lymphoid malignancies: Influence of antibody isotype, *Blood, 73*:1431–1442 (1989).

36.   A. A. Hertler and A. E. Frankel, Immunotoxins: A clinical review of their use in the treatment of malignancies, *J. Clin. Oncol., 7*:1932–1942 (1989).

37.   I. Pastan, M. C. Willingham, and D. J. FitzGerald, Immunotoxins, *Cell, 47*: 641–648 (1986).

38.   M. L. Grossbard and L. M. Nadler, Immunotoxin therapy of malignancy, in *Important Advances in Oncology* (V. T. DeVita, Jr., S. Hellman, and S. A. Rosenberg, eds.), J. B. Lippincott, Philadelphia, pp. 111–135 (1992).

39.   D. FitzGerald and I. Pastan, Targeted toxin therapy for the treatment of cancer, *J. Natl. Cancer Inst., 81*:1455–1463 (1989).

40.   J. M. Lambert, W. A. Blattler, G. D. McIntyre, V. S. Goldmacher, and C. J. Scott, Immunotoxins containing single-chain ribosome-inactivating proteins, *Cancer Treatment Res., 37*:175–209 (1988).

41.   Y. Endo, K. Mitsui, M. Motizuki, and K. Tsurugi, The mechanism of action

of ricin and related toxic lectins on eukaryotic ribosomes, *J. Biol. Chem.,* 262:5908–5912 (1987).

42. S. Olsnes and K. Sandvig, How protein toxins enter and kill cells, *Cancer Treatment Res., 37*:39–73 (1988).

43. R. J. Youle and J. D. M. Neville, Kinetics of protein synthesis inactivation by ricin-anti Thy 1.1 monoclonal antibody hybrids, *J. Biol. Chem., 257*:1598–1601 (1982).

44. R. J. Collier, Effect of diphtheria toxin on protein synthesis: Inactivation of one of the transfer factors, *J. Mol. Biol., 25*:83–98 (1967).

45. E. S. Vitetta, R. J. Fulton, R. D. May, M. Till, and J. W. Uhr, Redesigning nature's poisons to create anti-tumor reagents, *Science, 238*:1098–1104 (1987).

46. F. K. Jansen, H. E. Blythman, D. Carriere, et al., Immunotoxins: Hybrid molecules combining high specificity and potent cytotoxicity, *Immunol. Rev., 62*:185 (1982).

47. A. A. Hertler, D. M. Schlossman, M. J. Borowitz, H. E. Blythman, P. Casellas, and A. E. Frankel, An anti-CD5 immunotoxin for chronic lymphocytic leukemia: Enhancement of cytotoxicity with human serum albumin-monensin, *Int. J. Cancer, 43*:215–219 (1989).

48. G. Laurent, J. Pris, J. P. Farcet, et al., Effects of therapy with T101 ricin A-chain immunotoxin in two leukemia patients, *Blood, 67*:1680–1687 (1986).

49. A. A. Hertler, D. M. Schlossman, M. J. Borowitz, et al., A phase I study of T101-ricin A chain immunotoxin in refractory chronic lymphocytic leukemia, *J. Biol. Resp. Modif., 7*:97–113 (1988).

50. P. Casellas and F. K. Jansen, Immunotoxin enhancers, in *Immunotoxins* (A. E. Frankel, ed.), Kluwer, Norwell, MA, pp. 351–368 (1988).

51. F. LeMaistre, A. Deisseroth, B. Fogel, et al., Phase I trial of H65-RTA in patients with chronic lymphocytic leukemia, *Blood, 76*(suppl. 1):295a (1990).

52. B. J. P. Bourrie, P. Casellas, H. E. Blythman, and F. K. Jansen, Study of the plasma clearance of antibody ricin-A-chain immunotoxins. Evidence for specific recognition sites on the A-chain that mediate rapid clearance of the immunotoxin, *Eur. J. Biochem., 155*:1–10 (1986).

53. D. C. Blakey, G. J. Watson, P. P. Knowles, and P. E. Thorpe, Effect of chemical deglycosylation of ricin A chain on the in-vivo fate and cytotoxic activity and anti-Thy 1.1 antibody. *Cancer Res., 47*:947–952 (1987).

54. S. Siena, S. Villa, M. Bregni, G. Bonadonna, and A. M. Gianni, Amantadine potentiates T-lymphocyte killing by an anti-pan-T cell (CD5) ricin A-chain immunotoxin, *Blood, 69*:345–348 (1987).

55. R. O. Dillman, D. L. Shawler, R. E. Sobol, et al., Murine monoclonal antibody therapy in two patients with chronic lymphocytic leukemia, *Blood, 59*:1036–1045 (1982).

56. J. F. Agee, F. Garver, and G. B. Faguet, An antigen common to chronic lymphocytic and hairy cell leukemia not shared by normal lymphocytes nor by other leukemic cells, *Blood, 68*:62–68 (1986).

57. L. M. Nadler, B cell leukemia panel workshop: Summary and comments, *Leukocyte Typing II* (E. L. Reinherz, F. B. Haynes, L. M. Nadler, and I. D. Bernstein, eds.), Springer-Verlag, New York, p. 3 (1986).

58. K. C. Anderson, M. P. Bates, B. L. Slaughenhoupt, G. S. Pinkus, S. F. Schlossman, and L. M. Nadler, Expression of human B cell-associated antigens on leukemias and lymphomas. A model of human B cell differentiation, *Blood, 63*:1424–1433 (1984).

59. A. S. Freedman and L. M. Nadler, Cell surface markers in hematologic malignancies, *Sem. Oncol., 14*:193–214 (1987).

60. M. L. Grossbard, A. S. Freedman, J. Ritz, et al., Serotherapy of B-cll neoplasms with Anti-B4-blocked ricin: A Phase I trial of daily bolus infusion, *Blood, 79*:576–585 (1992).

61. P. Bacha, D. P. Williams, C. Waters, J. R. Murphy, and T. B. Strom, Interleukin-2 receptor cytotoxicity: Interleukin-2 receptor-mediated action of a diphtheria toxin-related interleukin-2 fusion protein, *J. Exp. Med., 167*:612–622 (1988).

62. K. Teshigawara, H. M. Wang, K. Kato, and K. A. Smith, Interleukin-2 high-affinity receptor expression requires two distinct binding proteins, *J. Exp. Med., 165*:223–238 (1987).

63. A. Rosolen, M. Nakanishi, and D. G. Poplack, Expression of interleukin-2 receptor β subunit in hematopoietic malignancies, *Blood, 73*:1968–1972 (1989).

64. F. Lemaistre, S. Maneghetti, M. Rosenblum, et al., A genetically engineered ligand-toxin, DAB_{486} IL-2 is active in the treatment of hematologic malignancies expressing the IL-2 receptor. *Anti. Immunocon. and Radiopharm., 4*(2): 205 (1991).

65. C. F. LeMaistre, M. G. Rosenblum, J. S. Reuben, et al., Therapeutic effects of genetically engineered toxin (DAB_{486}IL-2) in patient with chronic lymphocytic leukemia, *Lancet, 337*:1124–1125 (1991).

66. B. P. Cheson, J. M. Bennett, and K. R. Rai, Guidelines for clinical protocols for chronic lymphocytic leukemia: Recommendations of the National Cancer Institute-sponsored working group. *Am. J. Hematol., 29*:152–163 (1988).

67. R. E. Johnson, Total body irradiation: Relationship between therapeutic response and prognosis, *Cancer, 37*:2691–2696 (1976).

68. R. E. Johnson, Radiotherapy as primary treatment for chronic lymphocytic leukemia, *Clin. Hematol., 6*:237–244 (1977).

69. R. E. Johnson, Treatment of chronic lymphocytic leukemia by total body irradiation alone and combined with chemotherapy, *J. Radiat. Oncol. Biol. Phys., 5*:159–164 (1979).

70. E. E. Osgood, Treatment of chronic leukemias, *J. Nucl. Med., 5*:139 (1964).

71. E. E. Osgood, A. J. Seaman, and H. Tivey, Comparative survival times of X-ray treated versus ^{32}P treated patients with chronic leukemias under the program of titrated regularly spaced total body irradiation, *Radiology, 64*:373 (1955).

72. J. P. Lewis, G. L. DeNardo, S. J. Denardo, S. J. DeNardo, and L. F. O'Grady, Impact of Lym-1 radioimmuno-conjugate on refractory chronic lymphocytic leukemia (CLL), *Blood*, 295a (1990).

73. J. O. Armitage, Bone marrow transplantation in the treatment of patients with lymphoma, *Blood, 73*:1749–1758 (1989).

74. F. B. Petersen, F. R. Appelbaum, R. Hill, et al., Autologous marrow trans-

plantation for malignant lymphoma: A report of 101 cases from Seattle, *J. Clin. Oncol., 8*:638–647 (1990).

75. J. Ritz, T. Takvorian, L. M. Nadler, et al., Prevention of graft-versus-host disease by selective T-cell depletion of bone marrow with anti-T12 monoclonal antibody, *Blood, 72*(suppl. 1):403a (1988).

76. G. Bandini, M. Michallet, G. Rosgi, and S. Tura, Bone marrow transplantation for chronic lymphocytic leukemia, *Bone Marrow Transpl., 7*:251–253 (1991).

77. M. Michallet, B. Corront, D. Hollard, et al., Allogeneic bone marrow transplantation in chronic lymphocytic leukemia: 9 cases. *Bone Marrow Transpl., 4*(suppl. 2):12 (1988).

78. M. Michallet, B. Corront, D. Hollard, et al., Allogeneic bone marrow transplantation in chronic lymphocytic leukemia: 17 cases. Report from the EBMTG. *Bone Marrow Transpl., 7*:275–279 (1991).

79. J. S. Lee, D. O. Dixon, H. M. Kantarjian, M. J. Keating, and M. Talpaz, Prognosis of chronic lymphocytic leukemia: A multivariate regression analysis of 325 untreated patients, *Blood, 69*:929–936 (1987).

80. K. R. Rai, A. Sawitsky, E. P. Cronkite, A. Charana, R. N. Levy, and B. S. Pasternack, Clinical staging of chronic lymphocytic leukemia, *Blood, 46*:219–234 (1975).

81. J. Binet, A. Auquier, G. Dighiero, et al., A new prognostic classification of chronic lymphocytic leukemia derived from multivariate survival analysis, *Cancer, 48*: 198–206 (1981).

82. E. Montseratt, J. Sanchez-Bisono, N. Vinolas, and C. Rozmar, Lymphocyte doubling time in chronic lymphocytic leukaemia: Analysis of its prognostic significance, *Br. J. Haematol., 62*:567 (1986).

83. N. Vinolas, J. S. Reverter, A. Urbano-Ispizua, et al., Lymphocyte doubling time in chronic lymphocytic leukemia: An update of its prognostic significance, *Blood Cells, 12*:457 (1987).

84. G. Juliusson, D. G., Oscier, M. Fitchett, et al., Prognostic subgroups in B-cell CLL defined by specific chromosomal abnormalities, *N. Engl. J. Med., 323*: 720–724 (1990).

85. C. Rozman and E. Montserrat, Bone marrow biopsy in chronic lymphocytic leukemia, *Nouv. Rev. Fr. Hematol., 30*:369–371 (1988).

17

Diagnosis and Treatment
of CLL Variants

Daniel Catovsky
Royal Marsden Hospital, Institute of Cancer Research, London, England

INTRODUCTION

It has become apparent during the last decade that there is great heterogeneity within the lymphoid leukemias, a group of disorders that tend to center around chronic lymphocytic leukemia (CLL). These conditions were recognized when surface markers, chiefly monoclonal antibodies (MoAbs), were introduced for routine use in diagnosis and when greater attention was paid to morphologic detail and histologic patterns of infiltration. The FAB group acknowledged the new findings and published proposals aimed at classifying more objectively the B- and T-lymphoid leukemias (1). These have allowed a more objective evaluation of the clinical and therapeutic significance of the various disease entities.

In parallel with advances in diagnosis, a number of new and promising treatment modalities have emerged, chiefly interferon-α with activity in hairy cell leukemia (HCL) and a group of nucleoside analogs (2,3) with efficacy in selective lymphoid disorders, of which fludarabine monophosphate for the treatment of CLL is the best example (4).

This chapter will focus on the lymphoproliferative diseases that more often resemble CLL and that can loosely be described as "CLL variants," although they bear little resemblance to CLL on close analysis. Our group has been involved in clarifying the nature of some of the disorders that are often confused with CLL and has accumulated a large experience in their diagnosis over many years. As a result of this work, a number of discrete syndromes have emerged (5), such as three types of leukemic phase of non-Hodgkin's lymphoma (6–8), a form of splenic lymphoma with circulating villous lymphocytes (9,10), two different types of prolymphocytic leukaemia (B- and T-PLL) (4,11,12), large granular lymphocytic (LGL) leukemia (10), etc. In this context, it is important to recognize that there is clinical and morphologic heterogeneity even in bona fide CLL, on account not only of the well-known clinical stages but also on subtle degrees of transformation that are part of the natural evolution of the disease (5,13,14).

METHODOLOGY

Although relatively simple techniques are needed, high standards of excellence are required to produce the necessary results. The principal methods for the diagnosis of lymphoid leukemias are, in order of importance, (a) peripheral blood films; (b) membrane markers; (c) bone marrow aspirates and/or trephine core biopsies; (d) lymph node and/or spleen histology if such tissues are involved and available for study. Other investigations that

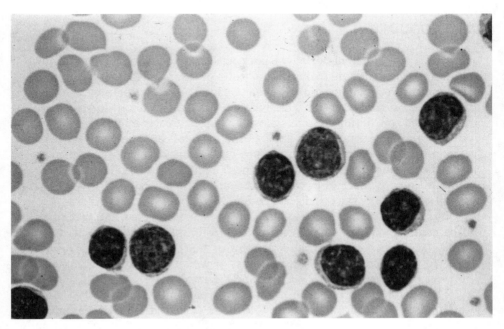

Figure 1   Peripheral blood film of a typical case of B-cell CLL.

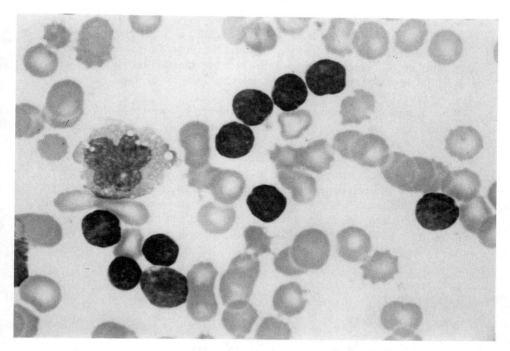

Figure 2 Peripheral blood film of a case of follicular lymphoma in leukemic phase. Note the very small cell size, by comparison with a monocyte, the lack of visible cytoplasm, and the cleaved nuclei in several cells.

may provide useful diagnostic information are cytochemistry, i.e., tartrate-resistant acid phosphatase (TRAP); protein electrophoresis and search for free light chains in the urine; imaging procedures, e.g., abdominal CT scans; etc. Rarely is one of the above tests sufficient for the correct diagnosis and classification. Often it is the combined information derived from them that provides the clues leading to a firm diagnosis.

The pathogenesis of lymphoid malignancies can now be studied with a new generation of research tools, some of which are also rapidly becoming routine diagnostic procedures, namely, chromosome analysis, immunoglobulin (Ig) and T-cell receptor (TCR) gene rearrangements, Southern blots, and PCR for the investigation of specific genes and chromosome breakpoint regions, i.e., c-myc, bcl-1, bcl-2, etc.

The careful preparation and examination of peripheral blood films is critical for the differential diagnosis between CLL (Fig. 1) and the seemingly similar blood picture of small-cell follicular lymphoma (FL) presenting with leukocytosis (6; Fig. 2), or for investigating the subtle changes in

CLL with an increased proportion of prolymphocytes, designated CLL/PL (13; Fig. 3), or of immunoblasts (Fig. 4). Because it is not possible to rely only on morphologic analysis in conditions that may resemble each other in a number of respects, a minimum number of immunologic markers is essential to determine, in the first instance, the B- or T-cell nature of proliferation (1,5,15).

When applying cell markers, it is important to be aware of some technical details that may alter the interpretation of results. For example, the density of Ig staining on the surface of B lymphocytes is weaker in B-CLL and strong in most other B-cell leukemias, but this can only be assessed with certainty if tests are performed on free-flowing cell suspensions rather than on cells fixed on tissues or on cytospin slides and tested by immunocytochemical methods. It is also necessary to know that some specific B- and T-cell antigens may be expressed differently, depending on the stages of cell maturation. For example, CD22, a B-cell antigen, and CD3, a T-cell antigen, are first detected on the cytoplasm, but not on the membrane, of

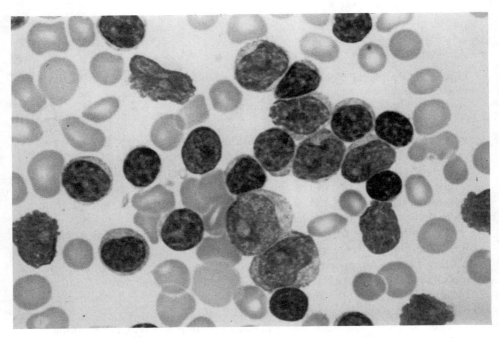

Figure 3 Peripheral blood film of a case of CLL/PL(B-CLL with more than 10% prolymphocytes); prolymphocytes are larger than lymphocytes and have a prominent nucleolus.

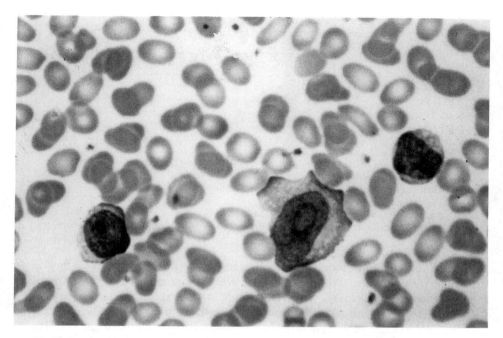

Figure 4 Blood film from a case of CLL in immunoblastic transformation. The large immunoblast has abundant basophilic cytoplasm and a prominent central nucleolus.

B and T cells, respectively, during the early maturation stages, and therefore will score as negative by flow cytometry analysis. On the other hand, these antigens are expressed in the membrane as well as in the cytoplasm in later stages of maturation. CD22, for example, is detected in the cytoplasm of early B-lineage lymphoblasts, in acute lymphoblastic leukemia (ALL), is weakly expressed (or negative) on the membrane of B-CLL lymphocytes, and is strongly expressed in the membrane of other neoplastic B cells (16; Table 1). Thus, for the differential diagnosis of B-CLL and related disorders, CD22 should be tested in suspension. In these diseases, cytoplasmic staining will be useful to ascertain that the cells are B and not T but will not differentiate CLL from its variants. Membrane staining will help distinguish CLL (weak or negative result) from other B-cell diseases (strong expression). The cytoplasmic detection of CD22 is important in ALL to determine the B lineage of immature lymphoblasts.

Bone marrow is the next key investigation. While aspirates provide additional morphologic information, particularly in cases with low white blood

Table 1 Differential Expression of Antigens in B- and T-Cell Leukemias

Antigen localization	CD22		CD3	
	Membrane[a]	Cytopl.[b]	Membrane[a]	Cytopl.[b]
ALL (B)	−	+	−	−
ALL (T)	−	−	−	+
B-CLL	+/−	+	−	−
B-PLL[c]	+	+	−	−
T-PLL[d]	−	−	+	+

[a]Cells in suspension tested by flow cytometry or fluorescence microscopy.
[b]Cells fixed in tissues or cytospin slides tested by immunocytochemistry (immunoperoxidase or immuno alkaline phosphatase anti-alkaline phosphatase) or by immunofluorescence.
[c]Prototype B disease; similar results in HCL and NHL (Table 4).
[d]Prototype T disease; similar results in other mature T-cell disorders (Table 9).

cell count (WBC), blood films are preferable for this purpose in cases with high WBC counts. Trephine biopsies will give details of the patterns of lymphocytic infiltration, which is variable in CLL according to the stage of the disease—e.g., interstitial, nodular, mixed, or diffuse—and has distinct features in some other processes—i.e., paratrabecular involvement in NHL, loose cell infiltration with increased reticulin in hairy cell leukemia (HCL), etc. Histology of the affected tissues (chiefly lymph nodes) is also an essential investigation for the differential diagnosis between CLL and the leukemic phase of NHL.

CLASSIFICATION OF B- AND T-CELL LEUKEMIAS

Here we will consider only leukemias arising from immunologically mature B and T cells. Lymphoblastic disorders (B- and T-lineage ALL) are not included. The first important distinction is between B and T disorders and the second, whether the disease is a primary leukemia or represents the leukemic phase of a NHL (leukemia/lymphoma syndrome). The most common conditions are listed in Tables 2 and 3. As the B-cell lymphoproliferative disorders are more common than the T-cell ones, these will be discussed in greater detail here.

THE MORPHOLOGIC HETEROGENEITY OF B-CLL

When considering the possible CLL variants, it should be borne in mind that CLL shows a degree of morphologic heterogeneity. Cases defined as CLL/PL have, by definition, more than 10% prolymphocytes (Fig. 3).

Table 2 Lymphoid Leukemias and Leukemia/Lymphoma
Syndromes of B-Cell Type

Primary leukemias
   Chronic lymphocytic leukemia (B-CLL)
   Prolymphocytic leukemia (B-PLL)
   Hairy cell leukemia (HCL)
   HCL variant
NHL in leukemic phase
   Splenic lymphoma with circulating villous lymphocytes (SLVL)
   Follicular lymphoma
   Intermediate (mantle zone)
   Large-cell lymphoma

Rare cases show a gradual increase in prolymphocytes, reaching close to the picture of B-PLL (13), which is defined as having more than 50% prolymphocytes. Evaluation of cell size by volume measurements always confirms in CLL/PL a dual cell population, which contrasts with the more uniform cell size of B-PLL. These studies have also shown that the size of the small-cell component is larger than the lymphocytes in uncomplicated CLL (14).

The typical membrane phenotype of B-CLL (Table 4) is also seen in most cases of CLL/PL, although in the latter it is not unusual to demonstrate some atypical findings, e.g., positive FMC7 or mCD22. An immunoblastic component (Fig. 4) is less frequent in peripheral blood films and, when present, often correlates with Richter transformation in lymphoid tissues (see below). When the large cells become a major feature, the differential diagnosis arises with large-cell NHL in leukemic phase (8).

The main diagnostic problem in CLL/PL is its distinction from the leukemic phase of mantle zone (or intermediate) NHL (1,7). The morphol-

Table 3 Lymphoid Leukemias and Leukemia/Lymphoma
Syndromes of T-Cell Type

Primary leukemias
   Large granular lymphocyte (LGL) leukemia
   Prolymphocytic leukemia (T-PLL)
NHL in leukemic phase
   Adult T-cell leukemia/lymphoma (ATLL) HTLV-I(+)
   Sezary syndrome
   Peripheral T-cell lymphoma HTLV-I(−)
   Large-cell lymphoma

Table 4 Differences in Immunophenotype Between CLL and Related B-Cell Disorders

Marker	B-CLL	B-PLL	NHL[a]	HCL
SmIg	Weak	←	Strong	→
CD5	+	−/+	−/+[b]	−
CD10	−	−	−/+[c]	−
CD11c	−[d]	−	−/+[d]	+ +
FMC7	−	+	+	+
mCD22	−	+	+	+
CD23	+	−	−	−
CD25/HC2	−	−	−	+ +[e]
B-ly-7	−	−	−	+ +[f]

[a]Follicular lymphoma, mantle-zone lymphoma, and SLVL.
[b]Positive in mantle-zone lymphoma and in 10% of SLVL.
[c]Positive in follicular lymphoma.
[d]Weakly expressed in 20% of B-CLL and 10% of SLVL.
[e]Negative in HCL variant
[f]Some HCL variant and occasional SLVL cases are B-ly-7 positive but never strongly positive as in HCL.

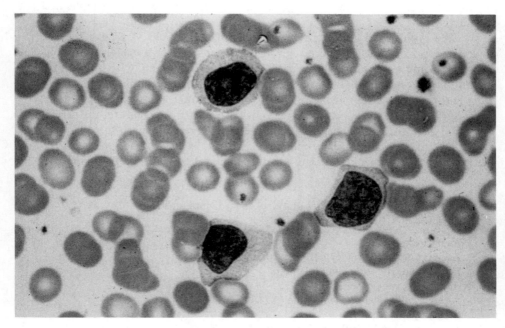

Figure 5 Blood film from a case of intermediate (mantle-zone) lymphoma. The cells are larger than those of CLL and follicular lymphoma and have more cytoplasm.

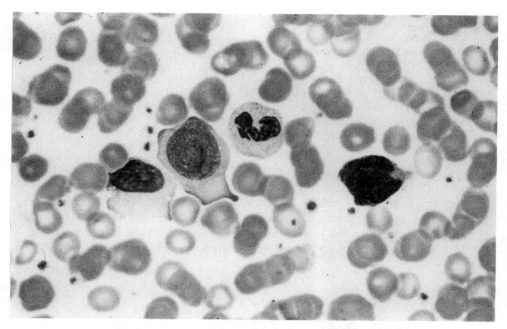

Figure 6 Circulating cells from another case of mantle-zone lymphoma. There is morphologic pleomorphism with medium and large size cells, some with irregular or indented nucleus.

ogy in such cases (Figs. 5 and 6) presents a degree of pleomorphism, with a mixture of medium and large cells, which can be confused with CLL of mixed cell type (1). This is compounded by the CD5 positivity of both these B-cell disorders, although other markers are different (Table 4).

The negative prognostic significance of the increased number of prolymphocytes in CLL/PL has been shown in two independent studies (17,18). It seems important when evaluating new therapies in CLL, such as fludarabine, to define the responses also according to this cytologic feature. Preliminary results from the M. D. Anderson group suggest a 50% response rate in CLL/PL with fludarabine phosphate (19).

B-CELL PROLYMPHOCYTIC LEUKEMIA

The classic definition of PLL by Galton et al. (11) referred to the B-cell form of the disease, which constitutes a distinct disease entity. The main features are summarized in Table 5 and the immunophenotype, by compari-

Table 5   Main Disease Features of B-PLL

Splenomegaly (> 10 cm b.c.m.)
No peripheral lymphadenopathy
Anemia (Hb < 10 g/dL)
Thrombocytopenia (platelets < 100 × 10^9/L)
High WBC (> 100 × 10^9/L)
No response to alkylating agents or prednisolone
Response to splenic irradiation, CHOP, and fludarabine
Worse prognosis than CLL

son with CLL, is listed in Table 4. Morphologically, B-PLL has a homogeneous picture (Figs. 7 and 8). The most characteristic feature of prolymphocytes is a prominent central nucleolus in a cell with relatively condensed
nuclear chromatin. The larger cell size of prolymphocytes, by comparison
with CLL lymphocytes, is best appreciated by cell volume estimations

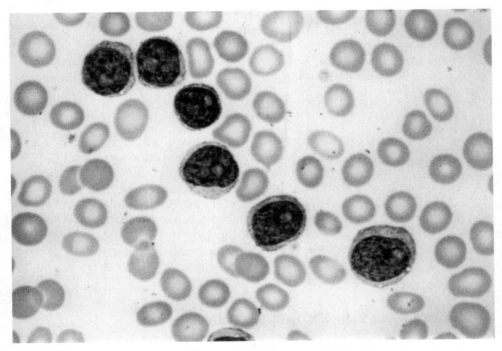

Figure 7   Peripheral blood film from a case of B-cell PLL. The prolymphocytes
are slightly larger than the CLL cells of Fig. 1, and each has a distinct nucleolus.

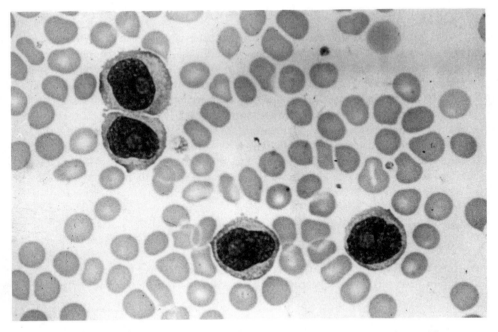

Figure 8 Blood film from another B-PLL; here the prolymphocytes are larger than those of Fig.7 and have a more abundant and moderately basophilic cytoplasm.

rather than in blood films, where the cell size may appear different according to the part of the film examined.

Therapy of B-PLL

B-PLL is, as a rule, refractory to alkylating agents and prednisolone, agents commonly used in CLL (5). Responses have been recorded to the combination CHOP, splenic irradiation, and splenectomy. The latter often needs to be followed by additional measures (5). We have observed partial responses to 2'-deoxycoformycin (DCF) in two of four patients (20). Kantarjian et al. reported responses with fludarabine in CLL/PL and some B-PLL, although they have defined the latter as having more than 30% prolymphocytes and cases with more than 50% prolymphocytes did not respond (19). A complete remission was reported by Whelan et al. (21) in a typical B-PLL, and we have recently documented a good partial remission in another. A further patient treated by us with very high WBC ($>500 \times 10^9/L$) and evidence of immunoblastic transformation in the bone marrow failed to respond.

HAIRY CELL LEUKEMIA AND HCL-VARIANT

It is beyond the scope of this chapter to describe in detail the main diagnostic features of HCL (5). The diagnosis of HCL can be made by peripheral blood films (Figs. 9 and 10), bone marrow biopsy (5), and immunophenotype (Table 4). The importance of HCL is that it shows the relevance of identifying discrete disease entities that respond selectively to some therapies and not to others. HCL shows exquisite sensitivity to interferon-α (5), DCF (2), and chlorodeoxyadenosine (3). It is of interest that a recently described variant form (HCL-V), which has morphologic features intermediate between HCL and B-PLL (Fig. 11), and has a number of other differences with typical HCL (Table 6), does not respond to interferon-α and very little to DCF (5,22).

SPLENIC LYMPHOMA WITH CIRCULATING
VILLOUS LYMPHOCYTES

Since the report by Neiman et al. (23), pathologists have become aware of patients treated by splenectomy with a diagnosis of HCL but with the

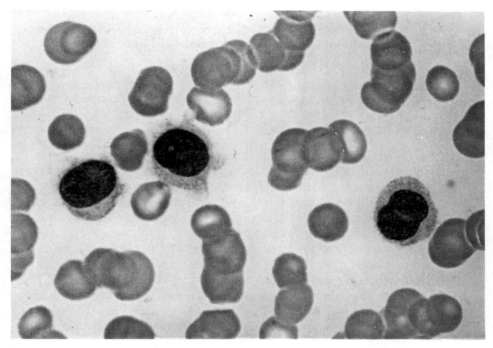

Figure 9   Circulating hairy cells from a case of HCL.

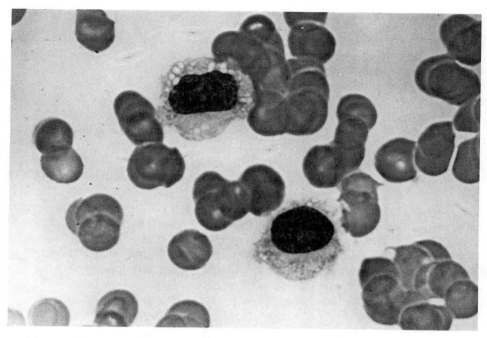

Figure 10 Blood film from another case of HCL with slightly larger hairy cells than those of Fig. 9.

spleen histology failing to demonstrate the typical features of the disease. The majority of such cases correspond to what we have described as SLVL (9,10), a disorder that is relatively frequent within the group of patients presenting with splenomegaly and lymphocytosis (Table 7).

The circulating lymphocytes in SLVL (Fig. 12) have fine villous projections, a moderately basophilic cytoplasm, and, depending on the cell size, small or medium, they tend to be confused with CLL or HCL. In half of the cases, SLVL cells have a visible nucleolus, but they rarely resemble prolymphocytes. The cytoplasm is less abundant than in hairy cells and tends to have the projections concentrated in one pole of the cell.

SLVL seems to affect primarily the spleen, with little or no bone marrow involvement in the early phases of the disease (9). The pattern of splenic infiltration is primarily in the white pulp (in contrast with HCL and HCL-V) but also showing spillover to the red pulp. Plasmacytic differentiation is observed in the spleen and in the peripheral blood. Therefore this condition can be classified as low-grade lymphoma, both in the Working Formulation (A, plasmacytoid) and in the Kiel classification (LP immunocytoma) (24). The plasma cell differentiation is supported by evidence of discrete mono-

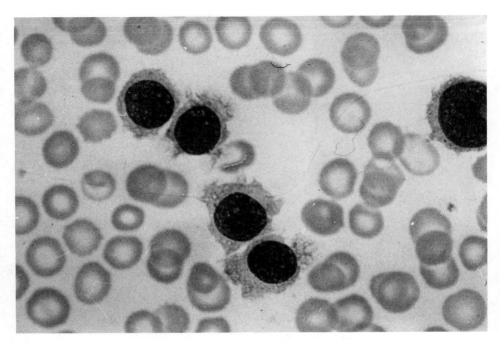

Figure 11 Peripheral blood film from a variant form of HCL. The nucleus is round, the nucleolus is visible but small; in cases the nucleolus is more prominent and resembles that of prolymphocytes.

Table 6 Features of HCL and Its Variant Form

Feature	HCL	HCL-V
Age (years)	40–50	>60
M : F ratio	5 : 1	1.4 : 1
WBC ($\times$ 10^9/L)	<10	>40
Monocytopenia	Present	Absent
HCL antigens[a]	Present	Only CD11c and B-ly-7 in some
Heavy-chain isotypes	IgM, D, G, A	IgC (IgA)
Response to IFN-α and 2′-deoxy-coformycin	Good	Poor

[a]CD11c, HC2, CD25, B-ly-7 (Table 4).

Table 7   Main Features of SLVL

Splenomegaly
WBC 10-30 $\times$ 10^9/L
M band and/or free light chains in the urine (65%)
No monocytopenia
Good response to splenectomy, sometimes to splenic irradia-
tion and, rarely, to alkylating agents
Good prognosis (median survival > 10 years)

clonal bands in the serum (usually less than 20 g/L) and/or of free light chains in the urine.

The membrane phenotype of SLVL cells is similar to that of other NHL and distinct from HCL. mainly by the lack of expression of the HCL "antigens" (Table 4), except for CD11c in 50% of cases. In contrast to CLL, most SLVL cases are CD5 − and CD23 − .

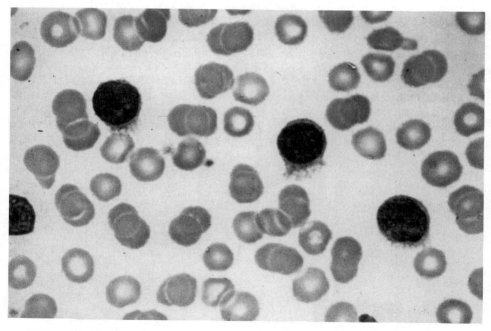

Figure 12   Peripheral blood film from a case of SLVL. The cells are smaller than both HCL and HCL-variant cells and have less abundant cytoplasm, which appears villous in one pole of the cell.

Cytogenetic analysis shows that 20% of cases have the translocation t(11;14)(q13;q32) (D. Oscier, E. Matutes, and V. Brito-Babapulle, personal communication), a feature seen also in intermediate (mantle-zone)/centrocytic NHL (25,26). Further studies are necessary to determine whether the break point in chromosome 11q13 involving the bcl-1 oncogene is similar in both these conditions.

Treatment of SLVL

The treatment of choice in SLVL is splenectomy, which further supports the concept of a primary splenic origin for the disease. Not infrequently, lymphocyte counts regress following splenectomy (10,24) together with the improvement of the Hb and platelet counts. We have reviewed our experience in 50 patients and shown that the disease has a very good prognosis, remaining stable for many years (10). Splenic irradiation may be indicated when splenectomy is contraindicated for medical reasons. The response to CLL-type therapy with chlorambucil or the combination COP (cyclophosphamide, oncovin, and prednisolone) is effective in only one-third of patients. Although not recognized initially, we have recently documented Richter-type transformation (large-cell lymphoma) in three patients, in one after 20 years of stable disease. There is no experience of the response of SLVL to interferon-α or to any of the new nucleoside analogs.

CLL/HCL "HYBRIDS"

Three recent reports in the American literature (27–29) have suggested the existence of "hybrid" lymphoproliferative disorders with features intermediate between CLL and HCL based largely on the expression of CD11c, a member of the family of cell adhesion molecules known as integrins (27–29). The CD11c antigen is not unique to HCL, as it is also expressed in CLL and SLVL, although infrequently (Table 4). Except for the case report of Sun et al. (27), none of the others (28,29) discuss the possibility that some of the CD11c+ cases were examples of SLVL. None of this group of patients represent, in fact, new disease entities. The case of Sun et al. (27) is compatible with the variant form of HCL (1,5,22; see above), which is supported by the expression of IgG as the main membrane immunoglobulin and the involvement of the splenic red pulp, characteristic of both HCL and its variant (22).

Hanson et al. (28) described 14 patients with splenomegaly, no lymphadenopathy, moderate lymphocytosis with B cells positive for CD11c (half of them CD5−). These features, and the presence of a monoclonal band in one of the five tested, suggest that some of these cases could have been diagnosed as SLVL (5,9, see above), a disease not considered by these authors, and others examples of CLL with expression of CD11c. Wormsley et al. (29) described 26 cases of CLL that were both CD5+ and CD11c+. Clinical and morphologic features were reviewed in 14, and only six had splenomegaly. This and the fact that CD5 is expressed only in 10% of SLVLs suggest that these cases were not examples of this disease. The overall phenotype of the circulating cells was more consistent with B-CLL (see Table 4), although half of the cases had strong expression of SmIg. The latter cases, together with the expression of CD5 and CD11c, are compatible with intermediate (mantle-zone) NHL in leukemic phase (see below), also suggested by the larger size of the circulating lymphocytes (19).

FOLLICULAR LYMPHOMA IN LEUKEMIC PHASE

Spiro et al. (30) described, in a seminal paper, the morphologic features of the most common form of leukemic phase in NHL, which is seen in one-third of cases of follicular lymphoma. This leukemia/lymphoma syndrome is often confused with, and should be distinguished from, CLL (6,27) and is defined by lymphocyte counts greater than $5 \times 10^9/L$. In the series by Spiro et al. (30), the highest lymphocyte counts were $30 \times 10^9/L$, but we have subsequently reported a series of patients with counts greater than $45 \times 10^9/L$ (6) and have since studied several other cases. It is precisely in the high-count cases where the diagnosis of CLL is always considered first. Cases of follicular lymphoma with blood involvement represent one extreme of the spectrum of this disease. In at least 50% of cases of follicular lymphoma there is evidence of bone marrow infiltration, usually paratrabecular deposits, as seen in trephine biopsies. In a proportion of these cases a degree of spillover to the blood can be demonstrated by flow cytometry analysis showing light-chain restriction even when WBC is normal and there is no apparent lymphocytosis.

The differential diagnosis between B-cell CLL and the leukemic phase of follicular lymphoma can easily be made if enough attention is paid to the morphology of the circulating NHL cells (Fig. 2). The cleaved cells of follicular lymphoma are very small, have little or no visible cytoplasm, have a smooth rather than clumped nuclear chromatin pattern (as seen in CLL), and have an irregular or angular nuclear outline with characteristic nuclear clefts or thin indentations (Fig. 2). The diagnosis should be suspected by the membrane phenotype, which characteristically shows a "non-CLL pattern" (1,6; Table 4): the small lymphoma cells express strongly SmIg, are CD5 and CD23 negative (in most cases) and are CD10, FMC7, and mCD22 positive. The immunologic findings are particularly useful in borderline cases and in those in which a lymph node biopsy is not available for study. Whenever possible, lymph node biopsy should be performed to confirm the diagnosis. In our experience, the small-cell type of follicular lymphoma predominates over the mixed small- and large-cell type (or centroblastic-centrocytic in the Kiel classification). The bone marrow trephine is no longer paratrabecular, but shows a more extensive diffuse pattern.

On clinical grounds, patients with follicular lymphoma in leukemic phase tend to be younger than those with CLL and, when WBCs are high, have bulky disease with hepatosplenomegaly and lymphadenopathy (Table 8).

This small-cell leukemic phase is not the only leukemia/lymphoma syndrome seen in follicular lymphoma. A blastic phase is also seen, but this is often a terminal event (30) and a manifestation of malignant transformation. Not infrequently, the blood picture in these cases resembles, and is confused with, acute lymphoblastic leukemia, although there is often a small cleaved cell population coexisting with the larger, often nucleolated blasts (centroblasts). This transformation should be considered with the leukemic phase of large-cell lymphoma (8) as, at this point, the lymph node appearances will have changed to those of a large-cell (high-grade) tumor.

In this context, it should be noted that another rather special form of acute leukemic transformation is seen in follicular lymphoma, with blasts resembling Burkitt cells, which have, in addition to the translocation t(14;18) characteristic of follicular lymphoma, one of the translocations associated with Burkitt's lymphoma, frequently t(8;14) (31) and, rarely, t(18:22).

The leukemic phase of follicular lymphoma can now be diagnosed more objectively by cytogenetic and/or DNA analysis, taking advantage of the fact that in 70–80% of cases the disease is associated with the translocation t(14;18)(q32;q21) with major or minor breakpoints in band q21 of chromo-

Table 8 The Leukemic Phase of B-Cell NHL
(Leukemia/Lymphoma Syndromes)

Disease features	Follicular lymphoma	Mantle zone	Large cell
Age[a]	51	66	71
Hb (g/dL)[a]	11.2	12	10.6
Platelets ($\times$ 10^9/L)[a]	147	200	129
WBC ($\times$ 10^9/L)[a]	103	45	56
Splenomegaly	100%	64%	62%
Hepatomegaly	80%	49%	44%
Lymphadenopathy	90%	82%	69%
Survival[a]	3 years	2 years	3.5 months

[a]Median values from our published cases (Refs. 6,7,8).

some 18 and the consequent rearrangement of the bcl-2 gene, which is localized in that region (32).

Treatment of Follicular Lymphoma in Leukemic Phase

Patients presenting with lymphocyte counts greater than $45 \times 10^9/L$ seem to respond poorly to the conventional alkylating agent/corticosteroid therapy that is effective in the less aggressive forms of follicular lymphoma. In our experience, combinations with anthracyclines, e.g., CHOP, or using mitozantrone instead of an anthracycline, are only partially effective. The new agent fludarabine (4) may hold promise in this area. We recently observed a good partial (PR) and a complete remission (CR) in two patients who were resistant to chlorambucil and CHOP, respectively. The partial response lasted unmaintained for 9 months, and the patient is currently responding to fludarabine a second time. The complete remission was documented by bone marrow biopsy, by cytogenetics, and by molecular analysis with the PCR method for the bcl-2 gene and has lasted, so far, 6 months unmaintained. The encouraging activity of fludarabine in previously treated low-grade NHL, including follicular lymphoma, was also documented in a collaborative series from London, showing 22% CR and 26% PR (21).

THE LEUKEMIC PHASE OF INTERMEDIATE (MANTLE-ZONE)/CENTROCYTIC NHL

The disorders grouped under the old term of "lymphosarcoma-cell leukemia" (1) included most of the leukemia/lymphoma syndromes listed in Tables 2 and 3. The most common of these is follicular lymphoma, discussed above. Another, less well-characterized disorder is the leukemic phase of intermediate (mantle-zone) lymphoma (1,7). One of the difficulties here is that this lymphoma is not specifically defined in the NCI Working Formulation, although in general it corresponds to group E or diffuse lymphoma of small cleaved cells. There is also some discrepancy about the identity of this disorder with mantle-zone NHL and the similarity and/or overlapping features with centrocytic lymphoma as defined by the Kiel classification (33). In addition to this, there are few reports documenting its leukemic phase, and there may also be problems in the differential diagnosis with CLL of mixed cell type, chiefly CLL/PL (1,7; Fig. 3), on account of the pleomorphic appearance on peripheral blood films (Figs. 5 and 6) and the CD5 reactivity (Table 4). The main morphologic difference from CLL and follicular center lymphoma is that small cells are scanty in intermediate lymphoma, the majority being medium or large in size with slight nuclear irregularity and moderate indentation. Histological examination of lymph nodes shows a diffuse pattern and could be distinguished from follicular lymphoma (33), but the histology of the spleen may be more difficult. The clinical and laboratory features of a series of cases that we have studied presenting with frank leukemia are listed in Table 8.

Up to one-third of cases with intermediate (mantle-zone) NHL may be associated with the chromosome translocation t(11;14) (q13;q34) that involves the candidate oncogene bcl-1 located at 11q13 (25,26). Thus, it is likely that molecular analysis will facilitate the diagnosis of this disorder, particularly to distinguish it from follicular lymphoma as it does not involve the bcl-2 gene. Unfortunately, other low-grade NHL, CLL/PL, and B-PLL may also carry the translocation t(11;14) (V. Brito-Babapulle, personal communication), although fine detail of the breakpoint regions in bcl-1 in these disorders is still not available and may conceivably disclose specific differences according to the particular disease group.

Treatment

In cases in leukemic phase, the disease is widespread (7) and the response of treatment and prognosis is worse than in low-grade NHL. The trend has been to use the combination CHOP or its variants, but there is no proven data of its efficacy. Fludarabine, in our experience based on two patients, appears not to be effective. Similarly, Whelan et al. failed to show a response in the three patients with a diagnosis of centrocytic lymphoma included in that series, contrasting with the good responses in follicular lymphoma (21).

THE LEUKEMIC PHASE OF LARGE-CELL LYMPHOMA

A leukemic phase is an uncommon complication of large-cell lymphoma (Tables 2 and 3). We have studied 24 cases over a period of 15 years (8). This syndrome should not be considered within the spectrum of "CLL variants," as the cells are large, blastic, and often resemble acute leukemia, more often monoblastic leukemia. The only "connection" with CLL is that it does include (and thus is indistinguishable from) CLL in immunoblastic transformation. The main clinical and laboratory features of B-cell large-cell lymphoma with leukemia are summarized in Table 8. Our series included two patients with a previous history of CLL (8). Occasionally, these cases are confused with PLL because of the prominent nucleolus, but the large-cell lymphoma cells are larger and more pleomorphic than either B or T-PLL (8) and have a larger cell volume (14).

RICHTER'S SYNDROME

Richter's syndrome is the best-known form of malignant transformation of CLL from a low-grade tumour to a high-grade NHL with diffuse large-cell/immunoblastic histology (5,34). The change can be a localized phenomenon, usually in one lymph node or a closely related group of nodes, or it can be a more generalized manifestation. As for other forms of large-cell NHL, a leukemic phase with peripheral blood and bone marrow involvement has been documented, with some cases resembling an acute leukemia. In some patients the presence of circulating immunoblasts (Fig. 4) may be the first indication of transformation. In others a well-known syndrome of fever, weight loss, sweating, and abdominal symptoms leads to the identification of large paraortic nodes with a transformed histology. In such cases the diagnosis may be difficult to make, and a laparotomy may be necessary. Extra nodal involvement is not rare. The diagnosis is usually made by lymph node aspirate and/or biopsy of the affected tissues.

The Richter cells are large immunoblasts with basophilic cytoplasm, vesicular nuclei, and prominent nucleolus. The aspect is often pleomorphic, and multinucleated cells resembling Reed-Sternberg cells can be seen. In the past a number of cases have been described as the association of CLL with Hodgkin's disease and it is possible that in many of them the pathological interpretation confused a pleomorphic large-cell lymphoma with Hodgkins's disease (5,34). This concept, however, has recently been revived by two reports (35,36), in which the Reed-Sternberg-like cells were shown by immunocytochemistry to have the phenotype of Hodgkin's cells, namely, CD15 (LeuM1) positive and CD45 (LCA) negative, rather than of large-cell NHL. In one of these cases the cells were shown to be CD20 (L26) positive, suggesting B lineage and thus to be related to CLL lymphocytes (36). Unfortunately, the light chains were not studied, and crucial investigations to determine whether the CLL and the large-cell NHL cells had the same or a different origin by means of the rearrangement of the Ig chain genes were not done.

Recent reports in which DNA analysis was performed suggest that in some patients, perhaps as many as 40%, the Richter's transformation represents a new malignancy (5,34). Immunologic studies by light-chain restriction analysis can often suggest whether the large cells are part of the same B-CLL clone. Richter cells often express strongly membrane and cytoplasmic Ig. In a recent case studied in our laboratory, a heavy-chain switch from IgM (in the CLL lymphocytes) to IgA (in the large-cell lymphoma) was documented but with both cells sharing the same light chain. DNA analysis (Martin Dyer, personal communication) showed a different pattern of heavy-chain gene rearrangement (consistent with the Ig switch) but the same rearrangement for the light-chain gene. It seems essential now to collect and study with DNA techniques the large-cell lymphoma and CLL cells in all cases to establish more clearly the nature of this transformation and its relation to CLL.

Treatment and Prognosis

Richter's syndrome is always associated with poor prognosis, and median survivals of 4–6 months are often quoted. The latter seem to relate directly to whether a response could be achieved with combination chemotherapy. In our experience, responses are better in patients with more localized transformation. CHOP or similar combinations as used in large-cell NHL are the treatments of choice. Complete remissions have been documented in a number of patients, and in these the outlook is more favorable. In cases with little or no response, the survival is very short.

HETEROGENEITY OF T-CELL LEUKEMIAS

The mature (post-thymic) T-cell leukemias and leukemia/lymphoma syndromes (Table 3) constitute a relatively rare group of diseases of great clinical and epidemiologic interest. On the assumption that membrane marker studies are one of the essential components of diagnosis (1), it will be immediately apparent that none of these disorders constitutes a variant form of CLL but, rather, distinct clinicopathologic entities (Table 9). The

Table 9 Immunophenotype in Mature[a] T-Cell Leukemias and Leukemia/Lymphoma Syndromes

MoAbs	LGL leukemia	T-PLL	ATLL	Sezary syndrome
CD2/3/5	+[b]	+	+	+
CD4	−[c]	+	+	+
CD7	−/+	+ +	−/+	−/+
CD8	+ +	−/+[d]	−	−
CD25	−	−	+ +	−/+
CD56/57	−/+	−	−	−

[a]Cells are always terminal deoxynucleotidyl negative and do not express the CD1a antigen.
[b]Half the cases are CD5 negative.
[c]Very rare cases positive.
[d]Negative in 70% of cases; co-expression of CD4 and CD8 or CD8+, CD4− in 30% of cases.

only confusion may arise from the use of the term T-CLL, by which some cases were described in the past (reviewed in Ref. 12). In more recent times this term has been replaced by one (or more) in which not only the T-cell nature but also the main morphologic characteristic of the cells is included in the disease definition. Thus, we now prefer the term "large granular lymphocytic leukemia" (12,37,38) for what has been described previously as T-CLL. T-PLL defines a T-cell leukemia in which the cells resemble prolymphocytes. Again, this disease has very little in common, in its natural history and pathogenesis, with B-PLL (5,39,40). When prolymphocytic leukemia was first described, there was no clear idea that it represented two diseases, as membrane markers were not universally applied at that time (11). The other components of the group correspond also to two other distinct disease entities: adult T-cell leukemia/lymphoma (ATLL), a disease associated with the retrovirus HTLV-I (5,37); and Sezary syndrome, one of the cutaneous T-cell lymphomas, and its rare variant, Sezary cell leukemia without erythroderma or other skin involvement (41). Some of the latter cases, as well as less common leukemic manifestations of peripheral T-cell lymphomas, bear some resemblance to ATLL but not to CLL. Large-cell lymphomas of T-cell type, which rarely evolve with a leukemic phase, are described in detail elsewhere (8).

LARGE GRANULAR LYMPHOCYTIC LEUKEMIA

We have discussed and illustrated elsewhere the characteristics of LGL leukemia (1,5,12,37). A comprehensive review has been published by Loughran et al. (38). Two problems have affected the recognition of this disease in the past: its benign nature in a significant majority, and the lack of clonal markers for T-cell proliferations. Both problems have now been overcome. The clonality of LGL leukemia has been shown by karyotype and DNA analysis. The slowly progressive or chronic nature of this condition does not conflict with the concept of a lymphoid leukemia, as is the case with the well-known cases of "smoldering B-CLL." The diagnosis should be suspected in cases with a persistent T-cell lymphocytosis greater than 5×10^9/L of several months' duration with no apparent cause. Confirmation is made by morphology which shows that more than 80% of the lymphocytes are granular, the patient has splenomegaly (Table 10) and/or a cytopenia (usually neutropenia), and the membrane phenotype (Table 9) shows the predominance of a distinct T-cell subset, infrequently represented in normal blood, e.g., CD3+,CD8+,CD56+,CD57. In such cases, evidence of T-cell clonality should be sought and is usually demonstrated. Only rare cases with a phenotype of natural killer cells, e.g., CD2+, CD3−,CD16+, will fail to show rearrangement of the T-cell receptor

Table 10 Main Features of Mature T-Cell Leukemias and
Leukemia/Lymphoma Syndromes

Feature	LGL	T-PLL	ATLL	Sezary
Splenomegaly	50%	90%	50%	40%
Lymphadenopathy	Rare	40%	60%	10%
Skin infiltration	Rare	20%	20%	100%
WBC ($\times\ 10^9$/L)	<20	>100	<50	<50
Hypercalcemia	−	−	65%	−
HTLV-I(+)	−	−	+ +	−

beta-, gamma-, and delta-chain genes. Often such cases have a more aggressive course; thus, the question of their benign or malignant nature rarely arises (5,12).

Therapy of LGL Leukemia

Many patients do not require therapy. Splenectomy will not correct the cytopenia(s). Some patients respond to alkylating agents and/or prednisolone (5). In others, the cytopenia may be corrected by means of cyclosporin A. Deoxycoformycin has not been very successful in our experience (42), and experience with other nuceloside analogs is not yet available.

T-CELL PROLYMPHOCYTIC LEUKEMIA

T-cell prolymphocytic leukemia (T-PLL) is characterized by organomegaly and frank leukemic manifestations (Table 10). Only in cases with a predominance of small prolymphocytes (20% of cases) could the diagnosis of CLL be considered. Even with available cell marker data, the lack of an easily recognized nucleolus in this subgroup of T-PLL has led to the wrong diagnosis of T-CLL. This is yet another reason to retain the term CLL only for the B-cell form of the disease (see above).

The membrane phenotype is similar to that of other mature (postthymic) T-cell leukemias (Table 9). The predominant phenotype is CD3 + ,CD4 + , CD7 + ,CD8 − . In one third of cases the cells co-express CD4 and CD8 or are CD4 − and CD8 + . No clinical differences have been recognized between these cases. In the last 10 years, we have collected data on 78 cases and have reached the conclusion that T-PLL constitutes a distinct form of T-cell leukemia (5,12,37). The diagnosis is made by the morphology of peripheral blood films and the immunologic profile. The skin deposits are characterized by dense infiltrates around the blood vessels and skin appendages in the dermis; epidermotropism is not a feature as seen in Sezary syndrome and rarely in ATLL. The content of acid hydrolases, e.g., acid phosphatase and alpha-naphthyl acetate esterase is, as a rule, higher in T-PLL cells than in cells from other T-cell disorders (5).

Work in our laboratory has disclosed a consistent chromosome abnormality with two breakpoints in chromosome 14 at 14q11 and 14q32. The former involves the locus for the T-cell receptor alpha- and delta-chain genes. The breakpoints at 14q32 are not homogeneous and span a region of at least 300 kilobases and do not involve the immunoglobulin heavy-chain gene (40).

Therapy of T-PLL

The prognosis of this disease is very poor (5,12,37), with a median survival of 7 months. Complete remissions have been documented with the combination CHOP in 6% and partial remissions in 27%. With 2′-deoxycoformycin (DCF) we have observed responses in 48% of patients (10% CR and 38% PR). The best responses were seen in cases with a CD4+,CD8− membrane phenotype (42). We have treated only two T-PLL patients with fludarabine. One of them was unresponsive to both DCF and fludarabine. The other had a prolonged CR with DCF but failed to respond upon relapse and was treated with fludarabine. With this agent a significant reduction in WBC from $300 \times 10^9/L$ to $6 \times 10^9 L$ was observed after three 5-day courses over 3 months, but the patient eventually died of an intercurrent complication.

ADULT T-CELL LEUKEMIA/LYMPHOMA

Adult T-cell leukemia/lymphoma has distinct geographic distribution, affecting the southwest islands of Japan, the Caribbean basin, and some areas of Brasil (5,37). There is evidence that this disease is caused by HTLV-I, which is integrated in the DNA of the leukemic cells. ATLL has a variety of clinical manifestations (Table 10). In one of them, chronic ATLL, seen in 3% of cases, the clinical picture may resemble CLL. Again, subtle morphologic details, immunophenotype, chiefly the reactivity with anti-Tac (CD25) (Table 9), and HTLV-I serology will suffice to establish the correct diagnosis, particularly in endemic areas.

Treatment of ATLL

The acute form of the disease has a median survival of 6.5 months. Good responses have been documented with a number of agents, particularly combinations used in high-grade NHL. However, remissions are of short duration. Opportunistic infections present a major challenge, as in AIDS. We have treated 20 patients with 2'-deoxycoformycin and documented only 15% responses (1 CR and 2 PR) with a median duration of 6 months (42). It is of interest that these responses were observed after previous therapy succeeded in reducing the tumor bulk. This suggests that the future approach to therapy in this disease may involve the sequential use of agents and/or combinations as the only way to secure more prolonged remissions.

REFERENCES

1. J. M. Bennett, D. Catovsky, M.-T. Daniel, G. Flandrin, D. A. G. Galton, H. R. Gralnick, and C. Sultan, Proposals for the classification of chronic (mature) B and T lymphoid leukaemias, *J. Clin. Pathol., 42*:567–584 (1989).
2. C. Dearden and D. Catovsky, Treatment of hairy cell leukemia with 2'-deoxycoformycin, *Leuk. Lymph., 1*:179–185 (1990).
3. L. D. Piro, C. J. Carrera, E. Beutler, and D. A. Carson, 2-chlorodeoxyadenosine: An effective new agent for the treatment of chronic lymphocytic leukemia, *Blood, 72*:1069–1073 (1988).
4. M. J. Keating, H. Kantarjian, S. O'Brien, C. Koller, M. Talpaz, J. Schachner, C. C. Childs, E. J. Freireich, and K. B. McCredie, Fludarabine: A new agent with marked cytoreductive activity in untreated chronic lymphocytic leukemia, *J. Clin. Oncol., 9*:44–49 (1991).
5. D. Catovsky and R. Foa, *The Lymphoid Leukaemias*, Butterworths, London, (1990).
6. J. V. Melo, D. S. F. Robinson, M. P. de Oliveira, I. W. Thompson, I. A. Lampert, J. P. Ng, D. A. G. Galton, and D. Catovsky, Morphology and immunology of circulating cells in leukaemic phase of follicular lymphoma, *J. Clin. Pathol., 41*:951–959 (1988).
7. M. S. Pombo de Oliveira, E. S. Jaffe, and D. Catovsky, Leukaemic phase of mantle zone (intermediate) lymphoma: Its characterisation in 11 cases, *J. Clin. Pathol., 42*:962–972 (1989).
8. B. Bain, E. Matutes, D. Robinson, I. A. Lampert, V. Brito-Babapulle, R. Morilla, and D. Catovsky, Leukaemia as a manifestation of large cell lymphoma, *Br. J. Haematol., 77*:301–310 (1991).
9. J. V. Melo, U. Hegde, A. Parreira, I. Thompson, I. A. Lampert, and D. Catovsky, Splenic B cell lymphoma with circulating villous lymphocytes: Differential diagnosis of B cell leukaemias with large spleens, *J. Clin. Pathol., 40*:642–651 (1987).
10. S. P. Mulligan, E. Matutes, C. Dearden, and D. Catovsky, Splenic lymphoma with villous lymphocytes: Natural history and response to therapy in 50 cases, *Br. J. Haematol., 78*:206–209 (1991).
11. D. A. G. Galton, J. M. Goldman, E. Wiltshaw, D. Catovsky, K. Henry, and G. J. Goldenberg, Prolymphocytic leukaemia, *Br. J. Haematol., 27*:7–23 (1974).
12. D. Catovsky and E. Matutes, Leukemias of mature T cells. Prolymphocytic

and large granular lymphocytic leukemia, in *Neoplastic Hematopathology* (D. M. Knowles, ed.), Williams & Wilkins, Baltimore, chap. 41 (1992).

13. J. V. Melo, D. Catovsky, and D. A. G. Galton, The relationship between chronic lymphocytic leukaemia and prolymphocytic leukaemia. II. Patterns of evolution of 'prolymphocytoid' transformation, *Br. J. Haematol., 64*:77–86 (1986).

14. J. V. Melo, J. Wardle, M. Chetty, J. England, S. M. Lewis, D. A. G. Galton, and D. Catovsky, The relationship between chronic lymphocytic leukaemia and prolymphocytic leukaemia. III. Evaluation of cell size by morphology and volume measurements, *Br. J. Haematol., 64*:469–478 (1986).

15. D. Catovsky, Overview, in *The Leukemic Cell* (D. Catovsky, ed.), Churchill Livingstone, Edinburgh, pp. 1–22 (1991).

16. S. Rani, M. de Oliveira, and D. Catovsky, Different expression of CD3 and CD22 in leukemic cells according to whether tested in suspension or fixed on slides, *Hematol. Pathol., 2*:73–78 (1988).

17. J. V. Melo, D. Catovsky, W. M. Gregory, and D. A. G. Galton, The relationship between chronic lymphocytic leukaemia and prolymphocytic leukaemia. IV. Analysis of survival and prognostic features, *Br. J. Haematol., 65*:23–29 (1987).

18. T. Vallespi, E. Montserrat, and M. A. Sanz, Chronic lymphocytic leukaemia: Prognostic value of lymphocyte morphological subtypes. A multivariate survival analysis in 146 patients. *Br. J. Haematol., 77*:478–485 (1991).

19. H. M. Kantarjian, J. R. Redman, and M. J. Keating, Fludarabine phosphate therapy in other lymphoid malignancies, *Sem. Oncol., 17*:66–70 (1990).

20. C. Dearden and D. Catovsky, Deoxycoformycin in the treatment of mature B-cell malignancies, *Br. J. Cancer, 62*:4–5 (1990).

21. J. S. Whelan, C. L. Davis, S. Rule, M. Ranson, O. P. Smith, O. B. Mehta, D. Catovsky, A. Z. S. Rohatiner, and T. A. Lister, Fludarabine phosphate for the treatment of low grade lymphoid malignancy, *Br. J. Cancer, 64*:120–123 (1991).

22. L. Sainati, E. Matutes, S. Mulligan, M. P. de Oliveira, S. Rani, I. A. Lampert, and D. Catovsky, A variant form of hairy cell leukemia resistant to α-interferon: Clinical and phenotypic characteristics of 17 patients, *Blood, 76*:157–162 (1990).

23. R. S. Neiman, A. L. Sullivan, and R. Jaffe, Malignant lymphoma simulating leukemic reticuloendotheliosis. A clinicopathologic study of ten cases, *Cancer, 43*:329–342 (1979).

24. P. Spriano, G. Barosi, R. Invernizzi, G. Ippolliti, A. Fortunato, R. Rosso, and U. Magrini, Splenomegalic immunocytoma with circulating hairy cells. Report of eight cases and revision of the literature, *Haematologica, 71*:25–33 (1986).

25. M. E. Williams, C. D. Westermann, and S. H. Swerdlow, Genotypic characterization of centrocytic lymphoma: Frequent rearrangement of the chromosome 11 bcl-1 locus, *Blood, 76*:1387–1391 (1990).

26. D. Leroux, F. Le Marc'Hadour, R. Gressin, M.-C. Jacob, E. Keddari, M. Monteil, P. Caillot, P. Jalbert, and J. J. Sotto, Non-Hodgkin's lymphomas

with t(11;14)(q13;q32): A subset of mantle zone/intermediate lymphocytic lymphoma?, *Br. J. Haematol., 77*:346–353 (1991).

27. T. Sun, M. Susin, N. Shevde, and S. Teichberg, Hybrid form of hairy cell leukemia and chronic lymphocytic leukemia, *Hematol. Oncol., 8*:283–294 (1990).

28. C. A. Hanson, T. E. Gribbin, B. Schnitzer, T. A. Schlegelmilch, B. S. Mitchell, and L. M. Stoolman, CD11c (LEU-M5) expression characterizes a B-cell chronic lymphoproliferative disorder with features of both chronic lymphocytic leukemia and hairy cell leukemia, *Blood, 76*:2360–2367 (1990).

29. S. B. Wormsley, S. M. Baird, N. Gadol, K. R. Rai, and R. E. Sobol, Characteristics of CD11c + CD5 + chronic B-cell leukemias and the identification of novel peripheral blood B-cell subsets with chronic lymphoid leukemia immunophenotypes, *Blood, 76*:123–130 (1990).

30. S. Spiro, D. A. G. Galton, E. Wiltshaw, and R. C. Lohmann, Follicular lymphoma: A survey of 75 cases with special reference to the syndrome resembling chronic lymphocytic leukaemia, *Br. J. Cancer, 31*(suppl. II):60–72 (1975).

31. V. Brito-Babapulle, A. Crawford, T. Khokhar, M. Laffan, E. Matutes, S. Fairhead, and D. Catovsky, Translocations t(14;18) and t(8;14) with rearranged bcl-2 and c-myc in a case presenting as B-ALL (L3), *Leukemia, 5*: 83–87 (1991).

32. E. Lipford, J. J. Wright, W. Urba, J. Whang-Peng, I. R. Kirsch, M. Raffeld, J. Cossman, D. L. Longo, A. Bakhshi, and S. J. Korsmeyer, Refinement of lymphoma cytogenetics by the chromosome 18q21 major breakpoint region, *Blood, 70*:1816–1823 (1987).

33. S. Jaffe, M. A. Bookman, and D. L. Longo, Lymphocytic lymphoma of intermediate differentiation. Mantle zone lymphoma: A distinct subtype of B-cell lymphoma, *Hum. Pathol., 18*:877–880 (1987).

34. G. Flandrin, Richter's syndrome, in *Chronic Lymphocytic Leukemia*, (A. Polliack and D. Catovsky, eds.), Harwood Academic Publishers, Chur, pp. 209–218 (1988).

35. M. Brecher and P. M. Banks, Hodgkin's disease variant of Richter's syndrome, *Am. J. Clin. Pathol., 93*:333–339 (1990).

36. J. Williams, A. Schned, J. D. Cotelingham, and E. S. Jaffe, Chronic lymphocytic leukemia with coexistent Hodgkin's disease, *Am. J. Surg. Pathol., 15*: 33–42 (1991).

37. E. Matutes and D. Catovsky, Mature T-cell leukemias and leukemia/lymphoma syndromes. Review of our experience in 175 cases, *Leuk. Lymp., 4*: 81–91 (1991).

38. T. P. Loughran and G. Starkebaum, Large granular lymphocytic leukemia. Report of 30 cases and review of the literature, *Medicine, 66*:397–405 (1987).

39. E. Matutes, J. Garcia-Talavera, M. O'Brien, and D. Catovsky, The morphological spectrum of T-prolymphocytic leukaemia, *Br. J. Haematol., 64*:111–123 (1986).

40. V. Brito-Babapulle and D. Catovsky, Inversions and tandem translocations involving chromosome 14q11 and 14q32 in T-prolymphocytic leukemia and

T-cell leukemias in patients with ataxia telangiectasia, *Cancer Genet. Cytogenet., 55*:1–9 (1991).

41. E. Matutes, D. M. Keeling, A. C. Newland, C. S. Scott, D. Mitchell, N. Traub, D. G. Wardle, and D. Catovsky, Sezary cell-like leukemia: A distinct type of mature T cell malignancy, *Leukemia, 4*:262–266 (1990).
42. C. Dearden, E. Matutes, and D. Catovsky, Deoxycoformycin in the treatment of mature T-cell leukaemias, *Br. J. Cancer, 64*:903–906 (1991).

18

Infection in Chronic Lymphocytic Leukemia: A Reappraisal

D. P. Kontoyianis, E. J. Anaissie, and G. P. Bodey
The University of Texas M. D. Anderson Cancer Center, Houston, Texas

The study of infectious complications in patients with chronic lymphocytic leukemia (CLL) is of great interest for two reasons: CLL is the most common hematologic malignancy in the Western world, accounting for 30% of all leukemias (1), and infection constitutes a major cause of morbidity and mortality in CLL, affecting 80% of patients in some series (2). In addition, the controversy surrounding the pathogenesis of these infections raises several questions related to their management.

The recent introduction of new and very promising therapeutic compounds such as fludarabine phosphate, 2'-deoxycoformycin (DCF), and 2-chlorodeoxyadenosine (CDA) has renewed the interest in clinical trials in CLL (3). But the successes achieved with these agents have come at the cost of more serious infections.

This chapter will delineate the magnitude of the problem of infections in CLL, review the abnormal host defenses against this disease, and focus on the evolving picture of the infectious complications and their association with the newer forms of therapy.

SPECTRUM OF INFECTIONS IN CLL

Infectious Complications Associated with Standard Cytotoxic Chemotherapy

Infection plays an important role in the mortality associated with CLL. However, neither the relative incidence of infection nor the infection-related mortality is known, despite numerous studies of infection in CLL. Table 1 summarizes the results of the largest reported series (4–17). Infection was the main cause of death for one-third of the patients referred to The University of Texas M. D. Anderson Cancer Center in the period 1970-1983 (18). In another large multicenter study of 660 patients from England, infection appeared to have contributed substantially to death (19). It is important to keep in mind, however, that most of these studies were retrospective in nature, with different criteria for infection diagnosis and cause of death. Furthermore, the aim of most of these studies was to analyze the leukemia status and not the infectious complications, and hence most of the studies did not take into consideration the stage of the underlying disease, neutrophil count, immunoglobulin levels, and whether or not patients were previously treated with cytotoxic agents (any of these factors may have an important impact on the nature and severity of infections in CLL). In addition, those reports tended to represent a selected patient population with advanced and refractory CLL such as are typically seen in tertiary-care centers.

Despite these limitations, it is clear from these studies that the incidence of infection in CLL patients is severalfold higher than that in the general population, and that this parallels the progression of the underlying leuke-

Table 1 Incidence of Infection in Patients with CLL

First author/year (ref.)	Patients with infections/ total patients	Total number of infections	Percent infections present at diagnosis of CLL	Death due to infection
Oswood/1952 (4)	30/102	—	—	11
Scott/1957 (5)	—	—	13	—
Pisciotta/1957 (6)	—	—	25	11
Ultmann/1959 (7)	19/33	—	—	—
Shaw/1960 (8)	25/42	50	—	—
Hudson/1960 (9)	15/40	—	—	—
Shaw/1961 (10)	12/18	13	—	66
Aroesty/1962 (11)	37/61	84	21	34
Boggs/1966 (12)	—	—	25	31
Zippin/1973 (13)	193/839	—	—	62
Hansen/1973 (14)	79/189	—	12	101
Twomey/1973 (2)	38/45	71	—	63
Travade/1986 (17)	—	159	38	47
Monserrat/1977 (18)	38/56	70	—	—
Revol/1974 (15)	104/266	132	—	—

mia. Also, it appears that a subset of patients may suffer recurrent infections (usually moderate upper respiratory tract or soft tissue infections) usually associated with hypogammaglobulinemia.

Table 2 summarizes the literature regarding the sites of involvement by infection. Pneumonia appeared to be the most frequent and severe infection, while bacteremia was typically seen in patients with profound neutropenia. The rate of nosocomial bloodstream infections was 9.4% in patients with CLL in a prospective surveillance study. In more than 50% of these patients, the polymorphonuclear leukocyte count at the time of bacteremia was less than 100/ml (20). Infections of the genitourinary tract system were also regularly noted.

Most of the classic associations between CLL and microbes have been derived from studies of specific pathogens rather than from studies aimed at the CLL patient population. However, it is clear from the literature that the majority of these infections are bacterial, and that infections with *Streptococcus pneumoniae* are not uncommon (6,10,17,21,22). Over a 6-year period, CLL was the underlying malignancy in 7 of 36 cases of pneumococcal bacteremia cared for in a cancer hospital (23). In another study of cancer patients, the estimated attack rate of pneumococcal bacteremia in patients with CLL was 10.8/1000 (24). *Staphylococcus aureus* infections were prominent in some series, while Gram-negative bacillary infections, particularly bacteremias, outnumbered Gram-positive infections in others (16,17). These latter series may represent patients with more advanced disease and profound myelosuppression. Fungal infections, particularly cryptococcal meningitis and disseminated histoplasmosis, have also been associated with CLL (25,26). Our recent experience at M. D. Anderson Cancer Center, though, indicates that the spectrum of fungal infections in patients with CLL has shifted from the endemic mycoses to infections with opportunistic fungi. For instance, mycoses caused by *Candida* and *Aspergillus* species represent a significant cause of death and tend to occur in patients with advanced disease and persistent profound neutropenia, conditions similar to those seen in patients with acute myeloid leukemia. Viral infections, particularly with herpes viruses, are reported to occur frequently in patients with CLL (2,7,16,26). Most of the herpes virus infections appear to be localized, although disseminated disease can be seen, particularly in patients with advanced disease and severe cell-mediated dysfunction (28,29). *Herpes simplex* virus (HSV) mucositis may follow a more chronic and indolent course in some CLL patients, in contrast with the more aggressive, recurrent behavior of this infection in patients with acute leukemia (30). However, viral infections do not seem to cause significant mortality, even though they are associated with substantial morbidity. On a historical note, vaccinia gangrenosa and generalized vaccinia have been reported in patients with CLL after smallpox vaccination (31,32).

Table 2 Infectious Site of Involvement[a]

Authors (ref.)	Oswood 1952 (4)	Ultmann 1959 (71)	Shaw 1960 (8)	Hudson 1960 (9)	Shaw 1961 (10)	Aroesty 1962 (11)	Twomey 1973 (2)	Revol 1974 (15)	Monserrat 1977 (16)	Travade 1986 (17)
Total PTS	102	33	42	40	18	61	45	266	56	60
Total PTS w/infect.	30	19	25	15	12	37	38	104	38	
Pneumonia	7	10	14	4	6	33	36	73	38	52
Head and neck	17	9	10	2	3	—	—	14	—	24
Bacteremia	—	6	7	—	—	8	4	5	2	15
Fever of unknown origin	—	2	—	—	—	—	—	—	—	14
Skin and soft tissue	—	6	10	2	3	24	14	25	12	28
Meningitis	—	—	—	—	—	—	1	1	—	2
Genitourinary	5	3	5	3	1	10	13	8	16	16
Miscellaneous	2	1	1	—	—	9	3	6	2	17

[a]Abbreviations: PTS, patients; infect., infection.

Other pathogens such as mycobacteria have rarely caused infections in patients with CLL. In fact, the prevalence of tuberculosis in CLL has been estimated to be only about 88 cases/10,000 patients (33). *Pneumocystis carinii* infections are exceedingly rare in CLL (34).

Infections Following Therapy with New Agents

Several clinical studies have now provided evidence that treatment with newer antineoplastic agents may be superior to conventional therapy in CLL. The most interesting of these compounds are three purine analogs: fludarabine phosphate, DCF, and CDA (3). The introduction of these newer therapeutic modalities, however, has been accompanied by an apparent increase in opportunistic infections caused by organisms such as *Pneumocystis carinii*, *Listeria monocytogenes*, and fungi. In addition, cases of disseminated herpes zoster may be occurring more frequently.

Fludarabine phosphate is a promising agent that has been investigated at our institution (35–37). When used as a single agent, fludarabine phosphate was well tolerated in previously untreated patients, except in elderly patients with advanced Rai stages who developed serious life-threatening opportunistic infections including pulmonary nocardiosis and disseminated candidiasis (36). On the other hand, previously treated patients who received fludarabine phosphate had a higher incidence of serious infections such as pneumonias, bloodstream infections, and exacerbation of dermatomal herpes zoster (36). The combination of fludarabine phosphate (30 mg/m^2 per day for 5 days, monthly) and prednisone (60 mg/m^2 per day for 5 days monthly) resulted in excellent response rates in refractory CLL, but was associated with more infections than the historical controls treated with conventional chemotherapy at M. D. Anderson Cancer Center. Most infections did not appear to correlate with absolute neutrophil count or immunoglobulin levels. On the other hand, advanced Rai stage, old age, low albumin and platelet values, and failure to achieve hematologic remission may indicate increased infectious risk (unpublished data). These infections may have been in part due to a significant reduction of CD4-positive circulating T lymphocytes and the reversal of the CD4 : CD8 ratio, frequently noted following fludarabine-plus-prednisone therapy (38,39). A few of our patients developed polymicrobial infections characteristically seen in patients with severe immune dysfunctions such as *Pneumocystis carinii* pneumonia (PCP), cytomegalovirus pneumonia, listeriosis, and disseminated mycoses (40).

Therapy with another promising agent, DCF, has been associated with the same pattern of infections (41,42). Thirty-four of 39 patients treated with DCF developed severe, life-threatening infections. These infections tended to occur in the first 6 weeks of therapy and were significantly more common in patients with advanced stage. Ten episodes of pneumonia and two fatal septicemias (*S. pneumoniae, pseudomonas*) were noted. Six patients were infected with HSV and three patients with varicella zoster. Disseminated candidiasis was noted in two patients and PCP in one. Therapy with DCF was resumed after resolution of these infections (41). In addition, a severe combined immunodeficiency (SCID)-like syndrome has been reported in CLL patients treated with DCF (43). This association is not surprising, since SCID is caused by the genetic absence of adenosine deaminase (ADA) activity and DCF is a potent lymphocytic agent that exerts its activity by tight binding of ADA (44). The inhibition of ADA by DCF therapy, together with impairment of lymphocytes, monocytes, macrophages, and natural killer (NK) cells, may explain this new spectrum of infections (45–48). T cells are typically more sensitive that B cells, and the CD4 subset is the most frequently affected (49). The similarity between the infectious complications of patients treated with fludarabine plus prednisone and those treated with DCF is striking and may be explained by the severe effect of these agents on CD4 cells.

While the experience with CDA is still quite limited, it appears that such therapy may also lead to infectious complications (50). In a small series of patients treated with this drug, pulmonary aspergillosis and disseminated varicella zoster virus were reported. In both cases of aspergillosis, the infection had been acquired on prior therapy with adrenal corticosteroids, and had worsened on CDA treatment.

Severe infections have not been a serious problem in patients treated with biologic-response modifiers such as the interferons, interleukin-2, or monoclonal antibodies (51–54). Unfortunately, to date these agents have not demonstrated substantial activity in CLL.

PATHOGENESIS OF INFECTION IN CLL

Hypogammaglobulinemia

Studies of gammaglobulin levels in patients with CLL and their relationship to infection are summarized in Table 3 (55–63). Most patients with CLL will ultimately develop significant hypogammaglobulinemia during the course of their illnesses (63). This defect is permanent and is generally not reversed by antileukemic therapy, even if complete remission is achieved (7,22). Patients with CLL and hypogammaglobulinemia seem to have a high propensity for developing bacterial infections, particularly recurrent ones (7,59). Bacteria classically associated with this setting include *Streptococcus pneumoniae* and *Hemophilus influenzae*. Not all studies have been

Table 3 Hypogammaglobulinemia and Infection in Patients with CLL

Author/year (ref.)	Patients with hypogamma-globulinemia/ total patients	Method of gammaglobulin assay	Correlation with infection	Comments
Rundles/1954 (56)	2/15	Paper electrophoresis and scanning	No	—
Ultman/1959 (7)	13/23	Paper electrophoresis	Yes	32 infections in 14 hypogammaglobulinemic patients versus 6 infections in 4 normogammaglobulinemic patients
Videback/1960 (57)	9/43	Paper electrophoresis	No	Increased frequency
Hudson/1960 (9)	27/40	Paper electrophoresis and scanning	Yes	14 infections in 29 hypogammaglobulinemic patients versus 1 infection in 11 normogammaglobulinemic patients
Creyssel/1958 (58)	31/61	Paper electrophoresis	Yes	Infections in 74% of the patients with hypogamma-globulinemia versus 36% of patients with normal IgG
Shaw/1960 (11)	23/36	Paper electrophoresis and scanning	Yes	Recurrent bacterial infections (32 in 14 hypogamma-globulinemic patients versus 6 infections in 4 normo-gammaglobulinemic patients)
Fairley/1961 (59)	74/110	Agar diffusion method	Yes	Strong correlation between hypogamma globulinemia and recurrent infections
Miller/1962 (22)	37/104	Immunoelectrophoresis	Yes	—
Klima/1962 (60)	51/103	Paper electrophoresis	Yes	—
Hansen/1973 (14)	54/138	Paper electrophoresis	No	Correlation between infection and neutropenia but not hypogammaglobulinemia
Monserrat/1977 (16)	?/56	Paper electrophoresis	No	—
Van Scoy/1981 (61)	20/43	Unspecified	Yes	12 of 17 patients with severe infections were hypogam-maglobulinemic
Chapel/1987 (55)	23/45	Unspecified	Yes	Correlation between low IgG level and recurrent infec-tions

able, however, to document this association. In addition, some questions remain: what would be the cutoff point of immunoglobulin levels below which the risk of infection increases significantly, and what is the relative importance of each immunoglobulin? Examining the natural history and the prognostic significance of serum immunoglobulins in B-cell CLL (B-CLL), Rozman et al. found that decreased IgA levels were the most significant prognostic factor, whereas IgM levels lacked any prognostic value (64). An attractive hypothesis is that a predominant IgA deficiency leads to an increased frequency of upper-respiratory-tract infections, similar to what is seen in patients with selective IgA deficiency and in CLL patients who suffer recurrent respiratory infections (65). Control of CLL has been associated with a decrease in the incidence and severity of infections in some patients, although no impact on immunoglobulin level could be detected (7,66). More recently, fludarabine therapy has been associated with a normalization of immunoglobulin levels in some hypogammaglobulinemic patients with CLL who achieved a complete remission (36). It is important to keep in mind, however, that patients with hypogammaglobulinemia may be free of infection, and, conversely, that CLL patients with a normal immunoglobulin level may suffer recurrent infections. This has led investigators to ask whether the inability of B cells to mount a specific antibody response against a pathogen may be more important than the hypoglobulinemia itself. The deficiencies of specific antibodies in patients with CLL has also been examined. Chapel looked at naturally occurring IgG antibodies against *Escherichia coli* and *S. pneumonia* in a selective group of 21 CLL patients with multiple infections or hypogammaglobulinemia (62). An association between low IgG titers to these two pathogens and repeated infections with these pathogens in CLL patients was found. Response to immunization has been shown to be defective in CLL patients (67–71).

Cell-Mediated Immunity

The literature provides ample in-vitro and in-vivo evidence of impaired cell-mediated immunity in CLL, even though the distinction between primary impairment and impairment secondary to cytotoxic chemotherapy is not always made (1). Effects on T-cell colony growth, increases in T-suppressor activity, decreases in T-helper activity, reversals of the CD4 : CD8 ratio, and defects in NK cells have all been reported (72–76). In addition, some investigators have reported decreased reactivity in their subjects to skin tests with recall antigens. However, the relationship of such defects to subsequent infection has not been established. It is likely, however, that the increased use of the purine analogs, which are known to cause severe CD4 depletion, will lead to an increase in the number of infections characteristically associated with dysfunction of cell-mediated immunity.

Neutropenia and Phagocytic Cell Defects

The association of neutropenia with infection-related morbidity and mortality in patients with CLL was reported as early as 1938, and the correlation between infection risk and neutropenia has been shown in other subsequent studies (10,14,16,21). In general, neutrophil count and function in patients with CLL appear to be normal, even in the presence of pronounced peripheral lymphocytosis (77,78). Recent reports, however, have indicated the presence of significant enzyme deficiencies (lysozyme and myeloperoxidase in particular), mainly in monocytes, but also in neutrophils of five untreated patients with CLL (79). These enzyme deficiencies were not, however, associated with an impairment of the monocyte transformation to macrophages. These defects were reversed when complete hematologic remission was achieved. Also, the serum of CLL patients has been reported to possess properties highly inhibitory to phagocytosis (80,81).

With the increasing use of combination cytotoxic chemotherapy in advanced CLL stages, it is likely that neutropenia will play a more and more important role in predisposing the patient to infection. It is interesting to note, for example, that the association between infection and hypogammaglobulinemia was less apparent in the studies in which neutropenia appeared to be a major predisposing factor to infection (mainly in patients with advanced disease). One could speculate, then, that hypogammaglobulinemia is associated with mild and moderate infections early in the course of CLL, while neutropenia is associated with more severe infections in patients with advanced disease.

Complement

No strong correlation between complement levels and infection has been established in CLL (55). Heath and Cheson have reported poor bacterial opsonization (particularly of *S. pneumoniae, S. aureus*, and *H. influenzae* in CLL, related to defective activation of complement. Hypogammaglobulinemia, which is common in these patients, was not sufficient to explain this defective complement activity, since it was not corrected by the addition of specific antibacterial antibodies.

Splenectomy

Splenectomy, which is occasionally performed in patients with CLL, could account for some of the infections with encapsulated bacteria associated with this malignancy (83). However, this procedure is performed infrequently at present.

Effects of Treatment

While, on the one hand, response to chemotherapy may result in a lower incidence of infections (8,22), on the other hand, chemotherapy and its associated neutropenia and T-cell dysfunction may further impair an already dysfunctioning immune system. In our experience with fludarabine phosphate, prior treatment with conventional chemotherapy may have been responsible for an increase in the incidence and severity of opportunistic infections. The impact of adrenal corticosteroids on the infectious risk in patients with CLL has also been investigated. In a study of 18 patients with "early" CLL (11), Shaw et al. randomly assigned nine patients to a regimen of 1 mg/kg of prednisone for 3 months followed by a 3-month rest period. This sequence was reversed in the remaining nine patients, who did not receive steroids during the first 3 months but followed the same dosage/ schedule of prednisone for the second 3-month period. More frequent and more severe infections were noted with prednisone therapy. The combination of steroids with fludarabine phosphate in patients with CLL treated at our institution was also associated with more severe opportunistic infections (particularly PCP and listeriosis) compared to therapy with fludarabine phosphate alone (unpublished data).

THERAPEUTIC STRATEGIES

There appear to be significant differences in the infection risk among patients with CLL according to the stage of disease and its treatment. Patients with early-stage disease do not usually require intensive chemotherapy, and thus antimicrobial prophylaxis may not be needed, unless the patients suffer repeated infections. On the other hand, patients with advanced disease receiving intensive cytotoxic chemotherapy are at higher risk for infection and should be considered for prophylaxis.

Infection Prophylaxis

Antibiotic Prophylaxis

The cost effectiveness of prophylactic antibiotics should be studied in patients with CLL who suffer recurrent respiratory tract or soft tissue infections. When no pathogen is identifiable, the ideal prophylactic agent should offer adequate coverage against commonly encountered upper-respiratory-tract pathogens such as *H. influenzae, S. pneumoniae,* and *S. aureus;* ampicillin/clavulanic acid would therefore seem to be a reasonable choice for countering most of these pathogens (84). On the other hand, the increased risk of acquiring certain bacterial, viral, and fungal infections occurring in patients treated with the new purine analogs would dictate another strategy, aimed at preventing infections with *L. monocytogenes, Pneumocystis carinii,* varicella zoster, and fungi.

Since immunization is usually ineffective in patients with CLL (66,67, 71), it is advisable that such patients be educated about their risk of overwhelming sepsis with encapsulated organisms and be supplied with an adequate amount of antibacterial agents, such as ampicillin/clavulanic acid, to be taken immediately in the event of fever.

Immunoglobulin Replacement

The early results of intravenous immunoglobulin (IVIG) administration in CLL patients with hypogammaglobulinemia and serious or chronic persistent infections were encouraging (85). The most important information, however, came from a large, randomized, double-blind, placebo-controlled multicenter trial of IVIG replacement (86). Eighty-four patients considered to be at increased risk of infection because of hypogammaglobulinemia, history of infection, or both, were randomly assigned a regimen of either IVIG (400 mg/kg) or an equivalent volume of normal saline at 3-week intervals for 1 year. Moderately severe bacterial infections were reduced by 50%, while minor and severe bacterial viral and fungal infections remained unchanged (Table 4). The reduction of bacterial infections was most dramatic in patients who completed the full year of study.

Despite these promising results, several questions remain regarding the role of IVIG therapy in these patients. Does IVIG replacement reduce the serious morbidity and mortality in patients with CLL? Based on the data from the above-mentioned study, only moderate bacterial infections were

Table 4   Incidence of Infections in the IVIG Trial (86)

	IVIG	Placebo	P value
Bacterial infections			
Major	8	11	0.25
Moderate	10	21	0.26
Trivial	5	10	0.10
Total	23	42	0.01
Viral infections			
Major	2	3	
Moderate	6	7	
Trivial	32	27	
Total	40	37	0.65
Fungal infections	3	2	
Patients free of infection	13	11	0.68

prevented. On the other hand, the more serious bacterial fungal and viral infections were not affected. Also, no reduction in mortality could be noted.

Is IVIG replacement cost-effective? The moderate bacterial infections that were prevented by IVIG could—very likely—have been prevented by less expensive oral antibacterials. Furthermore, a double-blind randomized trial comparing prophylaxis with IVIG and oral antibacterials could better delineate the role of these agents. Such a study could also address the role of prophylactic antibiotics in the prevention of more severe and potentially fatal infections not otherwise prevented by IVIG. The cost effectiveness of IVIG in patients with CLL was recently addressed by Weeks et al. (87). An expenditure of $6 million was necessary to achieve one quality-adjusted life-year, without any increase in life expectancy. Clearly, IVIG is an extremely expensive and not cost-effective approach to infection prophylaxis in this patient population. What is the exact mechanism of IVIG "protection" in CLL? Does IVIG help by "correcting" the existing hypogammaglobulinemia? Though the study mentioned above found no correlation between IgG levels and infectious risk, it is possible that an immunomodulator effect accounts for the observed benefit (85).

Which patients are most likely to benefit from IVIG prophylaxis, if any? This question needs to be urgently addressed, given the high cost of IVIG. At this point in time, there seems to be little justification for giving prophylactic IVIG to patients with early-stage CLL and no history of recurrent infections, even those with documented hypogammaglobulinemia. Also, patients with recurrent viral or fungal infections and patients with profound neutropenia are unlikely to derive great benefit from IVIG therapy. It is possible, though, that patients with IgG titers of <400 mg/dL or low antibody titers to encapsulated organisms and with a history of recurrent bacterial infections could potentially benefit from replacement therapy.

What is the optimum dosage/schedule for IVIG therapy? If IVIG replacement is considered, smaller doses given at longer intervals may be more cost-effective (88). Furthermore, since the greatest benefit was noted in patients who completed the full 1-year course of prophylaxis, patients who are unlikely to complete such a course should not be given IVIG (86).

How safe are human immunoglobulin preparations in terms of viral transmission? The potential risk of transmission of non-A, non-B hepatitis, while remote, still remains a concern, particularly if one considers long-term prophylaxis. However, no cases of IVIG-related hepatitis B or HIV virus have been reported thus far (89–93).

Vaccination

Antibody response to pneumococcal immunization in patients with CLL has been disappointing, particularly in patients with advanced disease. In addition, infections with serotypes that are not incorporated into the vaccine may also occur (94). While it is tempting to use multiple-dose immunization to improve serologic response, one should weigh this potential advantage against the risk of progression of the underlying disease if therapy is delayed.

Treatment of Infections

Febrile patients with CLL should be considered to have an infection until proven otherwise. As is done in all other febrile immunocompromised patients, a rigorous workup searching for the source of infection should be undertaken. In addition, treatment with broad-spectrum antimicrobial agents including a β-lactam antibiotic should be promptly instituted, particularly if the patient is neutropenic (95,96). Special consideration should be given to the patient undergoing therapy with the newer purine analogs: in such patients, Trimetoprime/sulfamethoxazole should probably be included in the initial regimen, particularly if the patient has signs and symptoms suggestive of PCP or meningitis, which may be caused by *L. monocytogenes*, or if the patient has risk factors for developing an infection such as extensive prior antileukemic therapy, advanced age and stage of disease, or treatment with continuous infusion fludarabine phosphate (97) or a combination of fludarabine and prednisone (36).

CONCLUSION

In conclusion, patients with CLL are at an increased risk of infectious morbidity and mortality. In early, untreated CLL patients, this risk may be related to hypogammaglobulinemia, but in patients with advanced disease, particularly those treated with the newer purine analogs, neutropenia and defects in cell-mediated immunity appear to be the major predisposing factors. IVIG, although it is of scientific interest, may be of little clinical relevance at the present time. In any case, the changing spectrum of infections in this latter group of patients mandates a newer approach to prophylaxis and therapy.

REFERENCES

1. K. A. Foon, K. R. Rai, and R. P. Gale, New insights into biology and therapy, *Ann. Intern. Med., 113*:525–539 (1990).
2. J. J. Twomey, Infections complicating multiple myeloma and chronic lymphocytic leukemia, *Arch. Intern. Med., 132*:562–565 (1973).
3. B. D. Cheson, Recent advances in the treatment of B-cell chronic lymphocytic leukemia, *Oncology, 4*:71–93 (1990).

4. E. E. Osgood and A. J. Seaman, Treatment of chronic leukemias: Results of therapy by titrated, regularly spaced total body irradiation phosphorus, or roentgen irradiation, *J. Am. Med. Assoc., 150*:1372–1379 (1952).

5. R. B. Scott, Chronic lymphatic leukemia, *Lancet 1*:1162–1167 (1957).

6. A. V. Pisciotta and J. S. Hirschbock, Therapeutic considerations in chronic lymphocytic leukemia, *Arch. Intern. Med., 99*:334–345 (1957).

7. J. E. Ultmann, W. Fish, E. Osserman, and A. Gellhorn, The clinical implications of hypogammaglobulinemia in patients with chronic lymphocytic leukemia and lymphocytic lymphosarcoma, *Ann. Intern. Med., 51*:501–516 (1959).

8. R. K. Shaw, C. Szwed, D. R. Boggs, J. L. Fahey, E. Frei, E. Morrison, and J. P. Utz, Infection and immunity in chronic lymphocytic leukemia, *Arch. Intern. Med., 106*:467–478 (1960).

9. R. P. Hudson and S. J. Wilson. Hypogammaglobulinemia and chronic lymphatic leukemia, *Cancer, 13*:200–204 (1960).

10. R. K. Shaw, D. R. Boggs, H. R. Silberman, and E. Frei, III, A study of prednisone therapy in chronic lymphocytic leukemia, *Blood, 17*:182–195 (1961).

11. J. M. Aroesty and F. W. Furth, Infection and chronic lymphocytic leukemia: A review of 61 cases, *N.Y. State J. Med., 62*:1946–1952(1962).

12. D. R. Boggs, S. A. Sofferman, M. M. Wintrobe, and G. E. Cartwright, Factors affecting the duration of survival of patients with chronic lymphocytic leukemia, *Am. J. Med., 40*:243–254 (1966).

13. C. Zippin, S. J. Cutler, W. J. Reeves, Jr., and D. Lum, Survival in chronic lymphocytic leukemia, *Blood, 42*:367–376 (1973).

14. M. M. Hansen, Chronic lymphocytic leukemia: Clinical studies based on 189 cases followed for a long time, *Scand. J. Haematol. Suppl., 18*:1–282 (1973).

15. L. Revol, R. Creyssel, P. A. Bryon, P. Coeur, and O. Gentilhomme, Leucemie lymphoide chronique, *Enc. Med. Chir.*, Paris, *Sang* 13013 B *20* (1974).

16. E. Monserrat-Costa, E. Matutes, C. Rozman, E. Feliu, A. Granena, L. Hernandez-Nieto, B. Momdedeu, and A. Urbano-Marquez, Infecciones en la leukemia linfoide cronica, *SNGRA (Sangre), 22*:968–975 (1977).

17. P. H. Travade, J. D. Dusart, D. Cavaroe, J. Beytout, and M. Rey, Les infections graves associees a la leucemie lymphoide chronique, *Presse Med., 15*:1715–1718 (1986).

18. J. S. Lee, D. Dixon, H. Kantarjian, M. J. Keating, and P. Talpaz, Prognosis of chronic lymphocytic leukemia: A multivariate regression analysis of 325 untreated patients, *Blood, 69*: 929–936 (1987).

19. D. Catovsky, J. Fooks, and S. Richards, Prognostic factors in chronic lymphocytic leukemia: The importance of age, sex, and response to treatment in survival. A report from the MRC CLL 1 trial, *Br. J. Haematol., 72*:141–149 (1989).

20. J. W. Mayo and R. P. Wenzel, Rates of hospital-acquired bloodstream infections in patients with specific malignancy, *Cancer, 50*:187–190 (1982).

21. M. M. Wintrobe and L. L. Hasenbush, Chronic leukemia. The early phase of chronic leukemia, the results of treatment and the effects of complicating infections: Study of 86 adults, *Arch. Intern. Med., 64*:701–718 (1939).

22. D. G. Miller and D. A. Karnofsky, Immunologic factors and resistance to infection in chronic lymphatic leukemia, *Am. J. Med., 31*:748–757 (1961).

23. C. H. Bernard, G. Mombelli, and J. Klastersky, Pneumococcal bacteremia in patients with neoplastic diseases, *Eur. J. Cancer Clin. Oncol., 17*:1041–1046 (1981).

24. M. Y. Chou, A. Brown, A. Blevins, and D. Armstrong, Severe pneumococcal infection in patients with neoplastic disease, *Cancer, 51*:1546–1550 (1983).

25. M. H. Kaplan, P. P. Rosen, and D. Armstrong, Cryptococcosis in a cancer hospital, *Cancer, 39*:2265–2274 (1977).

26. C. Kauffman, K. Israel, J. Smith, A. White, J. Schwarz, and C. Brooks, Histoplasmosis in immunosuppressed patients, *Am. J. Med., 64*:923–932 (1978).

27. M. S. Hirsch, Herpes group virus infections in the compromised host, in *Clinical Approach to Infection in the Compromised Host* (R. H. Rubin and L. S. Young, eds.), Plenum Medical Book Company, New York and London, pp. 347–362 (1981).

28. R. L. Marton and P. A. O'Leary, Herpes zoster generalisatus, associated with chronic lymphatic leukemia, Arch. Dermatol. Syphilol., 449:263–265 (1942).

29. V. J. Wile and H. H. Holeman, Generalized herpes zoster associated with leukemia, *Arch. Dermatol. Syphilol.,* 587–592 (1940).

30. A. Barrett, Chronic indolent orofacial herpes simplex virus infection in chronic leukemia: A report of three cases, *Oral Surg.*, 387–390 (1988).

31. J. E. Ultmann, Generalized vaccinia in a patient with CLL and hypo GG, *Ann. Intern. Med., 61*:728–732(1964).

32. F. R. FeKety, S. E. Malaivista, and D. L. Young, Vaccinia gangrenosa in CLL, *Arch. Intern. Med., 109*:205–208 (1967).

33. M. H. Kaplan, D. Armstrong, and P. Rosen, Tuberculosis complicating neoplastic disease, *Cancer, 33*:850–858 (1974).

34. A. Reed, B. Body, M. Austin, and H. Frierson, *Cunninghamella bertholletiae* and *pneumocystis carinii* pneumonia as a fatal complication of chronic lymphocytic leukemia, *Hum. Pathol., 19*:1470–1472 (1988).

35. J. J. Hutton, D. D. Von Hoff, J. Kuhn, et al., Phase I clinical investigation of 9-β-D-Arabinofuranosyl-2-fluoroadenine 5′-monophosphate (NSC 312887), a new purine antimetabolite, *Cancer Res., 44*:4183–4186 (1984).

36. M. J. Keating, Fludarabine phosphate in the treatment of chronic lymphocytic leukemia, *Sem. Oncol., 17*:49–62 (1990).

37. M. J. Keating, H. Kantarjian, M. Talpaz, et al., Fludarabine: A new agent with major activity against chronic lymphocytic leukemia, *Blood, 74*:19–25 (1989).

38. D. H. Boldt, D. D. Von Hoff, J. G. Kuhn, et al., Effects on human peripheral lymphocytes of in vivo administration of 9-β-D-arabinofuranosyl-2-fluoro-adenine-5-monophosphate (NSC 312887), a new purine antimetabolite, *Cancer Res., 44*: 4661–4666 (1984).

39. L. Robertson, Y. Huh, C. Hirsch-Ginsberg, H. Kantarjian, and M. J. Keating, Immunophenotypic assessment of response in CLL after fludarabine, *Proc. Am. Soc. Clin. Oncol., 9*:205 (1990).

40. P. J. Schilling and S. Vadhan-Raj, Concurrent cytomegalovirus and pneumocystis pneumonia after fludarabine therapy for chronic lymphocytic leukemia. *N. Engl. J. Med., 323*:833–834 (1990).

41. R. O. Dillman, R. Mick, and O. R. McIntyre, Pentostatin in chronic lymphocytic leukemia: A phase II trial of cancer and leukemia group B, *J. Clin. Oncol., 7*:433–438 (1989).

42. S. Riddell, J. B. Johnston, D. Bowman, R. Glazer, and L. G. Israels, 2′-Deoxycoformycin in chronic lymphatic leukemia and Waldenstrom's machroglobulinemia, *Proc. Am. Soc. Clin. Oncol., 4*:651 (1985).

43. P. J. O'Dwyer, A. S. Spiers, and S. Marsoni, Association of severe and fatal infections and treatment with pentostatin, *Cancer Treatment Rep., 70*:1117–1120 (1986).

44. E. R. Giblett, J. E. Anderson, F. Cohen, B. Pollara, and H. J. Meuwissen, Adenosine deaminase deficiency in two patients with severely impaired cellular immunity, *Lancet, 2*:1067–1069 (1972).

45. F. F. Snyder, M. S. Hershfield, and J. E. Seegmiller, Cytotoxic and metabolic effects of adenosine and adenine on human lymphoblasts, *Cancer Res., 38*:2357–2362 (1978).

46. M. R. Grever, M. A. Krause, and S. P. Balcerzak, Adenosine deaminase inhibition impairs monocyte cytotoxicity, *Clin. Res., 29*:368A (1981).

47. D. P. Gray, M. S. Coleman, and M. F. E. Siaw, Microphage biochemical abnormalities and impaired phagocytosis associated with 2′-deoxycoformycin and deoxyadenosine in culture, *Clin. Res., 30*:735A (1982).

48. M. R. Grever, M. F. E. Siaw, M. S. Coleman, et al., Inhibition of K and NK lymphocytote cytotoxicity by an inhibitor of adenosine deaminase and deoxyadenosine, *J. Immunol., 129*:365–369 (1982).

49. H. Ratech, W. K. Bell, R. Hirschhorn, et al., Effects of deoxycoformycin in mice. I: Suppression and enhanced in vivo antibody responses of thymus-dependent and independent antigens, *J. Immunol., 131*:3071–3076 (1984).

50. L. D. Piro, C. J. Carrera, E. Beutler, and D. A. Carson, 2-chlorodeoxyadenosine: An effective new agent for the treatment of chronic lymphocytic leukemia, *Blood, 72*:1069–1073 (1988).

51. M. Talpaz, M. Rosenblum, R. Kurzrock, J. Reuben, H. Kantarjian, and J. Gutterman, Clinical and laboratory changes induced by alpha interferon in chronic lymphocytic leukemia: A pilot study, *Am. J. Hematol., 24*:341–350 (1987).

52. S. Vadhan-Raj, A. Al-Katib, R. Bhalla, et al., Phase I trial of recombinant interferon gamma in cancer patients, *J. Clin. Oncol., 4*:137–146 (1986).

53. N. E. Kay, M. M. Oken, J. J. Maaza, and E. C. Bradley, Evidence for tumor reduction in refractory or relapsed B-CCL patients with infusional interleukin-2, *Nouv. Rev. Fr. Hematol., 30*:475–478, 1988.

54. A. A. Hertler, D. M. Schlossman, M. J. Borowitz, et al., A phase I study of T101-ricin: A chain immunotoxin in refractory chronic lymphocytic leukemia, *J. Biol. Resp. Med., 7*:97–113 (1988).

55. H. M. Chapel and C. Bunch, Mechanisms of infection in chronic lymphocytic leukemia, *Sem. Haematol., 24*:291–296 (1987).

56. R. W. Rundles, E. V. Coonrad, and T. Arends, Serum proteins in leukemia, *Am. J. Med., 16*:842–853 (1954).

57. A. Videbaek, Some clinical aspects of leukemia, *Acta Haematol., 24*:54–58 (1960).

58. R. Creyssel, R. Morel, M. Pellet, J. Medard, L. Revol, and R. Croizat, Deficit en gamma-globulines et complications infectieuses des leucemies lymphoides chroniques, *Sang, 29*:383–398 (1958).

59. G. H. Fairley and R. B. Scott, Hypogammaglobulinemia in chronic lymphocytic leukemia, *Br. Med. J., 4*:920–924 (1961).

60. R. Klima, H. Rettenbacher-Daubner, and H. Rieder, Elektrophoretisch und chemische Untersuchungen bei malignen Blutkrankheiten, *Wien Klin. Wschr., 74*:90–92 (1962).

61. M. B. Van Scoy-Mosher, M. Bick, V. Capostagno, R. L. Walford, and R. A. Gatti, A clinicopathologic analysis of chronic lymphocytic leukemia, *Am. J. Hematol., 10*:9–18 (1981).

62. H. M. Chapel, Hypogammaglobulinemia and chronic lymphocytic leukaemia, in *Chronic Lymphocytic Leukemia: Recent Progress, Future Advances* (R. P. Gale and K. R. Rai, eds.), Alan R. Liss, New York, pp. 383–389 (1987).

63. K. R. Rai and E. Montserrat, Prognostic factors in chronic lymphocytic leukemia, *Sem. Haematol., 4*:252–260 (1987).

64. C. Rozman, E. Montserrat, and N. Vinolas, Serum immunoglobulin and B-chronic lymphocytic leukemia, natural history and prognostic significance, *Cancer, 61*:279–283 (1988).

65. A. J. Amman and R. Hong, Selective IgA deficiency: Presentation of 30 cases and review of the literature, *Medicine, 50*:223–226 (1971).

66. D. L. Larson and L. J. Tomlinson, Quantitative antibody studies in man, III: Antibody response in leukemia and other malignant lymphomata, *J. Clin. Invest., 32*:317 (1953).

67. S. Saslaw, H. N. Carlise, and B. Bouroncle, Antibody response in hematologic patients, *Proc. Soc. Exp. Biol. Med., 106*:654–659 (1961).

68. M. Barr and G. H. Fairley, Circulating antibodies in reticuloses, *Lancet, 1*:1305–1309 (1961).

69. L. Cone and J. W. Uhr, Immunological deficiency disorders associated with chronic lymphocytic leukemia and multiple myeloma, *J. Clin. Invest., 43*:2241–2248 (1964).

70. R. B. Heath, G. H. Fairley, and J. S. Malpos, Production of antibodies against viruses in leukaemia and related diseases, *Br. J. Haematol., 10*:365–370 (1964).

71. J. I. Brody and L. H. Beizer, Immunologic incompetence of the neoplastic lymphocyte in CLL, *Ann. Intern. Med., 64*:1237–1245 (1966).

72. R. Foa, D. Catovsky, F. Lauria, and D. A. G. Galton, Reduced T-colony forming capacity by T-lymphocytes from B-chronic lymphocytic leukaemia, *Br. J. Haematol., 46*:623–625 (1980).

73. N. E. Kay, Abnormal T-cell subpopulation function in CLL: Excessive suppressor (T-gamma) and deficient helper (T-mu) activity with respect to B-cell proliferation, *Blood, 57*:418–420 (1981).

74. P. Hersey, J. Wotherspoon, G. Reid, and F. W. Gunz, Hypogammaglobulinemia associated with abnormalities of both B and T lymphocytes in patients with chronic lymphatic leukaemia, *Clin. Exp. Immunol., 39*:698–707 (1980).

75. C. D. Platsoucas, M. Galinski, S. Kempin, L. Reich, B. Clarkson, and R. A. Good, Abnormal T-lymphocyte subpoplations in patients with B cell chronic lymphocytic leukemia: An analysis by monoclonal antibodies, *J. Immunol.*, *129*:2305–2312 (1982).

76. C. D. Plastoucas, G. Hernandes, S. L. Gupta, S. Kempin, B. Clarkson, R. A. Good, and S. Gupta, Defective spontaneous and antibody-dependent cytotoxicity mediated by E-rosette-positive and E-rosette-negative cells in untreated patients with chronic lymphocytic leukemia: Augmentation by in vitro treatment with interferon, *J. Immunol.*, *125*:1216–1223 (1980).

77. P. Riis, *The Cytology of Inflammatory Exudate*, Munsgaard, Copenhagen, p. 80 (1959).

78. D. R. Boggs, Cellular composition of inflammatory exudates in human leukaemia, *Blood, 15*:466–475 (1960).

79. H. I. Zeya, E. Keku, F. Richards, and C. L. Spurr, Monocyte and granulocyte defect in chronic lymphocytic leukemia, *Am. J. Pathol., 95*:43–54 (1979).

80. A. J. Sbarra, W. Shirley, R. J. Selvaraj, E. Ouchi, and E. Rosenbaum, The role of phagocyte in host-parasite interactions, 1. The phagocytic capabilities of leukocytes from lymphoproliferative disorders, *Cancer Res., 24*:1959–1968 (1964).

81. K. Tornyos, Phagocytic activity of cells of the inflammatory exudate in human leukemia, *Cancer Res., 27*:1756–1760 (1967).

82. M. E. Heath and B. Cheson, Defective complement activity in chronic lymphocytic leukemia, *Am. J. Hematol., 19*:63–73 (1985).

83. J. H. Holt and L. J. Witts, Splenectomy in leukaemia and the reticuloses, *Quart. J. Med., 35*:369–384 (1966).

84. H. C. New, Progress and perspectives on beta-lactomase inhibition: a review of augmentin, *Am. J. Med., 79*(Suppl. 5B):39–43 (1985).

85. E. C. Besa, Use of intravenous immunoglobulin in chronic lymphocytic leukemia, *Am. J. Med. 71*:1035–1040 (1984).

86. C. Bunch, The co-operative group for the study of immunoglobulin in chronic lymphocytic leukemia, *N. Engl. J. Med., 319*:902–907 (1988).

87. J. C. Weeks, M. R. Tierney, and M. C. Weinstein. Cost effectiveness of prophylactic intravenous immune globulin in chronic lymphocytic leukemia, *N. Engl. J. Med., 325*:81–86 (1991).

88. J. Boelaert, A. Van Hoff, W. Willemarck, C. Eyndels, M. Delire, and A. Louwagie, Infection prevention by intravenous IgG in patients with myeloma or chronic leukemia. Abstracts of the 27th Annual Interscience Conference on Antimicrobial Agents and Chemotherapy, p. 264 (1987).

89. H. O. Ochs, S. H. Fisher, F. S. Virant, M. L. Lee, H. S. Kingdon, and R. J. Wedgwood (letter to the editor), Non-A, non-B hepatitis intravenous immunoglobulin, *Lancet, 1*:404–405 (1985).

90. M. L. Lee, S. G. Courter, D. Tait, and H. S. Kingdon, Long-term evaluation of intravenous immune globulin preparation with regard to non-A, non-B hepatitis safety, in *Viral Hepatitis and Liver Disease* (A. J. Zuckerman, ed.), Alan R. Liss, New York, pp. 596–599 (1988).

91. G. Mitra, M. F. Wong, M. M. Mozen, J. S. McDougal, and J. A. Levy,

Elimination of infectious retroviruses during preparation of immunoglobulins. *Transfusion, 26*:394–397 (1986).

92. Safety of therapeutic immune globulin preparations with respect to transmission of human T-lymphotropic virus type III/lymphadenopathy-associated virus infection, *MMWR, 35*:231–233 (1986).
93. S. A. Berkman, AIDS and plasma-derived products in the USA, in *Clinical use of Intravenous Immunoglobulins* (A. Morell, U. E. Nydegger, eds.), Academic Press, London, pp. 399–409 (1986).
94. Centers for Disease Control, Recommendation of the immunization practices advisory committee (ACIP): Pneumococcal polysaccharide vaccine, *MMWR*, 64–68, 73–76 (1989).
95. L. Young, Empirical antimicrobial therapy in the neutropenic host (editorial), *N. Engl. J. Med., 81*:237 (1986).
96. E. Anaissie, V. Fainstein, G. Bodey, et al., Randomized trial of β-lactam regimens in febrile neutropenic cancer patients, *Am. J. Med., 84*:581–589 (1988).
97. C. Puccio, A. Mittelman, S. Lichtman, et al., Phase II study of fludarabine phosphate (FAMP) in chronic lymphocytic leukemia (CLL), *Proc. Am. Soc. Clin. Oncol., 9*:206 (1990).

Index

About the Editor

BRUCE D. CHESON is Head, Medicine Section of the Clinical Investigations Branch, Cancer Therapy Evaluation Program, Division of Cancer Treatment, the National Cancer Institute, Bethesda, Maryland. The author or coauthor of more than 150 journal articles, book chapters, and abstracts, he is a Fellow of the American College of Physicians and a member of the American Society of Hematology, the American Society of Clinical Oncology, and the American Federation for Clinical Research. Dr. Cheson received the B.A. degree (1967) from the University of Virginia, Charlottesville, and the M.D. degree (1971) from the Tufts University School of Medicine, Boston, Massachusetts.